616.1 Jul

3403063354

CARDIOLOGY

EIGHTH EDITION

D0487312

Commissioning Editor: Laurence Hunter
Project Development Manager: Clive Hewat
Project Manager: Nancy Arnott
Designer: George Ajayi

CARDIOLOGY

EIGHTH EDITION

Desmond G. Julian MA MD FRCP FACC

Emeritus Professor of Cardiology
University of Newcastle-upon-Tyne, UK

J. Campbell Cowan MA DPhil FRCP

Consultant Cardiologist
Yorkshire Heart Centre, The General Infirmary at Leeds, Leeds, UK

James M. McLenachan MD FRCP

Consultant Cardiologist
Yorkshire Heart Centre, The General Infirmary at Leeds, Leeds, UK

with contributions from

William H.T. Smith MA PhD MRCP
Specialist Registrar in Cardiology
Yorkshire Heart Centre, The General Infirmary at Leeds, Leeds, UK

John D.R. Thomson BM BS BMedSci MRCP
Specialist Registrar in Paediatric Cardiology
Yorkshire Heart Centre, The General Infirmary at Leeds, Leeds, UK

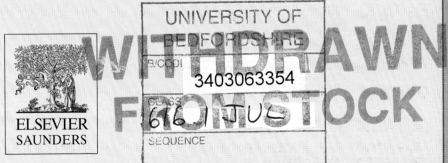

ELSEVIER
SAUNDERS

Edinburgh London New York Oxford Philadelphia St Louis Sydney Toronto 2005

ELSEVIER
SAUNDERS

Standard edition ISBN 07020 26956
International edition ISBN 07020 26948

British Library Cataloguing in Publication Data
A catalogue record for this book is available from the British Library

Library of Congress Cataloging in Publication Data
A catalog record for this book is available from the Library of Congress

Note
Medical knowledge is constantly changing. Standard safety precautions must be followed, but as new research and clinical experience broaden our knowledge, changes in treatment and drug therapy may become necessary or appropriate. Readers are advised to check the most current product information provided by the manufacturer of each drug to be administered to verify the recommended dose, the method and duration of administration, and contraindications. It is the responsibility of the practitioner, relying on experience and knowledge of the patient, to determine dosages and the best treatment for each individual patient. Neither the Publisher nor the authors assumes any liability for any injury and/or damage to persons or property arising from this publication.

The Publisher

 your source for books,
journals and multimedia
in the health sciences

www.elsevierhealth.com

The
publisher's
policy is to use
**paper manufactured
from sustainable forests**

Printed in China

Preface

The first edition of this book was published some 35 years ago in 1970. During this period the specialty of cardiology has evolved dramatically. Our understanding of the pathophysiology of cardiovascular diseases and of the therapies and interventions available for their treatment has changed radically. The pace of progress accelerates with time and the changes for this, the eighth edition, are the most extensive of any edition to date.

The text and illustrations have been extensively revised. The emergence of the concept of a spectrum of acute coronary syndromes has led us to amalgamate the clinical manifestations of coronary disease in a single chapter. We recognise that it is difficult for a small number of authors to provide an authoritative account covering the full breadth of a rapidly evolving specialty. For this edition, we have welcomed the involvement of Dr William Smith and Dr John Thomson as individual chapter authors, who have revised and updated the chapters on non-invasive imaging and congenital heart disease, respectively.

Despite the pace of change in the specialty, some aspects of an introductory text are relatively unchanging. The fundamentals of history taking and clinical examination, which have proved such a strength in previous editions, are retained for this edition. We do hope, however, that the more up-to-date layout and the addition of 'practice guidelines' will enhance the clarity of this edition.

As with previous editions, we hope that this edition will prove of value to a diverse readership, including medical students, nurses, junior doctors preparing for membership and general practitioners. We also recognise that the book retains an international readership in countries with a range of disease statistics and healthcare provision. We have endeavoured to retain the characteristics necessary to interest this diverse readership.

D.G. Julian

J.C. Cowan

J.M. McLenachan

Acknowledgements

We are grateful to the many colleagues who have contributed illustrations retained from earlier editions. We would particularly like to thank Jill Wharton, Alison Farrell, David Oxborough, Karen Sheard and Dr Mohan Sivananthan for contributing illustrations new to this edition.

Contents

1. THE ELECTRICAL ACTIVITY OF THE HEART: THE ELECTROCARDIOGRAM   1

The genesis of the electrocardiogram   1
The normal electrocardiogram   4
Abnormal electrocardiogram patterns   10
Electrocardiogram interpretation   14

2. THE SYMPTOMS OF HEART DISEASE   17

Dyspnoea   17
Cardiac pain   19
Palpitation   20
Oedema   21
Ascites   21
Cyanosis   22
Haemoptysis   22
Syncope   23

3. THE PHYSICAL SIGNS OF HEART DISEASE   25

The arterial pulse   25
Blood pressure measurement   27
The venous pulse and pressure   28
Inspection of the chest   30
Palpation of the chest   31
Auscultation: heart sounds and murmurs   32
General examination of patients with cardiac disease   42

4. NON-INVASIVE CARDIAC IMAGING   43

Plain radiography   43
Echocardiography   44
Cardiac magnetic resonance imaging   60
Non-invasive approaches to coronary heart disease   61

5. INVASIVE INVESTIGATIONS   70

Cardiac catheterization   70
Ventriculography and aortography   73
Coronary angiography   73
Invasive electrophysiological studies   76

6. DISEASES OF THE CORONARY ARTERIES – CAUSES, PATHOLOGY AND PREVENTION   78

The coronary circulation   78
Coronary artery disease   79
Public health approaches to prevention of ischaemic heart disease   88

7. CLINICAL PRESENTATIONS OF CORONARY DISEASE   90

Stable angina   90
Unstable angina, non-Q wave myocardial infarction and non-ST segment elevation myocardial infarction   105
ST segment elevation myocardial infarction   108
Cardiac rehabilitation   132

8. HEART FAILURE   135

The pathophysiology of heart failure   135
Clinical syndromes of heart failure   140
General management of heart failure   143
Pharmacological therapy   145
Ventricular resynchronization therapy   150
Arrythmia management   152
Acute left ventricular failure   152
Cardiogenic shock   153
Cardiac transplantation   155

9. DISORDERS OF RATE, RHYTHM AND CONDUCTION   159

Disturbances of rate and rhythm   159
Disorders of conduction   180
Investigation of rhythm abnormalities   185
Cardiac syncope   187
Management of bradyarrythmias – cardiac pacing   187
General management of tachyarrythmias   193
Practical arrythmia management   198
Cardiac arrest   202

10. DISEASES OF THE PERICARDIUM   208

Pathology   208
Acute pericarditis   208
Pericardial effusion   212
Pericardial tamponade   213
Pericardial constriction ('constrictive pericarditis')   216

11. CARDIOMYOPATHY AND MYOCARDITIS   220

Myocarditis   220
Cardiomyopathy   223

12. DISORDERS OF THE CARDIAC VALVES   234

Mitral valve disease   234
Aortic valve disease   252
Tricuspid valve disease   263
Pulmonary valve disease   265
Infective endocarditis   266

13. CONGENITAL HEART DISEASE   274

Varieties of congenital heart disease   274
Communications   275
Cyanotic lesions   286
Obstructive lesions   290
Complex conditions   296

14. HYPERTENSION AND HEART DISEASE   301

The concept of normal blood pressure   301
Measurement of blood pressure   303
Aetiology of hypertension   303
Pathophysiology of hypertension   309
Examination and investigation of the hypertensive patient   309
The decision to treat   312
Treatment of hypertension   314

15. DISEASES OF THE AORTA   319

The normal aorta   319
Imaging of the aorta   319
Dissecting aneurysm   320
Atypical aortic dissection   323
Aortic trauma   324
Chronic thoracic aneurysm   324
Aneurysms of the sinus of Valsalva   326

16. DISORDERS OF THE LUNGS AND PULMONARY CIRCULATION   328

Pulmonary embolism   328
Pulmonary hypertension   333
Pulmonary heart disease   337

17. SYSTEMIC DISORDERS AND THE HEART   341

Infections and the heart   341
Endocrine and metabolic disorders   347
Miscellaneous disorders   353
Normal physiological states   355

18. PSYCHOLOGICAL ASPECTS OF HEART DISEASE   361

Psychological factors in the genesis of hypertension and coronary
   disease   361
Anxiety state and the heart   361

19. SURGERY AND THE HEART   364

Anaesthesia and general surgery in patients with heart disease   364
Surgery for heart disease   367
Medical management of patients undergoing cardiac surgery   370
The replacement of heart valves   372

Index   377

The electrical activity of the heart: the electrocardiogram

Electrical activity is a basic characteristic of the heart and is the stimulus for cardiac contraction. Disturbances of electrical function are common in heart disease. Their registration as an electrocardiogram (ECG) plays an essential role in the diagnosis and management of heart disorders.

THE GENESIS OF THE ELECTROCARDIOGRAM

Pathways of conduction and the electrocardiogram

The sinus node is situated in the right atrium close to the entrance of the superior vena cava. The atrioventricular node lies in the right atrial wall immediately above the tricuspid valve. The fibres of the AV bundle (of His) arise from the atrioventricular node and run along the posterior border of the septum between the ventricles (Fig. 1.1). On reaching the muscular part of the septum, they split into right and left bundle branches and then spread out in the subendocardium of the ventricles as the Purkinje system. The right bundle is a slender, compact structure. The left bundle soon splits into two or more divisions or fascicles, one of which proceeds anteriorly, sharing the same blood supply as the right bundle, and another is directed posteriorly.

In the usual sequence of events, the electrical impulse arises in the sinus node and spreads across the atria to reach the atrioventricular node. It can then only reach the ventricles by passing into the rapidly conducting atrioventricular bundle and its branches.

The first part of the ventricles to be activated is the septum, followed by the endocardium. Finally, the impulse spreads outwards to the epicardium.

The spread of the cardiac impulse gives rise to the main deflections of the electrocardiogram: P, QRS and T waves (Fig. 1.2):

- *The P wave* represents atrial *depolarization*.
- *The PR interval* represents the time taken for the cardiac impulse to spread over the atrium and through the AV node and His–Purkinje system.
- *The QRS complex* represents ventricular depolarization.
- *The T wave* represents ventricular repolarization.

Electrodes and leads

A conventional ECG consists of tracings from 12 or more leads. The term 'lead' refers to the ECG obtained as a result of recording the difference in potential between a pair of electrodes.

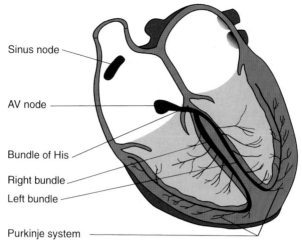

Fig. 1.1 The pathways of conduction.

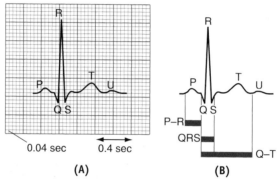

Fig. 1.2 (A) Normal ECG complexes. (B) PR, QRS and QT segments.

The bipolar (standard) leads

In these leads, the electrodes are attached to the limbs. In lead I the positive electrode is attached to the left arm and the negative to the right arm. In lead II the positive electrode is attached to the left leg and the negative to the right arm. In lead III the positive is attached to the left leg and the negative to the left arm. They may thus be depicted as:

- *lead I* = left arm minus right arm (LA–RA)
- *lead II* = left leg minus right arm (LL–RA)
- *lead III* = left leg minus left arm (LL–LA).

It can be deduced from these equations that lead II should be equal to the sum of leads I and III.

The position from which the heart is viewed by each of these leads is shown in Figure 1.3.

Unipolar leads

These have an exploring electrode placed on a chosen site linked with an indifferent electrode with a very small potential. In an attempt to obtain a

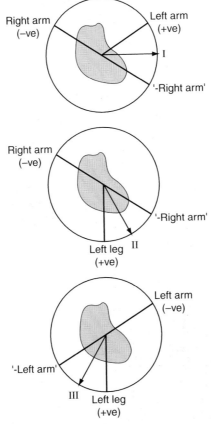

Fig. 1.3 Diagram of the effective position of the bipolar (standard) leads. In lead I, the positive electrode is attached to the left arm and the negative to the right arm. In effect, lead I is the sum of the potentials from the left arm with those that would be obtained from an electrode diametrically opposite the right arm. The resultant force is directed midway between these two points. Similar principles can be applied to derive the effective direction of the leads II and III.

central terminal with 'zero potential', Wilson connected all three limb electrodes through 5000 Ω resistances to form the indifferent electrode.

Unipolar chest leads
When unipolar leads are recorded from the chest wall, the exploring electrode is connected to the positive pole of the ECG and the negative to the central terminal of Wilson. By convention, the following sites are normally selected (Fig. 1.4):

- *V1*, the fourth intercostal space just to the right of the sternum
- *V2*, the fourth intercostal space just to the left of the sternum
- *V3*, midway betwen V2 and V4
- *V4*, the fifth intercostal space in the midclavicular line
- *V5*, the left anterior axillary line at the same horizontal level as V4
- *V6*, the left midaxillary line at the same horizontal level as V4.

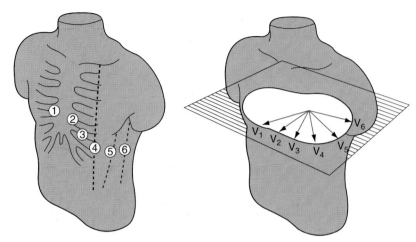

Fig. 1.4 The sites of electrode placement on the precordium.

Additional leads can be taken from V3R and V4R, sites on the right side of the chest equivalent to V3 and V4. Occasionally, leads may be placed at higher levels, for example the second, third or fourth intercostal spaces or further laterally (V7 and V8).

Unipolar limb leads

In these leads, the exploring electrode is placed on one limb, and the negative pole is connected to Wilson's central terminal, modified by the omission of the connection from the limb under study to the central terminal. This modification augments the voltage of the ECG, and the leads so derived are referred to as 'a' leads. They are designated as follows:

- *aVR*, right arm lead
- *aVL*, left arm lead
- aVF, left foot lead.

The resulting lead orientations and their relation to the standard bipolar leads are presented in Figure 1.15 on page 15.

THE NORMAL ELECTROCARDIOGRAM

Normally, ECGs are recorded at a rate of 25 mm/s and the ECG paper is printed with thin vertical lines 1 mm apart and thick vertical lines 5 mm apart (Fig. 1.5). The interval between the thin lines represents 0.04 s and that between two thick lines 0.20 s. If the heart rhythm is regular, the rate can be counted by dividing the number of small squares between two consecutive R waves into 1500 or large squares into 300.

There are also thin horizontal lines at 1-mm intervals and thick horizontal lines at 5-mm intervals. An ECG recording is standardized so that 1 mV gives a deflection of 10 mm on the paper. The height of a deflection therefore indicates its voltage.

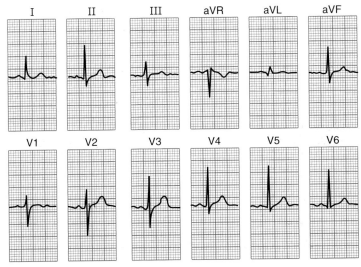

Fig. 1.5 Normal 12-lead electrocardiogram. Note the progression in the upright deflection from 'r' over the right ventricle (V1) to an 'R' over the left ventricle (V6).

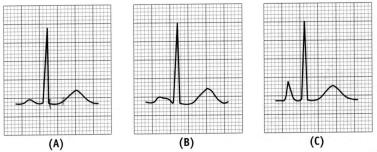

Fig. 1.6 P wave appearances in lead II. (A) Normal. (B) Broadened and notched (P mitrale). (C) Tall and peaked (P pulmonale).

The P wave

The normal P wave (Fig. 1.6A) results from the spread of electrical activity across the atria (the activity of the sinus node itself cannot be detected in the ECG). Because the impulse spreads from right to left, the P wave is upright in leads I, II and aVF, is inverted in aVR and may be upright, biphasic or inverted in lead III, aVL and V1. It should not be higher than 3 mm in the bipolar leads or 2.5 mm in the unipolar leads, or greater than 0.10 s in duration.

When abnormal, the P wave may become:

- *inverted* (i.e. negative in the leads in which it is usually positive). This indicates depolarization of the atria in an unusual direction, and that the pacemaker is not in the sinus node, but is situated either elsewhere in the atrium, in the AV node or below this; or there is dextrocardia
- *broadened and notched*, due to delayed depolarization of the left atrium when this chamber is enlarged (P mitrale) (Fig. 1.6B). In V1, the P wave is

then usually biphasic with a small positive wave preceding a deep and broad negative one

- *tall and peaked*, exceeding 3 mm, as a result of right atrial enlargement (P pulmonale) (Fig. 1.6C)
- *absent* or invisible due to the presence of junctional rhythm or sinoatrial block
- replaced by *flutter* or *fibrillation waves*.

PR interval

This is measured from the beginning of the P wave to the beginning of the QRS complex (i.e. to the onset of the Q wave if there is one, and to the onset of the R wave if there is not). This interval corresponds to the time taken for the impulse to travel from the sinus node to the ventricular muscle. There is an isoelectric segment between the end of the P wave and the beginning of the QRS, whilst the impulse is passing through the AV node and the specialized conducting tissue, as an insufficient amount of tissue is being electrically stimulated to produce a deflection detectable on the body surface.

The PR interval varies with age and with heart rate. The upper limit in children is 0.16, in adolescents 0.18 and in adults 0.20 s, although it may be even longer in a few normal individuals. The faster the heart rate the shorter is the PR interval. It is regarded as abnormally short if it is less than 0.10 s. A shortened PR interval is seen when the impulse originates in the junctional tissue and in the Wolff–Parkinson–White syndrome (see p. 165). The PR interval is prolonged in some forms of heart block (see p. 181).

The QRS complex

The QRS complex represents depolarization of the ventricular muscle. The components of the QRS complex are defined as follows (Fig. 1.7):

- The R wave is any positive (upward) deflection of the QRS. If there is more than one R wave, the second is denoted R′; an R wave of small voltage may be denoted r.
- A negative (downward) deflection preceding an R wave is termed Q.

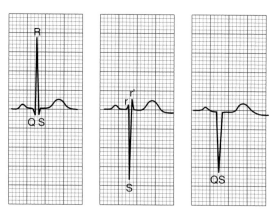

Fig. 1.7 Variations in the QRS complex (see text).

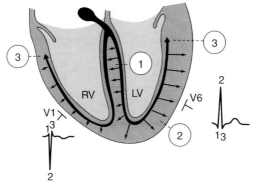

Fig. 1.8 Genesis of the QRS complex. Note that the first phase, directed from left to right across the septum, produces a Q wave in V6 and an R wave in V1. The second phase, due mainly to depolarization of the left ventricle from endocardium to epicardium, results in a tall R wave in V6 and a deep S wave in V1. Finally, depolarization of the basal parts of the ventricles may produce a terminal S wave in V6 and a terminal R wave in V1.

- A negative deflection following an R wave is termed S.
- If the ventricular complex is entirely negative (i.e. there is no R wave), the complex is termed QS.

The whole complex is often referred to as the QRS complex irrespective of whether one or two of its components are absent.

Ventricular depolarization starts in the middle of the left side of the septum and spreads across to the right (phase 1 of ventricular depolarization) (Fig. 1.8). Subsequently, the main free walls of the ventricles are activated, the impulse spreading from within outwards and from below upwards. Because of the dominating bulk of the left ventricle, the direction of the vector of phase 2 is to the left and posteriorly. Finally, the base of both ventricular walls and the interventricular septum are depolarized. The appearances of the QRS in different leads can be largely explained by the major vectors of these phases as is seen in Fig. 1.8. In leads facing the left ventricular surface, there is a small Q wave due to septal depolarization and a large R wave due to left ventricular depolarization. On the right side of the heart, as seen from V1, there is usually an r wave due to septal depolarization and a large S wave due to left ventricular forces directed away from the electrode.

Pathological Q waves

As mentioned, small, narrow Q waves are normally to be found in leads facing the left ventricle (e.g. lead I, aVL, aVF, V5 and V6). These Q waves do not normally exceed 2 mm in depth, or 0.03 s in width. It should be noted that QS waves are normal in aVR, and are common in V1. Abnormally broad and deep Q waves are often a feature of myocardial infarction (see p. 110). Q waves in lead III are difficult to evaluate but can be ignored if there are no Q waves either in lead II or in aVF, or if they do not exceed 0.03 s. Usually, a 'normal' Q wave in lead III diminishes or disappears on deep inspiration because of an alteration in the position of the heart, whilst the 'pathological' Q wave of infarction persists.

The QRS complex should not exceed 0.10 s in duration, and usually is in the range 0.06–0.08 s. Broad QRS complexes occur in bundle branch block (p. 12), in ventricular hypertrophy and in ventricular ectopic beats.

The T wave

The T wave is due to repolarization of the ventricles. If repolarization (the T wave) occurred in the same direction as depolarization (the QRS complex) the T wave would be directed in an opposite way to that of the QRS. In fact, depolarization takes place from endocardium to epicardium, whereas repolarization takes place from epicardium to endocardium. Because of this, the T wave usually points in the same direction as the major component of the QRS complex. Thus, the T wave is normally upright in leads I and II as well as in V3 to V6, is inverted in aVR, and may be upright or inverted in lead III, aVL, aVF and V1 and V2.

The T waves are usually not taller than 5 mm in standard leads and 10 mm in precordial leads. Unusually tall and peaked T waves may be seen in hyperkalaemia and in early myocardial infarction. Flattened T waves are seen when the voltage of all complexes is low, as in myxoedema, as well as in hypokalaemia and in a large number of other conditions in which it may be regarded as a nonspecific abnormality. Slight T wave inversion is also often non-specific, and may be due to such influences as hyperventilation, posture and smoking. The most important causes of T wave inversion are:

- myocardial ischaemia and infarction
- ventricular hypertrophy
- bundle branch block.

Detailed descriptions of T wave changes will be found in the subsequent section on abnormalities of the ST segment, and also under the subheadings dealing with ventricular hypertrophy, bundle branch block and myocardial infarction.

The QT interval

The QT interval represents the total time from the onset of ventricular depolarization to the completion of repolarization. It is measured from the beginning of the Q wave (or the R wave if there is no Q wave) to the end of the T wave. Its duration varies with heart rate, becoming shorter as the heart rate increases. In general, the QT interval at heart rates between 60 and 90 beats/min does not exceed in duration half the preceding RR interval. The measurement of the QT interval is often difficult as the end of the T wave cannot always be clearly identified, and the relationship between heart rate and duration of the QT is a complex one. Tables are available in textbooks of electrocardiography giving normal QT intervals. In practice, the main importance of a prolonged QT interval· is that it is associated with a risk of ventricular tachycardia (particularly torsades de pointes, p. 179) and sudden death. A long QT is sometimes an inherited abnormality but may result from such drugs as quinidine, procainamide, disopyramide, amiodarone and tricyclic antidepressants.

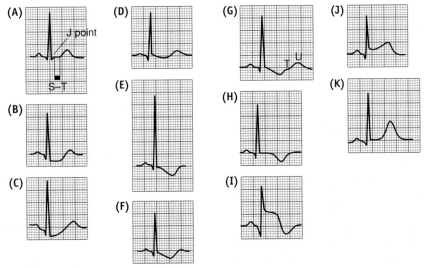

Fig. 1.9 Normal and abnormal ST segments and T waves. (A) Normal ST segment with J point. (B) Horizontal ST depression in myocardial ischaemia. (C) ST segment sloping upwards in sinus tachycardia. (D) ST sagging in digitalis therapy. (E) Asymmetrical T wave inversion associated with ventricular hypertrophy. (F) Similar pattern sometimes seen without voltage changes in hypertrophy – 'strain'. (G) ST sagging and prominent U waves of hypokalaemia. (H) Symmetrically inverted T wave of myocardial ischaemia or infarction. (I) ST elevation in acute myocardial infarction. (J) ST elevation in acute pericarditis. (K) Peaked T wave in hyperkalaemia.

The ST segment

The ST segment is that part of the ECG between the end of the QRS complex and the beginning of the T wave (Fig. 1.9). The point of junction between the S wave and the ST segment is known as the J point. The ST segment occurs during a period of unchanging polarity in the ventricles, corresponding with the plateau of the action potential. The normal ST segment is situated on the isoelectric line but curves upwards.

Displacements of the ST segment and variations in its shape are of great importance in electrocardiographic diagnosis. The characteristic abnormalities of the ST segment are illustrated in Fig. 1.9. In some normal individuals, particularly young people of African descent, slight ST elevation is seen. This may be up to 1 mm in standard leads and 2 mm in the right precordial leads. Depression of more than 0.5 mm is abnormal. When ST elevation occurs in normal individuals, it is often preceded by a slight notch on the downstroke of the R wave:

- *Acute myocardial infarction.* The ST segment is elevated with a curve which is convex upwards in the leads facing the infarct. At a later stage ST segment elevation becomes less pronounced as T wave inversion develops. These changes are considered in more detail on p. 110.
- *Pericarditis.* This also causes ST elevation, but the ST segments are concave upwards and the changes are widespread rather than localized as in myocardial infarction.

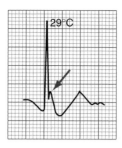

Fig. 1.10 ECG in hypothermia. The arrow indicates the characteristic prominent J wave.

- *Digitalis therapy*. This depresses the ST segment, particularly in leads II and III, so that there is a gentle sagging, but the T wave remains upright or flattened.
- *Ventricular hypertrophy*. ST segment depression may occur in leads facing the relevant ventricle and be accompanied by asymmetrical T wave inversion. This contrasts with the symmetrical T wave inversion seen in myocardial infarction and ischaemia.
- *Acute myocardial ischaemia*. The ST segment is horizontally depressed or slightly downward sloping from the J point onwards.
- *Sinus tachycardia*. There may be ST depression which slopes upwards from the J point.
- *Hypothermia*. There is a prominent J wave (the junction of the S wave and the ST segment) (Fig. 1.10).

The U wave

The U wave is a broad, low-voltage wave present in most normal ECGs. Its cause is unknown; it may become unusually prominent in hypokalaemia and with digitalis therapy.

ABNORMAL ELECTROCARDIOGRAM PATTERNS

Left ventricular hypertrophy (Fig. 1.11)

Hypertrophy of the left ventricle increases the amplitude of R waves in left chest leads and S waves in right chest leads. Where there is septal hypertrophy, deep but narrow Q waves are seen in left chest leads. When left ventricular hypertrophy becomes advanced, the T wave may become flattened in the leads in which the R wave is tall; eventually ST depression and T wave inversion may occur.

Many efforts have been made to lay down criteria for the diagnosis of left ventricular hypertrophy. None is satisfactory as many factors contribute to the amplitude of ECG waves, including the thickness of the chest wall and the age of the patient. The following criteria have gained wide acceptance:

- R in V5 or V6 plus S in V1 greater than 35 mm. This criterion applies only in individuals over 25 years of age. In younger persons, R in V5 or V6 plus S in V1 should exceed 40 mm before the diagnosis of left ventricular hypertrophy can be made

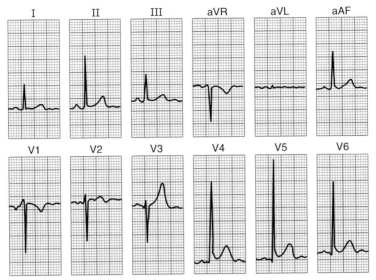

Fig. 1.11 Left ventricular hypertrophy. Note the deep S wave in lead V1 and the tall R waves in leads V5 and V6.

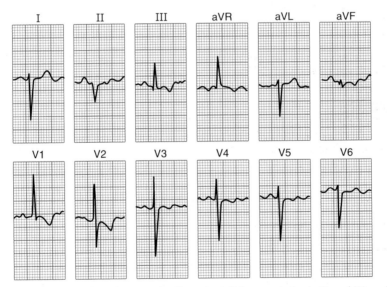

Fig. 1.12 Right ventricular hypertrophy. Note the tall R waves in leads V1 and V2, and associated T wave inversion extending across the chest leads to V5. There is right axis deviation.

- R in V5 or V6 greater than 25 mm
- R in aVL greater than 13 mm
- R in aVF greater than 20 mm.

Right ventricular hypertrophy (Fig. 1.12)

When the right ventricle becomes hypertrophied, the leads facing the right ventricle (particularly in V1, V3R and V4R) show dominant R waves instead of the usually dominant S wave. The diagnostic criterion for right ventricular hypertrophy is:

- R wave in V1 equal to or greater than the S wave and at least 5 mm tall.

As with left ventricular hypertrophy, ST depression and T wave inversion may develop in the leads with tall R waves.

Left bundle branch block (Fig. 1.13)

When the left branch of the bundle is blocked, the interventricular septum is activated from the right instead of from the left side and the initial vector (phase 1) is directed to the left. Because of this, the normal initial q wave in the left ventricular leads is lost, being replaced by a small r wave. Right ventricular depolarization, which follows, produces an r in V1 and an s in V6. The left ventricle is finally depolarized resulting in an R' in V6 and a broad S in V1. The QRS duration is increased to 0.12 s or more.

The abnormal left ventricular depolarization sequence in left bundle branch block causes secondary repolarization changes. Consequently, the ST segment and T wave are abnormal. This prevents interpretation of other factors causing ST and T wave changes, such as ischaemia and infarction.

Right bundle branch block (Fig. 1.14)

In this disorder, the right branch of the bundle is blocked, but the septum is activated from left to right, as in the normal heart. The left ventricular q wave is preserved, as is the initial r wave over right chest leads. The left ventricle is then depolarized, producing an S wave in right chest leads and an R wave in left chest leads. Finally, depolarization reaches the right ventricle, and so produces an R' in the right chest leads and a deep broad S wave in the left chest leads. An M pattern is thus seen in the right chest leads, such as V1. It is also common to see T wave abnormalities in leads V2 and V3.

The mean frontal QRS axis

The total electrical activity at any one moment of time can be summated and represented by a single electrical force of a certain magnitude and in a certain direction, termed the instantaneous vector. All the instantaneous vectors occurring during the inscription of the QRS complex can be averaged, the direction of the vector so derived being called the mean QRS axis. It is customary to measure this only in the frontal plane, based on the orientation of the limb leads (Fig. 1.15). The limb lead with the tallest R wave will be closest to the QRS axis.

An alternative method of deriving the mean frontal QRS axis is to find in which of the leads I, II, III, aVR, aVL and aVF, the deflections of the QRS above and below the line are most nearly equal. The mean frontal QRS axis is at right angles to this lead.

Left axis deviation is present when the axis is less than −30° and right axis deviation when the axis is greater than +110°.

(A)

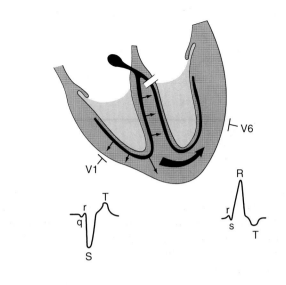

(B)

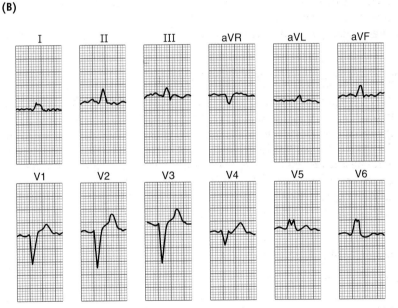

Fig. 1.13 Left bundle branch block. (A) The initial vector is abnormal in being from right to left across the septum, thus producing an initial r wave in V6 and a q wave in V1. (B) 12-lead ECG demonstrating features of left bundle branch block.

Calculation of the mean frontal QRS axis is of limited value except in a few conditions such as the differentiation of ostium primum from ostium secundum atrial septal defects (see p. 278).

Left axis deviation is often due to block in the anterior division (fascicle) of the left bundle branch, and when associated with right bundle branch block is a frequent precursor of complete heart block.

Right axis deviation commonly accompanies right ventricular hypertrophy, but may be due to block of the posterior fascicle of the left bundle.

(A)

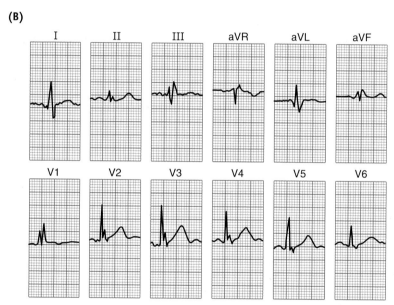

(B)

Fig. 1.14 Right bundle branch block. (A) The septum is depolarized normally from left to right and hence a small q is preserved in left ventricular leads and a small r in right ventricular leads. Left ventricular depolarization produces an s wave in V1 and an R wave in V6. Late depolarization of the right ventricle results in a prominent R′ wave in V1 and broad S wave in V6. (B) 12-lead ECG showing features of right bundle branch block.

ELECTROCARDIOGRAM INTERPRETATION

ECG interpretation is largely a matter of experience and pattern interpretation. However, while building experience, it is useful to develop a method of 'systematic' ECG analysis. This is most easily performed by asking oneself a number of questions in a logical sequence about P, QRS and T waves in turn. A simple system is presented in Box 1.1.

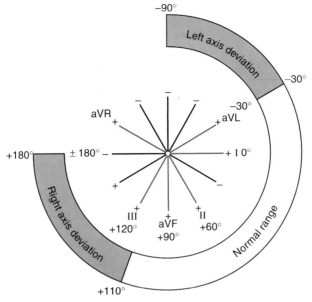

Fig. 1.15 Hexaxial reference system. The orientation of the limb leads in the frontal plane is shown, together with the normal range for the mean frontal QRS axis.

Box 1.1

A system of ECG interpretation

Rate and rhythm
What is the rate (see p. 4)?
Is it regular or irregular?

P wave
Are P waves present?
Is the P wave axis normal (p. 5)?
Is there evidence of left or right atrial enlargement (p. 6)?

PR interval *(normal range 0.12–0.20 s)*
Is the PR interval normal?
Is each QRS complex preceded by a P wave?
Is there evidence of a slurred QRS upstroke (delta wave) (p. 165)?

QRS complex
Is the QRS duration within normal limits (0.08–0.11 s)?
Is there evidence of bundle branch block (p. 12)?
Is the QRS axis normal (p. 12)?
Are pathological Q waves present (p. 7)?
Is there a normal R wave progression across the chest leads (p. 7)?

ST segment and T wave
Is there abnormal ST elevation or depression (p. 9)?
Are the T waves upright (except aVR and V1)?

QT interval
Is the QT interval normal (in general less than 0.44 s)?

FURTHER READING

Hampton, J. R. (1997) *The ECG in Practice*, 3rd edn. Edinburgh: Churchill Livingstone.

Mirvis, D.M. & Goldberger, A.L. (2001) Electrocardiography. In: Braunwald, E., Zipes, D.P., & Libby, P. *Heart Disease, A Textbook of Cardiovascular Medicine*. Philadelphia: Saunders.

Schamroth, L. (1989) *The 12 lead Electrocardiogram*. Oxford: Blackwell.

CHAPTER 2

The symptoms of heart disease

Heart disease may present in a wide variety of ways depending on the nature of the underlying disease process and whether this results in impaired cardiac function, coronary insufficiency or rhythm disturbance.

DYSPNOEA

Dyspnoea – difficulty with breathing – is the commonest symptom of heart failure. The term implies discomfort in the act of respiration, a consciousness of laboured breathing. It is, of course, also a symptom of respiratory disease and occurs in normal individuals on exercise.

No single explanation so far advanced accounts for all cases of dyspnoea. Furthermore, because it is subjective the degree of distress depends, in part, upon individual perceptions. Thus, some patients do not complain of breathlessness in spite of obviously laboured respiration, whereas others claim to be short of breath although their capacity for exercise is normal.

Mechanisms

The dyspnoea of cardiac disease may be due to the following factors:

- *Increased work of breathing*. It is probable that in most cases of cardiac failure the discomfort arises in overworked respiratory muscles. In left-sided cardiac failure, engorgement of the pulmonary veins and capillaries occurs; if the pulmonary capillary pressure exceeds 25 mmHg, fluid may exude from the alveolar walls or even into the alveoli. These changes make the lung more rigid (less compliant) and require more respiratory work for a given volume of air inspired.
- *Reduced vital capacity*. This is due to pulmonary venous congestion and, occasionally, to hydrothorax or ascites.
- *Reflex hyperventilation*. The pulmonary stretch receptors may be abnormally stretched by congestion of the lungs.
- *Bronchial narrowing*. Bronchial narrowing by spasm or fluid may occur in cardiac failure and adds to the work of breathing.
- *Hypoxaemia and carbon dioxide retention*. These may both contribute to dyspnoea. They are seldom important factors in patients with left-sided heart failure, in whom the carbon dioxide tension is normal or low as a

17

result of hyperventilation, and there is little hypoxaemia except when there is pulmonary oedema. In cyanotic congenital heart disease, hypoxaemia is severe.

Clinical features

Patients with cardiac dyspnoea breathe rapidly and shallowly. This pattern contrasts with that of anxious individuals who have deep and sighing respiration, and 'are unable to take a deep breath' or 'fill their lungs with air'. It also differs from the deep breathing of patients with diabetic keto-acidosis or renal failure.

Dyspnoea arising as a result of impaired cardiac function takes a number of forms according to the severity of the underlying problem:

Exertional dyspnoea

One of the earliest signs of left ventricular impairment is shortness of breath on exercise. If the disease is progressive, patients are likely to become increasingly limited until eventually they develop shortness of breath at rest.

Orthopnoea

Orthopnoea is dyspnoea when lying flat. There are several possible explanations for its occurrence in left heart failure:

- When an individual lies flat there is increased venous return, which in the patient on the verge of failure may increase pulmonary venous congestion, and thereby decrease pulmonary compliance and vital capacity.
- The vital capacity is reduced in the recumbent posture by the relatively high position of the diaphragm, which may be further displaced upwards by ascites or an enlarged liver.

Orthopnoea usually occurs when there is already a considerable limitation of exercise tolerance, but is occasionally an early symptom. Many patients learn for themselves that they are more comfortable propped up by three or four pillows.

Paroxysmal dyspnoea

In patients with left-sided cardiac failure, attacks of dyspnoea may develop without an obvious precipitating cause. They are most apt to occur during sleep (*paroxysmal nocturnal dyspnoea*). The mechanism is probably the same as that of orthopnoea, but the sensory unawareness of the sleeping state prevents the patient from correcting the situation by sitting up. Victims wake up intensely short of breath and frightened. They sit on the side of the bed or struggle to the window. The attack may pass off spontaneously within a few minutes, or progress to acute pulmonary oedema.

Acute pulmonary oedema

In this condition, fluid accumulates in the alveoli as a result of a high pulmonary capillary pressure. Such attacks occur in patients with mitral stenosis, acute myocardial infarction and other left-sided cardiac lesions. There is often a provoking factor such as an arrhythmia or respiratory infection.

The patient is intensely dyspnoeic with noisy breathing, cough and frothy sputum which is often blood-tinged. The skin is usually moist, cold and cyanosed. The pulse is fast and may be irregular. Crepitations may be heard throughout the chest in a severe attack. In some patients, rhonchi, due to fluid in the bronchi, predominate and the clinical picture may resemble bronchial asthma. Pulmonary oedema is usually visible on a chest radiograph.

Cheyne–Stokes respiration

In Cheyne–Stokes respiration, there is a periodic waxing and waning in the depth of respiration, over a period of about 1 min. This pattern of breathing is frequently an ominous sign, and is most often observed in moribund patients.

Functional capacity

On the basis of recommendations of the New York Heart Association, patients may be divided into four classes depending on the severity of their symptoms. This assessment of functional limitation is most often applied to the symptom of dyspnoea. The classification is as follows:

- *Class 1.* The patients, although they have heart disease, can withstand normal physical activity without symptoms.
- *Class 2.* The patient develops symptoms on moderate or severe exertion but not at rest or with mild exertion.
- *Class 3.* Symptoms are present even on mild exertion.
- *Class 4.* Symptoms are present at rest.

CARDIAC PAIN

There are two major causes of cardiac pain: myocardial ischaemia and pericarditis.

Myocardial ischaemia and infarction (see also Ch. 7)

A transient and reversible inadequacy of the coronary circulation gives rise to that type of chest pain known as angina pectoris. If the reduction in coronary blood flow is such as to cause death of an area of myocardium (myocardial infarction), the pain is usually more severe and prolonged.

The term angina pectoris was adopted by William Heberden, who in 1768 described the cardinal features of angina. These are:

- the *location* – in the retrosternal region, frequently radiating to the left arm or to the neck and lower jaw
- the *character* – often a strangling feeling, variously described by patients as a weight or pressure on their chest or as a tightness
- the *relationship to exertion*
- the *duration* (usually 1–10 min).

For a more detailed description of angina pectoris, see p. 90.

Angina pectoris most commonly occurs in response to exercise in patients with coronary artery disease. The same symptom can be provoked by paroxysmal tachycardia, when there is insufficient time during diastole for the coronary arteries to fill and meet the increased oxygen demands of the tachycardia. Angina is also a common symptom in aortic stenosis because of the inability of the coronary circulation to match the oxygen requirements of extreme left ventricular hypertrophy.

There seems little doubt that the cause of angina pectoris is myocardial hypoxia secondary to inadequate coronary blood flow. The site of angina appears to be the myocardium; the stimulus to the pain has not been determined but may be due to a chemical substance related to oxygen lack or to a phenomenon analogous to cramp. The impulses arising in the myocardium pass through afferent sympathetic fibres to reach the upper thoracic sympathetic ganglia and are then directed to the upper four or five thoracic spinal nerves. In this way, the same segments of the spinal cord receive sensations from the heart as receive sensory impulses from the anterior chest wall and the inner aspect of the arm, forearm and hand. The pain is perceived as arising in the territory supplied by the corresponding spinal somatic nerves, rather than in the organ itself.

The pain of myocardial infarction is similar to that of angina pectoris in its location and character, but its duration is longer (usually more than 30 min), it is usually more severe, and it has no relationship to exertion.

Pericarditis (see also Ch. 10)

Pain is a characteristic feature of pericarditis, and appears to arise in the parietal pericardium, the visceral pericardium being insensitive. It is usually sharp, but may be of an aching nature. It is situated in the retrosternal region, and radiates to the neck, back or upper abdomen, but rarely the arms. It may be exacerbated by inspiration, swallowing and movement, and may be worse in particular positions, such as when lying flat.

PALPITATION

The term palpitation means an awareness of the heart beat. In some cases it may be indicative of rhythm disturbance. In others it may merely indicate an awareness of normal rhythm.

It takes many different forms including a thumping sensation in the chest, a throbbing in the neck, a consciousness of missed or extra beats, or a racing of the heart. Anxious individuals are often distressed by the sinus tachycardia associated with emotion. Even normal individuals may be disagreeably conscious of their heart action when lying on the left side. Palpitation is, therefore, a common symptom in those without heart disease.

A careful history can sometimes help in distinguishing the cause:

- *Ectopic beats* frequently give rise to the sensation of jumping of the heart, missed beats or extra beats.
- Patients with *paroxysmal arrhythmias* are frequently aware of both the sudden onset and sudden termination of the arrhythmia.

- Patients with *atrial fibrillation* may be able to describe the chaotic irregularity of the heart beat.

Enquiry as to the mode of termination of a palpitation is particularly important in taking a history. By definition, all palpitations start suddenly when the patient is first aware of the symptom. However, the nature of the termination may provide some diagnostic clues as to the underlying heart rhythm. If the patient describes sudden termination, this is suggestive of some form of paroxysmal arrhythmia which has suddenly reverted to normal. If, by contrast, the palpitation subsides gradually, this would be more consistent with a sinus tachycardia which has gradually slowed down to normal.

In assessing the significance of palpitation it is important to enquire about associated symptoms such as dizziness, dyspnoea or chest discomfort as these may be features of a rapid arrhythmia causing haemodynamic compromise.

OEDEMA

Oedema – the accumulation of fluid in the interstitial tissues – is an important but relatively late manifestation of cardiac failure. It does not usually occur except in the presence of a raised venous pressure and salt and water retention. Oedema is preceded by a gain in body weight of some 3–5 kg due to an increase in the extracellular fluid.

Normally, fluid exudes into the tissues at the arterial ends of capillaries because the hydrostatic pressure of approximately 30 mmHg exceeds the colloid osmotic pressure of 25 mmHg. Fluid is reabsorbed at the venous ends because the hydrostatic pressure at this point is approximately 12 mmHg. Oedema occurs when there is inadequate reabsorption of fluid from the tissues. A high venous pressure alone can, by increasing the hydrostatic force at the venous ends of the capillaries, cause oedema, as it does, for example, in vena caval obstruction. Raised venous pressure is nearly always a factor in cardiac oedema, but is seldom the sole explanation, for the retention of salt and water almost invariably antedates the appearance of the oedema.

The location of oedema in cardiac failure is determined by local factors, particularly gravity. In the ambulant patient, it occurs bilaterally in the lower legs and feet; in those kept in bed, it accumulates in the sacral area. When the oedema is very great, it may affect the whole of the lower limbs, the genitalia, the abdominal and chest walls and even the face (anasarca).

In the oedema of cardiac failure, the tissues dimple ('pit') when pressure is applied to them by the thumb.

ASCITES

The intraperitoneal accumulation of fluid is a manifestation of advanced heart disease, usually occurring later than peripheral oedema but for similar reasons. In some conditions, however, such as tricuspid valve disease and constrictive pericarditis, ascites may be even more evident than oedema and is probably then, in part, a consequence of portal hypertension secondary to cardiac cirrhosis of the liver.

CYANOSIS

Cyanosis, a blue discoloration of the skin or mucous membranes, is more a sign than a symptom of heart disease and is often first noticed by relatives when the affected individual exercises or is exposed to cold temperatures. It is usually due to a large proportion of reduced haemoglobin in the superficial capillaries and venules. It has been observed that cyanosis appears when the amount of reduced haemoglobin in the blood of these vessels exceeds 5 g/100 ml.

Cyanosis results either from oxygen desaturation of the arterial blood or from an unusually large extraction of oxygen in the peripheral tissues. When the cyanosis is due to arterial oxygen desaturation, it is considered to be 'central' in origin because it is caused by a disorder in the heart or lungs. When the cause of the cyanosis is high oxygen extraction in the tissues, it is said to be 'peripheral'.

Central cyanosis is due either to blood bypassing the lungs as it is shunted from the venous side of the circulation to the arterial, as a result of congenital heart disease, or to inadequate oxygenation of the blood in the lungs, as in some varieties of lung disease. Clubbing of the digits is a common accompaniment of cyanotic congenital heart disease.

Peripheral cyanosis, a consequence of diminished blood flow through the skin and mucous membranes, occurs in normal people when they are cold, and in patients with a low cardiac output due to such conditions as mitral stenosis and acute circulatory failure.

The differentiation of central from peripheral cyanosis is usually not difficult. In peripheral cyanosis the skin is cold, and the cyanosis does not affect the warm mucous membranes such as those of the tongue. Furthermore, peripheral cyanosis can be abolished by warming the skin. The central origin of the cyanosis can be confirmed by measuring the arterial oxygen saturation which is usually less than 85%.

Rarely, central cyanosis may be due, not to arterial oxygen desaturation, but to methaemoglobinaemia or sulphaemoglobinaemia as a result of taking certain drugs.

HAEMOPTYSIS

The expectoration of blood is not uncommon in patients with heart disease. When it occurs it is a sign of advanced disease. Several mechanisms are involved; examination of the sputum may help to determine which of them is responsible.

Frank haemoptysis – the coughing up of pure blood – occurs in mitral stenosis, due to the rupture of pulmonary or bronchial veins, or to pulmonary infarction. When there is pulmonary infection, the sputum may be purulent or rusty in appearance. In pulmonary oedema, the frothy sputum may be pink or streaked with blood.

Of course, patients with heart disease may also have haemoptysis due to other types of lung disease such as tuberculosis, bronchiectasis and bronchial neoplasm.

SYNCOPE

Syncope is a transient loss of consciousness due to inadequate cerebral blood flow or perfusion pressure. Cerebral blood flow and perfusion pressure depend upon the cardiac output, the arterial blood pressure and the resistance of the cerebral circulation. Cerebral arteries are relatively uninfluenced by the autonomic system but are dilated by carbon dioxide.

Syncope can take on a number of different forms:

Vasomotor or vasodepressor syncope. The commonest type of syncope is that of the simple faint. It is often a response to emotion, but various physical factors such as blood loss, debility after infection and pain may contribute to its occurrence. It results from a combination of dilatation of the arterial resistance vessels in the muscles and a fall in heart rate. The resulting fall in blood pressure causes a diminished perfusion pressure in the brain and loss of consciousness.

Fainting of this kind usually develops when standing, rarely when sitting and virtually never when lying or walking. The first symptom is usually a sense of weakness, accompanied by yawning or sighing, sweating, nausea and 'a sinking feeling' in the stomach. After seconds or minutes, unconsciousness ensues; this is transient because the subject usually falls flat on the ground and this posture leads to an improvement in cerebral blood flow. In a severe attack, the face is pale, the pupils are dilated and respiration is slow. The heart rate is usually diminished and the radial pulse difficult to feel, although carotid artery pulsation can be detected without difficulty.

Micturition syncope. This occurs in adult men with nocturia. Consciousness is lost immediately after passing urine. It is particularly likely after considerable alcohol consumption. It may be due to reflex vasodilatation secondary to sudden relief of distension of the bladder combined with the vasodilator effects of alcohol and a warm bed.

Arrhythmias. This may result in syncope. A catastrophic fall in cardiac output may result if the heart rate is either extremely slow or very fast. In supraventricular and ventricular tachycardias the ventricular rate sometimes exceeds 180/min, leaving insufficient time for adequate filling of the heart. An important and dangerous form of syncope is the *Adams–Stokes attack*, which is a brief episode of cardiac arrest due to either asystole or ventricular fibrillation. This characteristically occurs in patients with heart block in whom either the ventricular pacemaker suddenly fails, or in whom ventricular arrhythmias are superimposed on the heart block. In most cases, effective cardiac action returns in 10–15 s, but if the attack is more prolonged, convulsions may occur. The return of consciousness is accompanied by flushing as blood flows once more through vessels dilated by hypoxia.

Syncope on exertion. This is a characteristic feature of severe aortic stenosis (see p. 255), and may be due to an inability of the heart to supply an adequate blood flow in the face of the increased demands of the muscles. Patients with aortic stenosis are also susceptible to syncope due to heart block or ventricular arrhythmias. Exertional syncope should also always raise suspicions of an exercise-induced tachyarrhythmia.

Carotid sinus syncope. This is a condition occurring in elderly individuals in whom light pressure on the carotid sinus produces extreme cardiac slowing or reflex hypotension.

Postural syncope. When a normal individual stands up, pooling of blood in the legs is prevented by arteriolar and venous constriction, and there is an acceleration of the heart rate together with an increase in plasma catecholamine levels. Postural syncope, due to orthostatic hypotension, occurs in patients with autonomic disorders, including diabetic neuropathy and tabes dorsalis, as well as in some otherwise normal elderly individuals in whom these compensatory mechanisms do not function. It also frequently arises in individuals treated excessively with diuretics or antihypertensive drugs.

FURTHER READING

Criteria Committee of the New York Heart Association (1964) *Diseases of the Heart and Blood Vessels (Nomenclature and Criteria for Diagnosis)*. Boston: Little, Brown.

CHAPTER 3

The physical signs of heart disease

Signs are small measurable things but interpretations are illimitable.

George Eliot, *Middlemarch*

THE ARTERIAL PULSE

The elastic structure of the aorta and its major branches enables them to act as both reservoirs and conduits. As a consequence, they are able to convert the highly pulsatile discontinuous blood flow from the ventricles into a more continuous flow in the peripheral vessels. The pressure pulse recorded a short distance above the aortic valve shows a sharp upstroke, produced by the rapid ejection of blood from the left ventricle, followed by a slower downstroke, as the rate of flow into peripheral arteries exceeds that from the left ventricle into the aorta (Fig. 3.1). This descending limb of the pulse wave is interrupted by the *dicrotic notch*, as the column of blood, briefly retreating towards the ventricle at the onset of diastole, is halted by aortic valve closure. As the main wave of the pulse travels peripherally, secondary waves are produced at the points of branching of the arteries. These are reflected backwards and summate with the main wave. Consequently, the peak systolic pressure in a peripheral artery may be higher than that in the central aorta.

When the arterial pulse is examined, the following characteristics should be noted:

- rate
- rhythm
- amplitude
- character or wave form.

It is customary to feel the right radial artery to determine the rate and rhythm of the heart, but the amplitude and quality of the pulse is better appreciated in the branchial or carotid arteries.

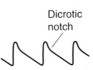

Dicrotic notch

Fig. 3.1 The normal arterial pulse wave.

One should also search for pulsation in the radial, brachial, carotid, femoral, dorsalis pedis and posterior tibial arteries on both sides.

The heart and pulse rate

The rate of the pulse, if regular, can be calculated by multiplying the number of beats in 15 s by 4. If it is irregular, the number of beats in 30 s should be doubled. The pulse rate in normal resting adults ranges from 60 to 100/min. A rate of less than 60/min is most commonly due to sinus bradycardia (see p. 160), but may also be due to junctional rhythm or heart block. Rates in excess of 100/min (tachycardia) are most often due to sinus tachycardia associated with emotion or exercise; the heart rate may exceed 200 beats per minute on vigorous exercise. If the rate exceeds 120/min at rest in adults, some form of arrhythmia is likely (see Ch. 9).

Pulse rhythm

The normal pulse is regular or exhibits sinus arrhythmia, which is a rise in rate with inspiration and fall in rate with expiration. In the case of irregular rhythms, the nature of the irregularity may suggest the underlying cause:

- An occasional irregularity in an otherwise regular pulse suggests ectopic beats.
- A totally irregular pulse suggests atrial fibrillation.

The amplitude and character of the pulse

The amplitude of the pulse depends on the pulse pressure, i.e. the difference between the systolic and diastolic pressures. Different types of pulse are as follows:

- *Small volume pulse.* This is the case when there is a low stroke volume and peripheral vasoconstriction as occurs in acute myocardial infarction, the shock syndrome, mitral stenosis and pericardial constriction or tamponade.
- *Anacrotic pulse.* This may occur in aortic stenosis; the pulse is small and prolonged and has a slow upstroke. (Fig. 3.2).
- *Pulsus bisferiens.* This is another possible pulse abnormality in aortic valve disease; the pulse is of moderate or large volume in which a double beat can be felt. This sign suggests a combination of aortic stenosis and regurgitation.
- *Large volume pulse.* This occurs in aortic regurgitation, anaemia, pregnancy and thyrotoxicosis.

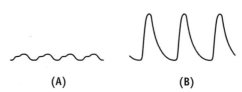

(A)   (B)

Fig. 3.2 (A) The pulse of severe aortic stenosis. (B) The rapidly rising and collapsing pulse of aortic regurgitation.

- *Collapsing pulse*. When a large volume pulse rises rapidly and collapses suddenly (Fig. 3.2) it is described as a *collapsing* pulse; this is also called a *waterhammer* pulse after a Victorian toy of this name. This type of pulse is encountered when there is a rapid runoff of blood during diastole as in aortic regurgitation, persistent ductus arteriosus and arteriovenous fistulae. It is best felt by placing the palm of the hand on the patient's vertically elevated forearm, thereby increasing the retrograde flow of blood during diastole.
- *Respiratory pulse variation*. A reduction in systolic pressure of up to 10 mmHg may occur on inspiration in normal people, probably because the capacity of the pulmonary vascular bed enlarges and reduces the return of blood to the left ventricle. This is partly compensated for by a simultaneous increase in right ventricular output.
- *Pulsus paradoxus*. A more substantial inspiratory fall, which occurs in obstructive airways disease, especially asthma, and pericardial constriction, produces *pulsus paradoxus*. In obstructive lung disease, the reduction in arterial pressure is the consequence of the increased negativity of the intrathoracic pressure. In pericardial constriction and tamponade, an inspiratory increase in the right ventricle occurs at the expense of the left ventricle, as they are both confined within an indistensible pericardium.
- *Pulsus alternans*. In this, the beats are evenly spaced in time but are alternately large and small in volume. This is most readily detected when the blood pressure is being measured, for as the cuff is being deflated, only alternate beats are heard at first. After a fall of a further 5 or 10 mmHg, every beat is audible. Pulsus alternans is frequently a sign of severe left ventricular failure.
- *Absence of a peripheral pulse*. This indicates an anatomical aberration, or narrowing or occlusion of the artery proximal to it. In coarctation of the aorta (p. 291), pulsation of the femoral arteries is delayed compared with that of the radial arteries.

BLOOD PRESSURE MEASUREMENT

Precise measurement of the blood pressure can be obtained only by intraarterial catheterization but a sphygmomanometer is sufficiently accurate for clinical purposes. This instrument consists of a manometer linked to an inflatable bag, surrounded by an inelastic cuff. The size of bag and cuff is of importance in ensuring accuracy, large cuffs being required for the obese and small for children. The cuff must fit around the arm snugly, being neither loose nor touching any article of clothing. It should be applied about 2 cm above the antecubital space with the rubber bag over the medial aspect of the arm.

Guidelines for practice:

- It is best for the patient to be reclining comfortably, but the blood pressure can be taken satisfactorily with the patient sitting or standing provided the limb is supported and at the same level as the heart.
- The patient should be warm, comfortable and in a quiet environment, and should have stayed in the same position for 5 min before the blood pressure recording; if in doubt, several recordings should be made.

PRACTICE GUIDELINES

- The cuff should be inflated until the pulsations of the brachial artery can no longer be felt. The pressure is then raised by a further 20 mmHg.
- The diaphragm of the stethoscope is placed over the brachial artery in the antecubital fossa, just below the cuff.
- The pressure in the cuff is gradually reduced at about 2 mmHg per second. As the pressure falls, sounds (Korotkoff sounds) are heard. The pressure at first appearance of the sounds (phase 1) is the *systolic pressure*.
- As the pressure falls further the sounds muffle (phase 4) and then disappear altogether (phase 5). *Diastolic pressure* is usually taken as phase 5, because measurement is more consistent than phase 4 and because phase 5 more closely represents the intravascular diastolic pressure.
- Sometimes there is a period of silence (phase 2) after the first appearance of the sounds before they reappear (phase 3). This is known as the auscultatory gap. It is important not to mistake phase 2 or phase 5 or indeed phase 3 for phase 1.

Occasionally it may be of value to measure blood pressure in the leg; the patient should be lying on the abdomen, with a large cuff covering the mid-thigh region, and the stethoscope placed in the popliteal fossa.

Certain circumstances make blood pressure estimations difficult. In atrial fibrillation and other arrhythmias, the blood pressure may vary from beat to beat; the average of a number of beats should be taken for both the systolic and diastolic pressures.

THE VENOUS PULSE AND PRESSURE (FIG. 3.3)

Inspection of the veins in the neck is an essential but often neglected part of cardiac diagnosis. The external jugular vein is easily seen, but is so often obstructed as it passes through the fascial plane that it cannot be relied upon as a guide to the true venous pressure. The internal jugular vein cannot be directly visualized, but it imparts a broad pulsation to the tissues of the neck overlying it. Its undulations can be seen in virtually all individuals, if the correct technique of examination is used; occasionally, especially in the obese or bullnecked, it cannot be identified.

There are normally three peaks:

- 'a' corresponding to atrial systole
- 'c' occurring at the time of tricuspid valve closure
- 'v' at the time of tricuspid valve opening.

There are two troughs:

- 'x' corresponding to the descent of the tricuspid valve ring as the right ventricle contracts
- 'y' trough representing the fall in pressure as blood flows into the right ventricle.

As it is usually not possible to see the 'c' wave in the jugular pulse, the normal venous pulse in the neck is composed of two positive and two negative waves (Fig. 3.3).

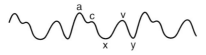

Fig. 3.3 The venous pulse. Note the 'a' wave due to atrial systole and the 'c' wave occurring at the time of tricuspid valve closure. The upstroke of the 'v' wave occurs as the atrium is filling passively during ventricular systole; the descent from the peak of 'v' to 'y' occurs as blood flows from the atrium to the ventricle after tricuspid valve opening.

It is important to observe both the *waveform* and the *pressure level* of the jugular venous pulse.

PRACTICE GUIDELINES

The patient should be reclining with the chest, head and neck at 45°, and with the muscles of the neck relaxed. A number of points aid in distinguishing a venous from an arterial pulse:

- The venous pulse normally shows two positive pulsations in each cardiac cycle compared with the single pulsation in the arteries.
- The venous pulse cannot usually be felt, although it can be readily seen, whereas the arterial pulsation is more easily felt than seen.
- The venous pulse waves can be obliterated by light pressure at the root of the neck.
- Pressure on the abdomen, by increasing venous return to the thorax, increases the venous pressure in the neck transiently and permits it to be visualized more easily.

The venous pressure

The venous pressure is assessed as the vertical height of the top of the venous column above the sternal angle. In normal individuals, this does not exceed 2 cm. If venous pulsation cannot be seen with the patient at 45°, the patient should be placed more horizontally until it can. In some patients the venous pulse may be so elevated that the level of the pulse only becomes apparent with the patient sitting fully upright.

Venous waveform

The timing of venous waves may be difficult to assess; it is essential either to feel the carotid artery pulsation on the other side of the neck or to listen for the first heart sound in order to allow identification of the 'a' wave which precedes these two events.

In pathological states a number of abnormal waveforms may be observed:

- *Giant 'a' wave* (Fig. 3.4). This develops when the right atrium contracts forcefully against the increased resistance provided by a stenotic tricuspid valve, or hypertrophied right ventricle.
- *Cannon waves*. These are large venous pulsations due to atrial contraction against a closed tricuspid valve. They occur intermittently in complete heart block and in ventricular tachycardia when atrial and ventricular systoles coincide (Fig. 3.4). In junctional rhythms, atrial and ventricular

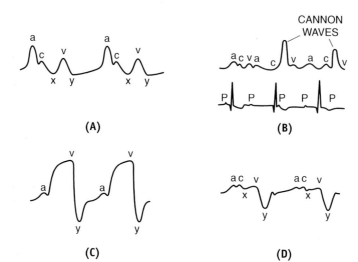

Fig. 3.4 (A) The giant 'a' wave. (B) Intermittent cannon waves in complete heart block, occurring at the time of synchronous atrial and ventricular contraction. (C) The systolic venous pulsation of tricuspid regurgitation. (D) The venous pulse in pericardial constriction, showing the rapid 'y' descent, followed by a plateau.

contractions are synchronous and cannon waves occur with every heart beat.

- *Systolic venous pulsation ('v' wave).* This is due to blood regurgitating into the venous system during ventricular systole and is characteristic of tricuspid regurgitation (Fig. 3.4).
- *Pericardial constriction.* In this, the venous pressure is greatly raised, and there is a sharp 'y' descent as blood rushes into the right ventricle in the early part of diastole (Fig. 3.4). Another feature of this condition is elevation of venous pressure during inspiration because the increase in venous return at this time cannot be accommodated by the constricted right ventricle.

INSPECTION OF THE CHEST

Abnormalities of the thorax and lungs may cause changes in the position of the heart; they may also result from or cause heart disease. Funnel chest (pectus excavatum) and kyphoscoliosis may lead to displacement of the heart. Cardiac enlargement associated with advanced congenital heart disease in childhood may cause deformity of the sternum and ribs.

The rate and pattern of breathing should be noted. The respiratory rate is often increased in left ventricular failure. Prolonged expiration suggests obstructive airway disease.

The cardiac impulse is frequently visible, particularly when there is heart disease. It is often possible to see the exaggerated apical impulse of left ventricular hypertrophy, the displaced apex of left ventricular dilatation, the left parasternal pulsation of right ventricular hypertrophy or the abnormal pulmonary arterial pulsation in the second and third left interspaces in pulmonary hypertension.

PALPATION OF THE CHEST

The apex beat

In the normal individual, the maximal thrust of the left ventricle – the apex beat – can be felt at or just internal to the mid-clavicular line in the fifth intercostal space. If it is displaced, one should determine whether this is due to abnormalities of the thoracic cage or lungs. After the apex beat has been located and assessed, the whole precordium should be explored with the palm of the hand in the search for abnormal pulsation.

PRACTICE GUIDELINES

The ventricular impulse may be abnormal in a number of different ways:
- Left ventricular hypertrophy produces a sustained heaving or thrusting apex beat.
- Left ventricular dilatation displaces the apex downwards and outwards. If there is a large left ventricular stroke volume, as in aortic regurgitation, the impulse is vigorous, but when myocardial contractility is impaired as by ischaemic heart disease, it may be diffuse and feeble.
- In mitral stenosis, the apex beat often has a characteristic abrupt tapping quality due to the vibrations associated with the loud first sound.
- In patients with a left ventricular aneurysm, the outward movement of the aneurysmal segment during systole gives rise to an abnormal sustained apical impulse.
- In patients with hypertrophic obstructive cardiomyopathy, a characteristic double impulse can sometimes be palpated, the first phase representing the onset of systole and the second contraction against an obstructed outflow.

Right ventricular impulse

The right ventricular impulse in the left parasternal region is not usually palpable in health, except in children and thin adults.

PRACTICE GUIDELINES

- In right ventricular hypertrophy, as occurs in pulmonary stenosis and pulmonary hypertension (particularly secondary to mitral stenosis), there is a sustained lifting impulse along the left sternal edge.
- When there is right ventricular dilatation associated with a high right ventricular output (as in atrial septal defect), the impulse is vigorous but less sustained.
- Pulmonary arterial pulsation can quite often be felt in the second left intercostal space when there is pulmonary hypertension or high pulmonary blood flow.
- Occasionally, the pulsation of an aneurysm can be detected in the aortic area.

Thrills

Thrills are the tactile equivalent of murmurs. They do not occur in the absence of loud murmurs and have no significance beyond that possessed by the murmur. Thrills are usually best felt by the palm of the hand when patients are sitting upright and holding their breath in full expiration. The commonest thrills are the following:

- an apical systolic thrill corresponding with the loud systolic murmur of mitral regurgitation
- a systolic thrill between the apex and the left sternal edge in ventricular septal defect
- a systolic thrill in the second right intercostal space, occasionally over the sternum and the third or fourth left intercostal space, in aortic stenosis. This is often associated with a systolic thrill over the carotid arteries
- a systolic thrill in the second or third left intercostal spaces in pulmonary stenosis
- diastolic and presystolic thrills at the apex in mitral stenosis (best felt with the patient rotated to the left)
- a continuous systolic and diastolic thrill below the left clavicle in persistent ductus arteriosus.

It is rare for the murmurs of aortic or pulmonary regurgitation to be accompanied by a thrill.

After the chest has been palpated, the opportunity should be taken to palpate the abdomen. Particular attention should be paid to the liver. Enlargement, often tender, is a characteristic feature of rightsided heart failure. Systolic pulsation may be felt in tricuspid regurgitation.

Percussion of the heart

Although originally described as a means of estimating size and position of the heart, estimates are crude and have no place in an era when echocardiography can provide the same information both easily and accurately.

AUSCULTATION: HEART SOUNDS AND MURMURS

Vibrations within the heart give rise to sounds which are loud enough to be audible through a stethoscope and to be registered graphically by a phonocardiogram. If the noise is brief and transient, it is termed a heart sound; if more prolonged, it is a murmur. Careful auscultation, combined with the other methods of physical examination, provides information about the heart which even the most sophisticated modern techniques of investigation can scarcely match.

Physicians should always use stethoscopes with which they are familiar. The earpieces should fit comfortably; the tubing should be short (not greater than 30 cm) and thick-walled. Both types of endpiece (diaphragm and bell) are necessary:

- The rigid diaphragm is best for hearing high-frequency sounds and murmurs such as the second heart sound and the diastolic murmur of aortic regurgitation.
- The bell pressed *lightly* on the chest is superior to the diaphragm for the low-pitched third and fourth heart sounds and the mid-diastolic and presystolic murmurs of mitral stenosis.

Traditionally, there are four areas of auscultation:

- aortic (right second intercostal space)
- pulmonary (left second intercostal space)
- tricuspid (lower sternal)
- mitral (apex beat).

These designations are somewhat misleading, especially with regard to the aortic valve, because aortic murmurs (especially if diastolic) are often maximal at the left sternal edge at the level of the fourth intercostal space. The opening snap of mitral stenosis is also best heard in this area. Auscultation should never be restricted to the traditional areas; one should start on one side of the precordium and gradually move the stethoscope towards the other areas.

Guidelines for practice:

- Palpate the carotid artery during auscultation to identify the first and second heart sounds – carotid pulsation occurs just after the first heart sound.
- Begin in the pulmonary area. The aortic area may be listened to next, before moving obliquely across the sternum to the lower left sternal edge, thence to the tricuspid area, to the mitral area and into the axilla.
- Initially, the first heart sound should be identified and assessed before turning one's attention to the second heart sound and to any additional sounds.
- Having noted any normal or abnormal sounds, one should then listen for systolic and, later, for diastolic murmurs.
- One should then listen particularly in the aortic, pulmonary and lower left sternal edge areas with the patient sitting up and holding the breath in full expiration.
- The apical area should be listened to with the patient rotated into the left lateral position.
- If mitral stenosis is suspected, the patient should exercise by sitting forward and backwards several times, and then lie down again in the left lateral position.

The heart sounds

The first sound

The first sound occurs at the time of closure of the atrioventricular valves. Although some have attributed the sound to the impact of closure, it seems more likely that it is due to the tensing of the cusps as they are projected into the atrium at the beginning of ventricular systole. Both tricuspid and mitral valves contribute to the sound. As these valves close slightly asynchronously, the first heart sound, in health, may be narrowly split. As the mitral component is louder, the first heart sound is usually best heard at the apex.

The intensity of the first heart sound is related to the extent of upward movement of the cusps when the ventricles contract. In the normal resting heart the valve cusps come into light contact with each other before the onset of ventricular systole which, therefore, projects them only a short distance. Characteristics associated with different sounds are as follows:

- If the cusps are well down in the ventricular chamber, ventricular systole forces them rapidly upwards and causes a loud sound. This situation arises when the atrium contracts immediately before the ventricle (short PR interval) and when the left atrial pressure is abnormally high, as in mitral stenosis.
- In complete heart block, the relationship between atrial and ventricular systole changes from cycle to cycle, and the first sound varies in intensity accordingly.
- When the cusps are rigid, as in calcific mitral valve disease, the first sound is soft or inaudible.

The second sound

The second heart sound is related to the closure of the semilunar valves. Normally, it is single on expiration but splits into its aortic and pulmonary components during inspiration (Fig. 3.5). This phenomenon is accounted for by the prolongation of right ventricular systole associated with the increased flow into the right side of the heart occurring with inspiration. Splitting is best heard in the second left intercostal space and can occur as follows:

- Abnormally wide splitting of the second sound, due to delay in pulmonary valve closure, occurs when the right ventricle is over-burdened by either a volume load (as in atrial septal defect) or a pressure load (as in pulmonary stenosis), or when there is a delay in electrical activation of the right ventricle (as in right bundle branch block).
- In atrial septal defect, there is usually 'fixed' splitting of the second heart sound because the increase in venous return on inspiration affects the filling of both ventricles.
- When there is left bundle branch block and when the left ventricle is over-burdened, as by systemic hypertension or aortic stenosis, the aortic component of the sound may be delayed. This produces 'reversed' splitting; the sound being single on inspiration and split on expiration (Fig. 3.6).

The intensity of the second heart sound may be increased by systemic or pulmonary hypertension, but this is not a reliable sign. The aortic component of the second sound may be reduced or inaudible in aortic stenosis, particularly if the aortic valve is calcified, and the pulmonary component may be soft or absent in pulmonary stenosis. Both first and second sounds may be

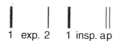

1   exp. 2   1 insp. ap

Fig. 3.5 Normal splitting of the second heart sound during inspiration, with the aortic component preceding the pulmonary.

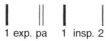

1 exp. pa   1 insp. 2

Fig. 3.6 'Reversed' splitting of the second sound. Due to delay in left ventricular emptying, the aortic component follows the pulmonary component of the second sound on expiration. On inspiration, the pulmonary component is, as usual, delayed and is superimposed on the aortic component.

soft when the heart is separated from the chest wall by fat, pericardial effusion or emphysematous lung, or when the cardiac output is low as in shock.

The third sound (Fig. 3.7A)

The third sound occurs at the end of the period of rapid filling of the ventricles. It is probably due to sudden tensing of the valve structures and ventricular walls at this time. It is usually generated in the left ventricle and is best heard at or internal to the apex. The sound is low-pitched and distant, and is often heard only with the lightly applied stethoscope bell. Although normal in the young, it is a pathological finding in the middle-aged and elderly. Its presence implies either left ventricular failure or abnormally rapid filling of the ventricle, as in mitral regurgitation, pregnancy or anaemia. Occasionally, a third heart sound can be heard over the right ventricle in right ventricular failure. In pericardial constriction, there is a very early third heart sound of higher frequency associated with the sudden limitation to ventricular filling.

The fourth or atrial sound (Fig. 3.7B)

This sound resembles the third heart sound in being low-pitched and best heard at the apex, and probably has a similar mechanism. In this instance, the ventricular distension results from atrial contraction; the fourth sound immediately precedes the first heart sound. It is rarely heard in health, and is usually a sign of either ventricular failure or hypertrophy. Thus, a fourth heart sound is heard over the left ventricle in some cases of aortic stenosis, hypertension and ischaemic heart disease. A right ventricular fourth heart sound may be heard at the left sternal edge in pulmonary stenosis and pulmonary hypertension.

Gallop rhythm

This term is applied to a cadence of three heart sounds which may be heard in the presence of tachycardia. It may be due to a third heart sound, to a fourth heart sound or to the superimposition of the two ('summation gallop').

Additional sounds in systole

Early systolic sounds (ejection sounds or clicks) occur at the time of aortic and pulmonary valve opening (Fig. 3.7C). The clicks may arise from sudden

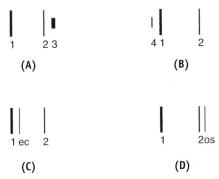

Fig. 3.7 (A) The third heart sound. (B) The fourth or atrial sound. (C) The ejection click (ec). (D) The opening snap.

tensing of the opening cusps or from distension of the great vessels. Aortic clicks are almost invariable in valvar aortic stenosis provided the cusps are not calcified, and may be present in systemic hypertension. Pulmonary systolic clicks occur under conditions in which the pulmonary artery is dilated, as it is in valvar pulmonary stenosis and in pulmonary hypertension. They are usually heard best in held expiration.

Clicks occurring later in systole are usually due to ballooning of a mitral valve cusp (mitral valve prolapse). A systolic clicking or crunching may occur in pneumothorax.

The opening snap (Fig. 3.7D)

This is one of the most important signs in auscultation and is virtually diagnostic of mitral stenosis. It occurs at the time of mitral valve opening and is presumed to be due to sudden tension of stenosed but pliant cusps. It is soft or absent if the mitral valve is rigid from fibrosis or calcification. It is heard best at the left sternal edge in the fourth intercostal space or between this point and the apex beat and has a snapping quality. Unlike splitting of the second sound and the third heart sound with which it may be confused, it can often be heard widely over the precordium (see Table 3.1).

Heart murmurs

Murmurs appear to result from vibrations set up by turbulent blood flow. Turbulence is encouraged by high velocity of flow, by abrupt change in the calibre of a vessel or chamber and by reduced blood viscosity.

Table 3.1 The differentiation of splitting of the second heart sound, the opening snap, and the third heart sound (of the left ventricle)

	Splitting of second sound (normal)	Splitting of second sound (fixed)	Splitting of second sound (reversed)	Opening snap	Third heart sound
Interval between first component of second sound and 'extra' sound	0–0.05 s (maximal on inspiration)	0.03–0.08 s (at all phases)	0.01–0.03 s (maximal on expiration)	0.03–0.12 s	0.10–0.16 s
Effect of inspiration	Widens	Unaffected	Narrows	None	None
Character		Abrupt – heard best with diaphragm		'Snap' – heard best with diaphragm	Low-pitched – heard best with bell
Site of maximal intensity		Second left intercostal space		Lower left sternal edge	At apex
Radiation		Left sternal edge		All cardiac areas	Localized (usually)

Murmurs therefore develop when there is rapid flow through a valve, valvar narrowing, or anaemia.

The following features of a murmur should be noted:

- its timing in the cardiac cycle
- its location and radiation
- its intensity and its quality.

Murmurs may occur either in systole or in diastole; they may continue from one into the other.

Murmurs are usually best heard at the place on the chest wall closest to their site of origin or in the direction of blood flow. Thus, the murmur of aortic stenosis is loudest over the aortic valve (the third left intercostal space), or in the second right intercostal space, or in the neck. On the other hand, the diastolic murmur of aortic regurgitation is usually maximal at the fourth left intercostal space and is less well heard in the 'aortic area'.

The intensity of murmurs can be classified in six grades:

- *Grade 1* Only just audible, even under good auscultatory conditions
- *Grade 2* Soft
- *Grade 3* Moderately loud
- *Grade 4* Loud and accompanied by a palpable thrill
- *Grade 5* Very loud but not audible with the stethoscope away from the chest
- *Grade 6* So loud as to be audible with the stethoscope lifted from the chest wall.

In practice only systolic murmurs are ever loud enough to achieve grades 5 and 6; diastolic murmurs are classified using the 4 grades, 1 to 4.

The quality of a murmur may be 'blowing', 'rumbling', 'harsh' or 'musical'. These are poor descriptions of what is heard; only with experience can one appreciate what is meant by such terms. Murmurs may also be described as low, medium or high pitched.

Systolic murmurs

These murmurs are usually midsystolic or pansystolic (holosystolic) in timing.

Midsystolic murmurs

These murmurs start after the opening of the aortic and pulmonary valves, increase in intensity to a maximum in midsystole and decrease and disappear before the second heart sound (Fig. 3.8A). Because of their configuration, they are sometimes called 'diamond-shaped', and are also termed 'ejection systolic murmurs' because they arise during ejection of blood from the ventricles into great arteries. Murmurs arising at the aortic and pulmonary valves are characteristically midsystolic. Other characteristics and locations of these murmurs are as follows:

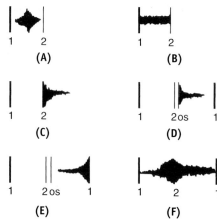

Fig. 3.8 (A) A midsystolic murmur. (B) A pansystolic murmur. (C) An early diastolic murmur. (D) A mid-diastolic murmur, following an opening snap in mitral stenosis. (E) The presystolic murmur of mitral stenosis. (F) The continuous murmur of a persistent ductus arteriosus.

- The murmur of *aortic stenosis*, which is often harsh, is usually best heard in the second right intercostal space, although sometimes it is maximal at the lower left sternal edge or even at the apex. It frequently radiates to the neck. The murmur of subaortic stenosis is loudest at the lower left sternal edge.
- The murmur of pulmonary valve stenosis is maximal at the second left intercostal space, that of infundibular pulmonary stenosis most intense at the third or fourth left intercostal space.
- A systolic murmur due to high flow in the pulmonary artery is characteristic of atrial septal defect but also occurs in conditions associated with a high cardiac output such as pregnancy, thyrotoxicosis and anaemia. These murmurs are usually of no more than grade 3 intensity and are not associated with thrills.
- Quite frequently, particularly in children, midsystolic murmurs may be heard in the pulmonary area for which no organic cause can be found. These may be termed 'functional' or 'benign'. Such murmurs are neither intense nor accompanied by a thrill. They usually vary with position and respiration.

Pansystolic (holosystolic) murmurs

These murmurs persist from the first to the second heart sound and only occur as a result of mitral regurgitation, tricuspid regurgitation or ventricular septal defect, for it is only in these conditions that a pressure difference exists across the defective valve or septum throughout systole (Fig. 3.8B). The characteristics and locations of these murmurs are as follows:

- In mitral regurgitation, the murmur is maximal at or just internal to the apex beat, and radiates into the axilla. It may be maximal in late systole.
- The murmur of tricuspid regurgitation is usually loudest in the xiphisternal region, or at the lower left sternal edge. It frequently radiates to the apex and may therefore be readily confused with that of mitral

regurgitation, but differs in becoming louder on inspiration, due to the increase in venous return at this time. In practice, tricuspid regurgitant murmurs are rare.

- The murmur of ventricular septal defect is usually loud and is maximal at the lower left sternal edge.

Late systolic murmurs

In addition to midsystolic and pansystolic murmurs, murmurs can be confined to late systole; this is generally a sign of a prolapsed mitral cusp and characteristically follows a midsystolic click.

Assessing the significance of a systolic murmur

This is a very common clinical problem. Systolic murmurs are commonplace, particularly amongst the elderly. While echocardiography may be necessary for a definitive opinion as to the significance of a murmur, a reasonable judgement can generally be reached on clinical grounds, based on a murmur's timing, location, radiation, intensity and character in association with other abnormal findings.

- In *aortic stenosis*, there is usually a loud murmur at the lower left sternal edge and aortic area, which frequently radiates to the carotids. There may be additional clues as to the diagnosis with an associated thrill, a small flat pulse and left ventricular hypertrophy. If the valve cusps are not calcified, there is an early systolic ('ejection') click; if the stenosis is severe, there may be reversed splitting of the second sound.
- In *aortic valve sclerosis*, a common finding in the elderly, there is an aortic systolic murmur in the absence of any of the other features of aortic stenosis.
- In *pulmonary stenosis*, the loud murmur in the pulmonary or lower left sternal area is accompanied by right ventricular hypertrophy, a soft and late pulmonary component of the second sound and a systolic thrill.
- In severe *mitral regurgitation*, the apical systolic murmur, which is well heard from cardiac apex to axilla, is usually accompanied by left ventricular enlargement. It may be accompanied by a third heart sound and a mid-diastolic flow murmur.
- *Tricuspid regurgitant* murmurs are rare, but if present are usually increased by inspiration. However, it is generally of greater value to search for associated signs of tricuspid regurgitation, a prominent systolic 'V' wave in the jugular venous pulse and a pulsatile liver.
- *Benign systolic murmurs* are seldom of more than grade 2 intensity, are never pansystolic, are usually best heard in the pulmonary area and are not associated with cardiac enlargement or with abnormal heart sounds. Similar murmurs are encountered in pregnancy, thyrotoxicosis and anaemia, and these conditions should be excluded before a murmur is accepted as being of no significance.
- The pulmonary systolic murmur of atrial septal defect resembles a benign systolic murmur but is accompanied by wide splitting of the second heart sound, and often by a mid-diastolic murmur due to high flow across the tricuspid valve.

Diastolic murmurs

Diastolic murmurs are of three main varieties: early diastolic, mid-diastolic and presystolic.

Early (immediate) diastolic murmurs

These murmurs occur shortly after closure of the aortic or pulmonary valves at the beginning of diastole (Fig. 3.8C). They are due to regurgitation through one or other of these valves when pressure in the aorta or pulmonary artery exceeds that of the related ventricle. The murmur decreases in intensity as diastole continues. The murmur is usually soft, high-pitched and blowing, and is best heard by using the diaphragm chest piece with the patient sitting forward, in full expiration. The locations of these murmurs are as follows:

- The murmur of *aortic regurgitation* is usually loudest at the third or fourth left intercostal space close to the sternum, but is occasionally maximal in the second right intercostal space.
- The uncommon early diastolic murmur of *pulmonary regurgitation* (the Graham Steell murmur) is best heard in the left second, third and fourth intercostal spaces. It is similar in character to that of aortic regurgitation but is increased by inspiration and is accompanied by signs of pulmonary hypertension.

Mid-diastolic murmurs

Mid-diastolic murmurs are associated with flow through the atrioventricular valves and necessarily start an appreciable time after the second heart sound. The causes of mid-diastolic murmurs are as follows:

- The most important cause is *mitral stenosis*, in which there is a low-pitched murmur maximal in a localized area at or internal to the apex beat. The murmur is most easily heard with the bell of the stethoscope and with the patient lying in the left lateral position, preferably after exercise (Fig. 3.8D). It is frequently associated with an opening snap, a presystolic murmur and a loud first heart sound.
- In tricuspid stenosis, a murmur due to a similar mechanism occurs, but in this condition it is maximal in the xiphisternal or lower left sternal region. This murmur is often of a rather scratchy character and is accentuated by inspiration. It is a very rare finding.
- Mid-diastolic murmurs may also occur when there is a *high blood flow* through atrioventricular valves. Such flow murmurs in the mitral area occur in association with mitral regurgitation, ventricular septal defect and persistent ductus arteriosus. A high-flow tricuspid murmur occurs in atrial septal defect. Another mid-diastolic murmur is that due to rheumatic valvulitis (the Carey Coombs murmur).
- A mid-diastolic murmur may also be heard, in the absence of mitral valve disease, in patients with severe aortic regurgitation (the Austin Flint murmur). This may be due to the aortic regurgitant flow pushing the aortic cusp of the mitral valve across the mitral valve orifice, thereby causing turbulence as blood is also flowing simultaneously from the left atrium to the left ventricle.

Presystolic murmurs

Presystolic murmurs are produced when atrial systole propels blood through narrowed mitral or tricuspid valves. The causes of presystolic murmurs are as follows:

- The *presystolic murmur of mitral stenosis* leads up to the loud first sound of that condition (Fig. 3.8E); it is most easily heard with the patient lying in the left lateral position with the bell of the stethoscope placed at or internal to the apex beat.
- The *presystolic murmur of tricuspid stenosis* is maximal in the xiphisternal region or at the lower left sternal edge and is accentuated by inspiration. It is rarely heard.

- Diastolic murmurs are in general more difficult to hear than systolic murmurs.
- They require 'focusing' one's attention on sounds of a specific frequency, high-pitched in the case of an early diastolic murmur and low-pitched in the case of a mid-diastolic murmur.
- In contradistinction to systolic murmurs, diastolic murmurs are always of pathological significance and should prompt further investigation.

Continuous murmurs

The term 'continuous' is applied to a murmur which starts during systole and continues into diastole; it is not necessarily continuous throughout the cardiac cycle. The commonest types are the venous hum and the murmur of persistent ductus arteriosus:

- The *venous hum* is common in childhood, but may be heard in anaemic or pregnant adults. It is due to high blood flow in the jugular veins and can be diminished or abolished by lying the patient flat, or by constricting the veins by pressure. It is usually loudest in the neck, but may be audible over the upper chest.
- The murmur in *persistent ductus arteriosus* is caused by the flow of blood from the high-pressure aorta into the low-pressure pulmonary artery. It is maximal in the left second intercostal space or under the left clavicle. It increases in intensity throughout systole, is maximal at the time of the second heart sound, and diminishes during diastole (Fig. 3.8F). It often has a 'machinery' or whirring quality.
- Similar murmurs are caused by systemic, pulmonary and coronary arteriovenous fistulae, and by rupture of an aneurysm of a sinus of Valsalva (see p. 326).

Pericardial friction rub

As roughened visceral and parietal layers of pericardium slide over one another, they produce a harsh creaking sound which may be likened to the noise made by two pieces of sandpaper rubbing together. As the movement occurs during ventricular systole, ventricular diastole and atrial systole, the rub may be present at one or all of these times. It may be heard all over the precordium, or only at a localized site. It usually sounds superficial and can be accentuated by leaning the patient forward or by pressing the stethoscope diaphragm firmly on the chest. It can occur in acute pericarditis of any cause, as well as in uraemic pericarditis and during the course of acute myocardial infarction. In the latter condition, it is often evanescent, lasting for only a few minutes or hours.

GENERAL EXAMINATION OF PATIENTS WITH CARDIAC DISEASE

In addition to a detailed examination of the heart, a more general examination may reveal useful additional clues regarding underlying cardiac problems. The systemic manifestations of cardiac disease are considered later in the relevant chapters, but include:

- cyanosis and clubbing in congenital heart disease (Ch. 13)
- splinter haemorrhages, clubbing, Osler's nodes and splenomegaly in patients with subacute bacterial endocarditis (Ch. 12)
- xanthelasma and tendon xanthomata in patients with hyperlipidaemia.
- an assessment of additional features of right heart failure, assessing the presence of ankle oedema and hepatomegaly (Ch. 8).

FURTHER READING

Boudreau Conover, M. & Tilkian, A.G. (1993) *Understanding Heart Sounds and Murmurs with an Introduction to Lung Sounds*. Philadelphia: Saunders.

Perloff, J.K. (1986) *Physical Examination of the Heart and Circulation*. Philadelphia: Saunders.

Turner, R.W.D. & Gold, R.G. (1984) *Auscultation of the Heart*. Edinburgh: Churchill Livingstone.

CHAPTER 4

Non-invasive cardiac imaging

W.H.T. Smith

Definitive cardiac investigation often involves invasive techniques with inherent risks and discomfort to the patient. Non-invasive techniques can either select patients for invasive investigation, or in many conditions, provide information that is complementary or superior to that obtained invasively. Invasive techniques will always exist to facilitate interventional treatments but soon it may be possible to fully investigate many patients non-invasively.

PLAIN RADIOGRAPHY

Plain radiographs are usually taken in posteroanterior and lateral views.

The normal cardiac contour

In the posteroanterior projection, the patient faces the X-ray cassette. In this view (Fig. 4.1) the right border of the heart consists of the (from above downwards):

- superior vena cava
- ascending aorta
- right atrium
- inferior vena cava.

The left border of the heart is formed by the:

- aortic arch
- pulmonary artery and its left main branch
- left ventricle.

Between the left ventricle and the diaphragm, there may be a small triangular shadow due to an epicardial fat pad. In this view, the maximum transverse diameter of the heart does not usually exceed 50% of the chest, measured from the inner aspects of the ribs, although 'cardiothoracic ratios' greater than this are sometimes seen in normal individuals.

In the lateral view (Fig. 4.2), the anterior border of the heart is formed by the:

- pulmonary artery
- right ventricle.

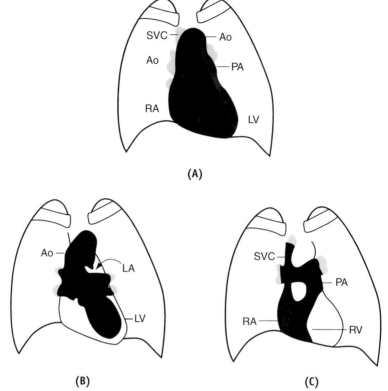

Fig. 4.1 The posteroanterior view. (A) The normal chest radiograph. (B) Appearances of the left side of the heart, after injection of radio-opaque material into the left atrium, showing the positions of the left atrium (LA), the left ventricle (LV) and the aorta (Ao). (C) Appearances of the right side of the heart after injection of radio-opaque material into the superior vena cava (SVC). The positions of the right atrium (RA), the right ventricle (RV), and the pulmonary artery (PA), are shown.

The posterior border is formed by the:

- left atrium
- left ventricle.

ECHOCARDIOGRAPHY

Echocardiography or cardiac ultrasound provides both anatomical and physiological information using widely available and portable equipment. Live moving images are obtained and interpreted by the operator, without the need for lengthy postprocessing. Cardiac anatomy is most commonly evaluated by two dimensional (2D) or B-mode imaging, where a 2D image or 'slice' through the heart is obtained from a probe held on the patient's chest. The two main 'windows' to view the heart from are the parasternal (2nd to 4th left intercostal space, adjacent to the sternum – Fig. 4.3) and apical (5th intercostal space, mid clavicular line – Fig. 4.4). For both these windows, images are often best with the patient rolled to the left to bring the heart

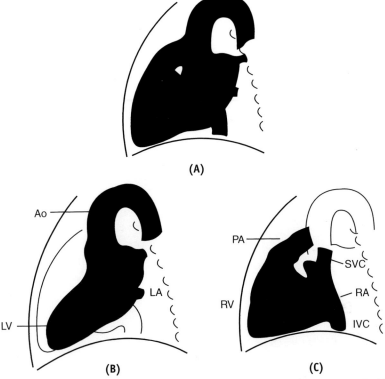

(A)

Ao

LA

LV

(B)

PA

RV

SVC

RA

IVC

(C)

Fig. 4.2 The lateral view. (A) Normal chest radiograph. (B) Appearances of the left side of the heart, after injection of radio-opaque contrast medium into the left atrium, showing the positions of the left atrium (LA), left ventricle (LV) and aorta (Ao). (C) Appearances of the right side of the heart after injection of contrast medium into the right atrium showing positions of superior and inferior venae cavae (SVC, IVC), right atrium (RA), right ventricle (RV) and pulmonary artery (PA).

closer to the chest wall. By changing the angle or position of the probe against the patient's chest, the 'slice' can be varied to examine the entire heart. This modality is useful in all conditions but especially in the evaluation of left ventricular function and valve morphology. Due to advances in 2D imaging, M-mode imaging (one dimension only plotted against time – Fig. 4.5) is less commonly employed but it does allow temporal information to be represented on a still image and is ideal for accurate measurements and analysing rapidly moving structures in relation to events on the ECG.

Doppler echocardiography

The use of Doppler allows information about blood flow within the heart and blood vessels to be obtained. Just as the pitch of a sound rises if it moves towards the observer, the frequency of reflected ultrasound increases if it is reflected off red blood cells moving towards the transducer. Conversely, the reflected frequency is lower than that emitted if the red cells are moving

(A)

(B)

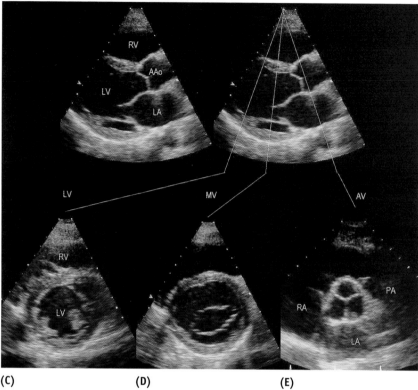

(C)　　　　　**(D)**　　　　　**(E)**

Fig. 4.3 Normal parasternal echo views. The parasternal long (A and B) and short (C–E) axes are perpendicular (i.e. the probe is rotated 90° clockwise). The different short axis views are obtained by varying the probe angulation. Right ventricle (RV), left ventricle (LV), left atrium (LA), right atrium (RA), pulmonary artery (PA) and ascending aorta (AAo).

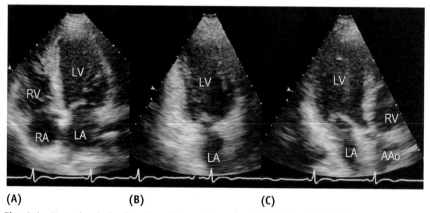

(A)　　　　　**(B)**　　　　　**(C)**

Fig. 4.4 Normal apical echo views. These views should all include the left ventricular apex and the mid-point of the mitral valve and be perpendicular to the left ventricular short axis. (A) apical 4 chamber view (analogous to the horizontal long axis in SPECT). (B) Apical 2 chamber view (rotate the probe 60° anticlockwise from the 4 chamber view). (C) Apical long axis view (a further 60° anticlockwise rotation). Right ventricle (RV), left ventricle (LV), left atrium (LA), right atrium (RA) and ascending aorta (AAo).

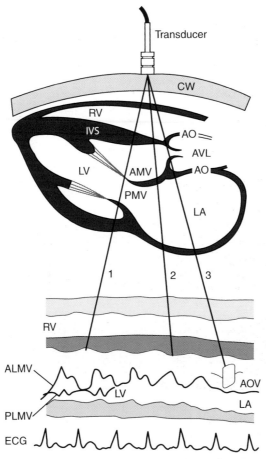

Fig. 4.5 The transducer is angled in different directions to permit study of the various cardiac structures. (1) The beam traverses the right ventricle (RV), interventricular septum (IVS), and anterior and posterior leaflets of the mitral valve (ALMV and PLMV). These leaflets separate abruptly as the blood flows rapidly from the left atrium to the left ventricle. As the flow decreases they approximate only to be separated again when atrial contraction propels more blood into the ventricle. (2) Provides good views of the RV, septum, ALMV and left atrium. (3) Shows separation of the aortic valve cusps in systole.

away from the probe. The degree of this 'Doppler shift' in frequency can be measured and allows the velocity of red cells to be calculated, as the greater the velocity, the greater the Doppler shift. This information is represented as a spectral trace where velocity of blood is plotted on the Y axis against time on the X axis. Different types of Doppler include:

- *Pulse wave Doppler* which measures velocity at a specific depth along a scan line. This is particularly useful in measuring flow characteristics through the mitral valve (Fig 4.6A) and in the left ventricular outflow tract.
- *Continuous wave Doppler* which measures velocity at all depths along the scan line but is able to measure higher velocities (Fig. 4.6B). This is particularly useful in quantifying valvular stenoses (Fig. 4.7) where the relationship between the pressure gradient across the valve and the

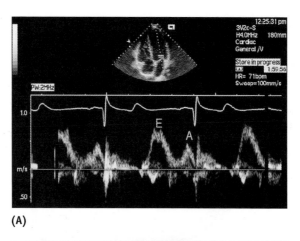

(A)

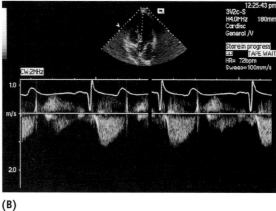

(B)

Fig. 4.6 Normal Doppler. Pulse wave Doppler through the mitral valve (A) demonstrates biphasic left ventricle filling with the passive early E wave (E) followed by the active filling caused by atrial contraction or A wave (A). As pulse Doppler samples velocity at a specific depth, only one velocity is recorded giving the linear spectral trace. Continuous wave Doppler through the aortic valve (B) measures the velocity of red cells at every point along the scan line. Many different velocities up to the maximum are sampled resulting in a solid spectral trace. As a rule, normal velocities (through adult valves) at rest are approximately 1 m/s (0.7 to 1.4 m/s).

velocity of blood flowing through it is given by the Bernoulli equation which can be simplified to:

Peak pressure gradient (mmHg) = $4 \times (\text{Velocity (ms}^{-1}))^2$

- *Colour flow Doppler* which superimposes Doppler information on top of the 2D image. Different velocities are colour coded according to a scale displayed on the monitor with blood flow towards the probe traditionally shown as red and that away from the transducer as blue. This modality is useful in identifying small, high velocity jets such as in aortic regurgitation (Fig. 4.8), mitral regurgitation (Fig 4.9) and ventriculoseptal defects (Fig. 4.10). Data from all modalities are combined to fully evaluate abnormalities.

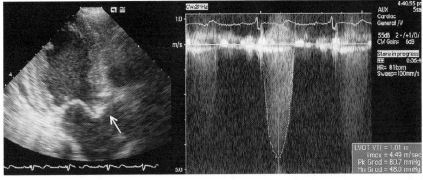

Fig. 4.7 Severe aortic stenosis. Apical long axis view (left) shows that the aortic valve is heavily calcified (arrow) and immobile with evidence of LVH. The CW Doppler trace (right) shows high velocity (4.5 m/s) in the proximal aorta. Calculations therefore suggest a peak pressure gradient of around 80 mmHg (4×4.5^2).

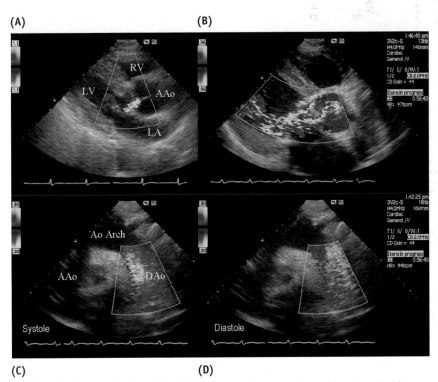

Fig. 4.8 Aortic regurgitation (AR). (A) Parasternal long axis view with colour Doppler demonstrating a thin, short jet of mild AR. (B) Similar view demonstrating a broad jet of severe AR extending well back into the left ventricle. In severe AR, flow reversal in the aortic arch in diastole can be demonstrated. (C) Systolic forward flow in the decending aorta is blue (away from the probe positioned in the suprasternal notch). (D) In diastole, flow reversal (i.e. blood flowing retrogradely back up the descending aorta) is seen in the descending aorta as red.

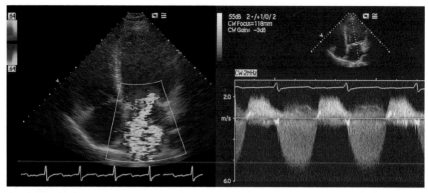

Fig. 4.9 Mitral regurgitation. The apical 4 chamber view with colour Doppler (left) shows a broad jet of severe mitral regurgitation reaching the back and swirling around the LA. An area of flow acceleration can be seen on the ventricular side of the mitral valve. There is a strong CW Doppler signal (right).

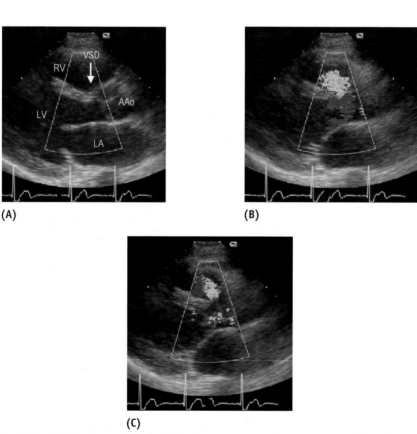

Fig. 4.10 Ventriculoseptal defect (VSD). These parasternal long axis views with colour flow Doppler at (A) end diastole, (B) mid systole, and (C) early diastole, show flow from the high pressure left ventricle to the low pressure right ventricle is present in systole and early diastole. Ventricular septal defects are commonly associated with aortic regurgitation (C) as part of the aortic valve can prolapse due to lack of support from below. A high velocity jet (>5 m/s) confirms significant systolic pressure gradient between the two ventricles and excludes significant pulmonary hypertension.

Utility of echocardiography

The role of echocardiography (echo) has expanded rapidly from being a specialist tool to a basic cardiac investigation. Echo can be helpful in the evaluation of any condition which affects the structure or function of the heart:

- *Evaluation of left ventricular function.* Rotation of the probe to examine the left ventricle in every axis allows assessment of overall left ventricular function, and importantly, allows identification of differences in regional wall motion which is the hallmark of coronary artery disease. An indication of which coronary artery is responsible for left ventricular impairment can be inferred from the affected segment of left ventricle (Fig. 4.11). Other abnormalities of the left ventricle such as hypertrophic cardiomyopathy are demonstrated (Fig 4.12).
- *Abnormalities of the right ventricle* such as right ventricular dilatation and hypertrophy are less commonly noted. Pulmonary hypertension can be identified by the finding of a high velocity jet of tricuspid regurgitation (Fig. 4.13).
- *Heart valves* move very quickly and the high temporal resolution of ultrasound makes this modality ideal for their assessment (Fig 4.14). See also Chapter 12.

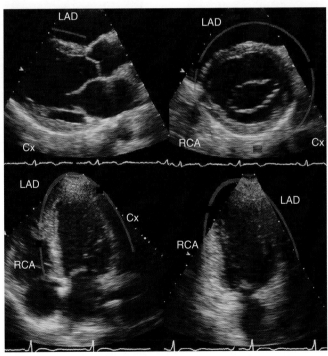

Fig. 4.11 Arterial supply of the left ventricle. In general, the left anterior descending (LAD) artery supplies much of the left ventricle from the anterior septum to the anterolateral wall basally to the entire circumference of the left ventricle at the apex where it wraps around the apex. The relative contribution of the right coronary artery (RCA) and circumflex (Cx) varies, but in general, the right coronary artery supplies the basal inferior septum and inferior wall while the circumflex supplies the posterior and lateral walls.

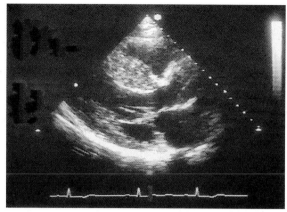

Fig. 4.12   Parasternal long axis showing marked thickening of the interventricular septum in a patient with hypertrophic cardiomyopathy.

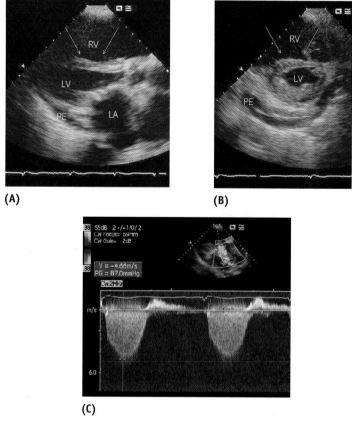

Fig. 4.13   Pulmonary hypertension. The relationship of the left and right ventricles is altered due to the pressure-overloaded right ventricle which has eventually dilated. The septum is flattened (arrowed) in parasternal long (A) and short (B) axis views. There is also a small pericardial effusion (PE). The high velocity of the jet of tricuspid regurgitation (C) suggests a pressure gradient of 85 mmHg between right ventricle and right atrium, which in the absence of significant pulmonary valve disease, implies pulmonary hypertension.

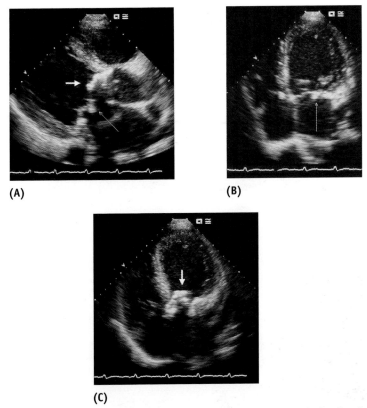

Fig. 4.14 Aortic and mitral endocarditis. Parasternal long axis (A), apical 4 chamber (B) and angled apical 4 chamber (C) views showing large vegetations on the aortic valve (broad arrows) with consequent valvular destruction. This was associated with severe regurgitation (Fig. 4.8B–D). A smaller vegetation is seen on the mitral valve (fine arrows). Both vegetations are on the 'downstream' side of the valve as is characteristic in endocarditis.

- *The pericardium* is rarely seen unless abnormal but significant effusions (Fig. 4.15) or pericardial thickening is commonly identified.
- *Extra-cardiac structures* can be demonstrated (Fig 4.16) but the limited field of view of echo makes this technique less applicable than cardiac magnetic resonance imaging (MR) or computed tomography (CT) for this purpose.

Transoesophageal echocardiography (TOE)

In this technique, the ultrasound probe is mounted on a modified gastroscope and is passed into the oesophagus under conscious sedation. The technique offers a posterior, and in the transgastric position, an inferior 'window' in which to image the heart. The proximity of the probe to the heart, and the lack of lung and chest wall for ultrasound to penetrate, allows the use of higher frequency ultrasound than the conventional transthoracic approach (7 Hz cf 3–4 Hz). This typically results in clearer images (Fig. 4.17). Transoesophageal echo complements but does not replace transthoracic echo. Although the images of the left heart are often superior to transthoracic

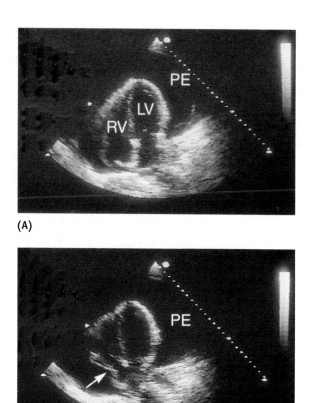

(A)

(B)

Fig. 4.15 (A and B) Massive pericardial effusion (PE) which appears as an echo-free space around the heart. (B) Diastolic 'collapse' of the free wall of the right atrium (arrowed). This is a non-specific sign. Diastolic collapse of the right ventricle, if present, is a sign of cardiac tamponade.

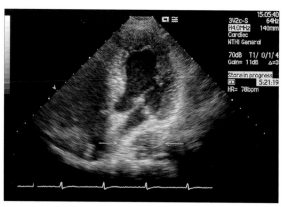

Fig. 4.16 Echocardiogram demonstrating extrinsic compression of the left atrium by oesophageal tumour (arrows).

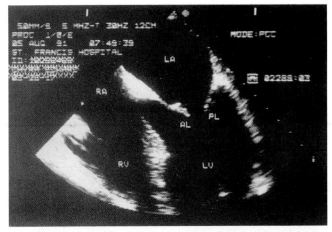

Fig. 4.17 Four-chamber view from the transoesophageal approach showing the left atrium (LA), left ventricle (LV), right atrium (RA) and right ventricle (RV). Note the close proximity of the probe to the anterior and posterior mitral valve leaflets (AL and PL), making transoesophogeal echo an important investigation in patients with mitral valve disease.

images, the tricuspid valve and other anterior structures are often better visualized via the transthoracic approach.

Indications for TOE
- Unexplained stroke or systemic emboli
- Confirmed or suspected endocarditis especially prosthetic valves
- To rule out significant left atrial thrombus before d.c. cardioversion or trans-septal puncture for mitral valve or electrophysiological intervention (Fig. 4.18)
- Clarify anatomy to determine suitability
  - of atrial septal defect for percutaneous closure (Fig. 4.19)
  - of the mitral valve for repair or valvuloplasty (Figs 4.20, 4.18)
- Suspected atrial masses not clearly seen on transthoracic echo (Fig. 4.21)
- Suspected aortic dissection (Fig. 4.22)
- To guide operations/procedures, e.g. mitral valve repair, percutaneous ASD closure
- Assessment of prosthetic mitral valves, particularly if regurgitation is suspected
- When transthoracic imaging has failed to produce diagnostic information.

Indications for TOE in suspected cardiac source of embolus
Indications for TOE in this setting vary between institutions. In general, the detection rate of TOE is greatest, and is most likely to lead to a change in management, when there are multiple emboli in different arterial territories and when there are no other likely causes. Identifiable causes include:

- thrombus in the left atrium, left atrial appendage (Fig. 4.18), or ventricle
- patent foramen ovale (PFO) (Fig. 4.23)

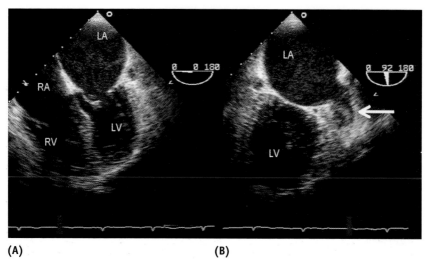

(A) **(B)**

Fig. 4.18 Transoesophageal echo. A multiplane probe allows the 4 chamber (A) and 2 chamber (B) views to be obtained by rotating the transducer at the tip of the probe by 90° without moving the probe physically within the patient. This example shows mitral stenosis with left atrial dilatation. Spontaneous contrast is seen in the left atrium due to slow flow of blood and thrombus has formed in the left atrial appendage (arrow).

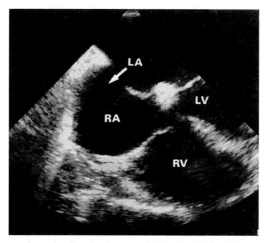

Fig. 4.19 Transoesophageal echo showing an atrial septal defect. The communication between the left atrium and right atrium is arrowed. (LA: left atrium; RA: right atrium; RV: right ventricle; LV: left ventricle.)

- aortic or mitral endocarditis
- left-sided cardiac tumours (Fig. 4.21)
- pedunculated aortic atheroma (>4 mm).

Indications for TOE in suspected endocarditis (see also Chapter 12)
- Prosthetic valves
- *Staphylococcus aureus* – greater likelihood of abscess or perforation
- Failure to respond to appropriate antibiotics

(A)   (B)

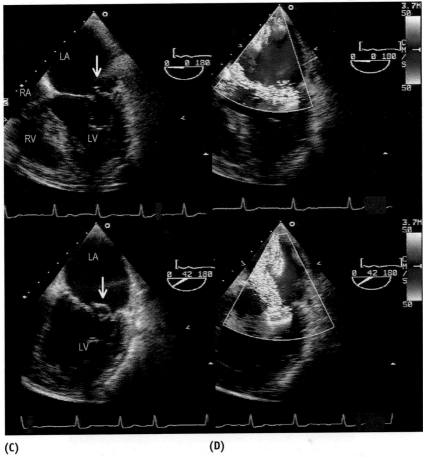

(C)   (D)

Fig. 4.20 Transoesophageal echo showing prolapse of the middle scallop of the posterior mitral valve leaflet (arrow) in the 4 chamber view (A) and with the transducer rotated 40° (C). The corresponding colour Doppler images (B and D) illustrate the consequent mitral regurgitation. Mitral prolapse is often amenable to surgical repair. Note the eccentric nature of the 'jet' of mitral regurgitation directed away from the prolapsing leaflet.

- Clinically suspected diagnosis but normal transthoracic echo
- Aortic valve endocarditis (greater likelihood of abscess).

Contrast media in echocardiography

The simplest contrast agent used in echocardiography is agitated saline. Here, 1 ml of air is vigorously mixed with 9 ml saline to produce tiny bubbles of air and is rapidly injected into a proximal vein. When this enters the right heart, ultrasound is scattered more intensely by the bubbles than the red blood cells, and consequently, the signal from the 'blood pool' is increased. The bubbles are destroyed by their passage though the pulmonary vascular bed, and consequently, none are seen in the left heart chambers. This technique is very helpful for detection of patent foramen ovales (PFO). In

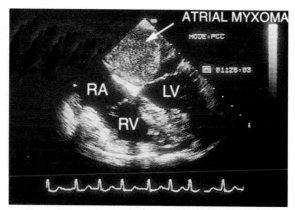

Fig. 4.21 A large left atrial myxoma seen on transoesophageal echo. This is attached to the interatrial septum and fills most of the left atrial cavity.

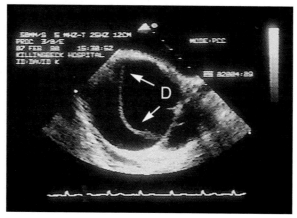

Fig. 4.22 Dissection of the ascending aorta. The dissection flap (D) is clearly visible.

this setting, even small shunts are made apparent by the passage of a few bubbles across the intra-atrial septum (Fig. 4.23).

The expanding application of echo especially in the assessment of myocardial ischaemia, demands clear delineation of the endocardial border. Bubble contrast media capable of crossing the pulmonary vascular bed have been developed to achieve left heart opacification following intravenous injection. These agents are most widely used in stress echo, where clear endocardial definition is essential, but they also have a role in defining left ventricular geometry and function when conventional signals are poor, and in augmenting the strength of Doppler signals.

Myocardial contrast echocardiography (MCE) enables assessment of myocardial perfusion (Fig 4.24). Currently, this pushes technology to the limit as only a small proportion of the intravenously injected contrast reaches the myocardium and once there, it is destroyed by pressure changes and the ultrasound itself. Nevertheless, there is great potential for this technique, not just in stress echo to detect ischaemia, but also to determine whether reperfusion has occurred following thrombolysis for myocardial infarction.

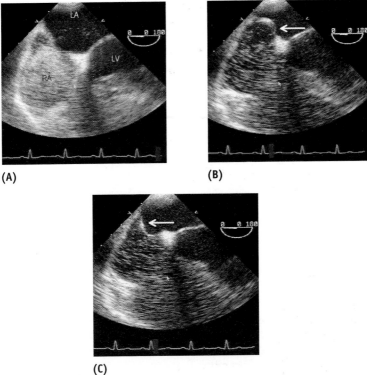

Fig. 4.23 Transoesophageal echo showing a patent foramen ovale and atrial septal aneurysm. Agitated saline contrast is seen opacifying the right atrium. A few bubbles are seen passing into the left atrium (A). The degree of redundant tissue in the atrial septum is demonstrated by the billowing of this structure throughout the cardiac cycle (B and C). The combination of a PFO and atrial septal aneurysm carries a greater risk of emboli than either finding alone.

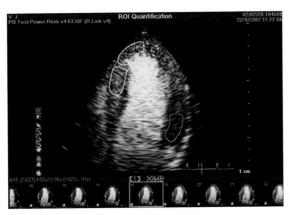

Fig. 4.24 Myocardial contrast echo. The perfusion of microbubbles into different myocardial segments is assessed by their reflected signal at rest and under stress. (Image courtesy of Philips Medical Systems.)

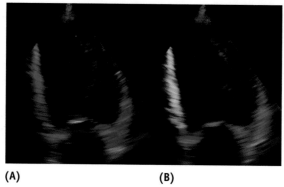

(A)   **(B)**

Fig. 4.25 Tissue Doppler echo illustrating asynchronous left ventricular contraction. (A) early in systole, the septal wall contracts and is displayed red as it moves towards the transducer. At the same time, depolarization has not yet reached the lateral wall, which consequently is pushed out by septal contraction and appears blue as it is moving away from the transducer. (B) Later in systole, the delayed depolarization reaches the lateral wall which contracts and appears red, but by this time, the septum is beginning to relax and appears blue as the lateral wall contraction pushes it away from the transducer.

Tissue Doppler

This technique allows the motion of individual segments of the myocardium to be analysed and compared. Its utility is in providing information about patterns of relaxation and contraction that cannot be appreciated by the naked eye from real time 2D images. Impaired left ventricular relaxation (diastolic dysfunction) can be identified this way. Recently, interest in resynchronization therapy or biventricular pacing (see also Chapter 8) has led to tissue Doppler being used to identify asynchronous contraction of the septum and lateral walls of the left ventricle (Fig. 4.25). This can be resynchronized by correctly timed pacing signals from the right ventricular apex and typically the lateral left ventricular wall (via a wire positioned in the coronary sinus).

CARDIAC MAGNETIC RESONANCE IMAGING

Cardiac MRI, like echo, can evaluate both cardiac structure and function. Consequently it can be of use in any condition affecting the heart. Although patients with pacemakers, implantable defibrillators or cerebral aneurysm clips should not be imaged, prosthetic valves, sternal wires and coronary stents can be safely imaged, albeit with significant signal 'drop-out' around these objects.

Advantages of cardiac MRI over echo:

- greater resolution
- wider field of view
- images degraded less by obesity or lung disease.

Disadvantages of cardiac MRI compared to echo:

- lengthy imaging and processing
- less widely available
- not portable and claustrophobic.

Table 4.1 Indications for cardiac MRI

Indication	Particular advantage of cardiac MRI
Congenital heart disease	Wider field of view than echo with ability to visualize pulmonary arteries without angiography Shunt calculation and 3D reconstruction possible
Cardiomyopathies	Can identify specific features suggesting an aetiology: • Late enhancement after gadolinium injection of infarcted areas in coronary disease (Fig. 4.26) • Gadolinium enhancement of the central longitudinal myocardial layer in some forms of dilated cardiomyopathy • Fibro-fatty infiltration of the right ventricle – arrhythmogenic right ventricular cardiomyopathy (Fig 4.27) • Iron overload in thalassaemia, haemochromatosis, sickle cell anaemia, can be identified • Myocardial involvement – sarcoid
Pericardial constriction	Identifies pericardial thickening enabling distinction from restrictive cardiomyopathy (Fig 4.28)
Aortic pathology	Wide field of view and ability to image in any plane allows assessment of coarctation and dissection. Avoids X-rays cf CT if follow up required (Fig 4.29)
Cardiac tumours and masses	Wide field of view demonstrating involvement of neighbouring structures (Fig 4.30) Offers some degree of tissue characterization by comparing signal in different modalities, e.g. T1, T2, fat suppressed, after gadolinium contrast
Coronary arteries	Technique of choice for determining path of anomalous coronary arteries. The risk of sudden death is greater when the left coronary artery passes between the aorta and main pulmonary artery, where it can be compressed. Other anomalies are more benign
Left ventricular dimensions and function	High reproducibility enables small changes to be reliably identified with treatment. This can reduce the number of patients required for a research study to be adequately powered.

Currently due to limited availability, cardiac MRI is reserved for conditions where it has particular superiority over other modalities (Table 4.1).

NON-INVASIVE APPROACHES TO CORONARY HEART DISEASE

The exercise electrocardiogram (ECG) (see Chapter 7) remains the usual first line non-invasive investigation for coronary disease. It is physiological and readily available but its sensitivity and specificity are limiting in certain situations. In these cases non-invasive imaging modalities can be helpful.

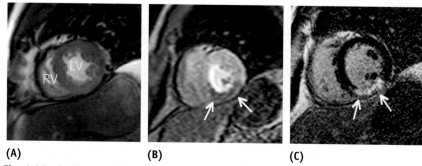

(A)   (B)   (C)

Fig. 4.26 Cardiac MRI illustrating acute inferior myocardial infarction. (A) Left ventricular geometry in short axis is normal acutely (wall thinning occurs chronically) but wall motion and thickening is reduced. (B) Intravenous gadolinium contrast is slow to enter the infarcted tissue and a perfusion defect (dark area) is seen inferiorly (arrows). (C) After 15–20 min, gadolinium has washed out of normal myocardium but is slow to clear from the area of infarction, resulting in 'delayed enhancement' (arrows).

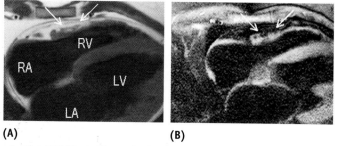

(A)   (B)

Fig. 4.27 Cardiac MRI illustrating arrhythmogenic right ventricular cardiomyopathy. (A) 'black blood' sequence shows areas of high signal infiltrating the right ventricular free wall (arrows). (B) 'Fat suppressed' imaging demonstrates areas of signal suppression in the same area confirming the fatty nature of the infiltration (arrows).

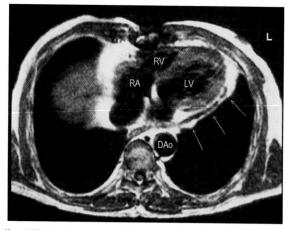

Fig. 4.28 Cardiac MRI showing pericardial constriction. The thickened pericardium (dark rim) is highlighted within epicardial fat (bright). Area of interest is arrowed. Cardiac MRI can also demonstrate abnormal ventricular filling patterns in these patents.

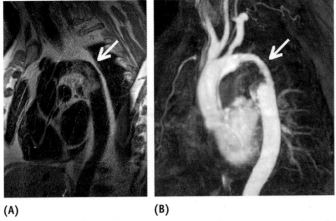

(A) **(B)**

Fig. 4.29 Cardiac MRI (A) and MR angiogram (B) showing compression of the aortic arch by extrinsic tumour The MR angiogram can be reconstructed in three dimensions and rotated to fully appreciate the extent of pathology.

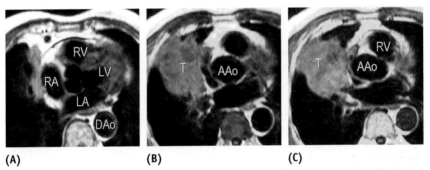

(A) **(B)** **(C)**

Fig. 4.30 Cardiac MRI showing tumour involvement of the heart. Lung tumour (T) invading the pericardium and right atrium in (A) inferior, (B) middle and (C) superior axial slices through the thorax. (DAo: descending aorta; AAo: ascending aorta.)

Non-invasive imaging modalities

- Stress echo
- Nuclear cardiology
- Magnetic resonance imaging.

Indications

- Detect ischaemia in patients with uninterpretable ECGs
- Detect ischaemia in patients who cannot exercise maximally
- Exclude significant coronary heart disease without angiography
- Evaluating the significance of anatomically borderline coronary stenoses
- Localize ischaemia to a particular coronary territory
- Detecting the presence of 'hibernating' myocardium.

The ischaemic cascade

From Figure 4.31 it is clear that techniques able to detect abnormal perfusion or function will detect lesser levels of ischaemia than those reliant on the

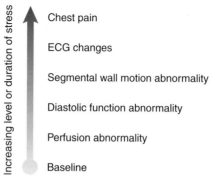

Fig. 4.31 Ischaemic cascade.

ECG and symptoms, and therefore offer greater sensitivity. They are also less influenced by other factors such as blood pressure or conduction system disease which profoundly alter the ECG.

Stress agents

The choice of how ischaemia is induced depends on which imaging modality is used, patient factors and local expertise. Options include:

- exercise (usually treadmill)
- inotrope infusion (e.g. dobutamine)
- vasodilator infusion (e.g. adenosine).

PRACTICE GUIDELINES

Stress echo and cardiac MRI perfusion are usually performed under dobutamine stress as exercise is inconvenient due to the need for the patient to lie still for imaging at peak stress. Vasodilators produce relative changes in regional perfusion and do not readily induce abnormalities in wall thickening and motion.

Most nuclear medicine departments will try to use exercise stress if possible as it is the most physiological. There is no need to image during exercise as the distribution of technetium is determined by myocardial perfusion at the time of injection and this remains fairly constant for the next few hours allowing imaging to occur after exercise. If patients cannot exercise, a vasodilator such as adenosine is usually chosen for simplicity and lower risk of complications unless there is a history of bronchospasm, when dobutamine stress is used. Often a small amount of exercise such as leg raising or pumping up a blood pressure cuff is used to augment pharmacological stress even in patients who are 'unable to exercise'.

Stress echocardiography

In the detection of ischaemia, stress echo relies principally on detecting abnormalities in wall thickening and wall motion in response to stress. An initial study is performed at rest and compared to subsequent studies repeated under increasing levels of pharmacological stress (usually dobutamine 10–40 μg/kg/min). A normal segment of myocardium contracts and thickens more vigorously with increasing stimulation. Ischaemic myocardium typically becomes more active under minimal stimulation (5–15 µg/kg/min) but at maximal stimulation, wall motion and thickening are reduced. This biphasic response offers the greatest specificity but it is difficult to identify and often simply a reduction in wall motion with peak stress is the only abnormality detected in ischaemic regions. If a significant proportion of the total myocardium is ischaemic, this can result in an increase in the end systolic volume with stress and this is associated with adverse prognosis. This assessment is simplest when resting ventricular function is normal. The evaluation of a ventricle with abnormal resting function is more complex, (see Table 4.2). Areas of full thickness infarction should remain thin and akinetic both at rest and under stress. Often there are adjacent regions with partial thickness infarction, normally functioning myocardium which may or may not become ischaemic under stress, and myocardium which is viable but chronically ischaemic to the extent that its resting contraction is depressed (hibernating). Assessment of such patients can be extremely difficult even with optimal imaging.

Harmonic imaging, particularly when used in conjunction with contrast agents, has revolutionized stress echo. These developments allow clearer definition of the endocardium, which is essential for assessment of wall thickening. This greatly improves the diagnostic yield of stress echo and

Table 4.2 Typical findings of stress echocardiography in ischaemic heart disease

	Resting	Low dose	High dose
Normal	Normal diastolic wall thickness, left ventricular wall thickens and moves in systole	left ventricular thickening and wall motion increase	Further increase in wall thickening and motion
Ischaemic	As normal	Wall thickening and motion may initially increase	Reduced wall thickening and motion compared to adjacent normal regions
Full thickness myocardial infarction	Thin, fails to thicken, akinetic*	No change	No change
Partial thickness myocardial infarction	Some thinning. Reduced wall thickening Reduced wall motion	Wall thickening and motion increase but not as much as normal	Wall thickening and motion continue to increase but not as much as normal
Hibernation	Normal thickness Reduced wall thickening and motion	Wall thickening and motion initially increase	Wall thickening and motion reduce or become dyskinetic

* Akinetic segments may appear to move if they are pulled by adjacent segments of myocardium. This can be distinguished by their failure to thicken in systole.

increases its applicability to include patients with suboptimal conventional images.

Nuclear cardiology

This technique, also known as single photon emission computerized tomography or SPECT, relies on the injection of a radioactive substance which is taken up by the myocardium. This is then detected by a gamma camera to provide information about myocardial perfusion and ventricular function. SPECT images are usually displayed as a series of consecutive slices through the heart in short axis (as for echo), horizontal long axis (analogous to the echo 4 chamber view) and the perpendicular, vertical long axis (between the long axis and 2 chamber views on echo) (see Fig 4.32).

The most commonly used agents are thallium 201 and technetium 99. Thallium is a potassium analogue, which is taken up by viable myocardial cells in proportion to blood flow. Thallium injection is performed at peak stress. At this point, hypoperfused myocardium will have less uptake (and therefore less of a signal detected by the gamma camera) than normally perfused myocardium. Over the next few hours, thallium redistributes so that its concentration in hypoperfused but viable myocardium becomes equal to normal regions over time. The ischaemic defect is therefore referred to as 'reversible'. Areas of infarction have reduced uptake initially that does not change over time (no reversibility).

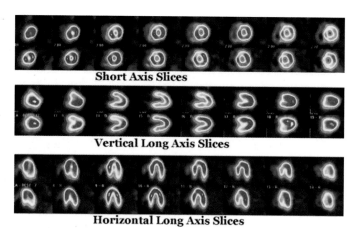

Short Axis Slices

Vertical Long Axis Slices

Horizontal Long Axis Slices

Fig. 4.32 Normal SPECT scan. Three mutually perpendicular imaging planes are shown. In each view, the images performed under stress are shown above, and those performed at rest are below. The different images in each row represent sequential slices through the heart in that plane. In the short axis slices, the left ventricle appears as a complete 'doughnut' with the anterior wall at the top, and the inferior wall below with the septum on the left and lateral wall on the right. In the vertical long axis views, the left ventricular anterior wall is above and the inferior wall below with the apex to the right. In the horizontal long axis views, the left ventricular septal (left) and lateral (right) walls are seen. The right ventricle is less well seen due to its lesser muscle mass but occasionally right ventricular pathology can be evident in the short and horizontal long axis views (to the left of the left ventricle in both views).

The technetium labelled agents, (tetrofosmin and sestamibi), also distribute to viable myocardium in relation to blood flow. Both agents are bound within the myocardial cell irreversibly and consequently have far less redistribution than thallium. Therefore, rest and stress studies need to be performed separately, usually on consecutive days.

Advantages of thallium
- Cheaper
- Greater evidence base
- Potential for assessing lung uptake.

Advantages of technetium
- Improved image quality
- Faster imaging allows ventricular function to be assessed
- Better quantification.

In most laboratories, the superior image quality and the ability to simultaneously assess ventricular function are the overriding factors for why technetium is increasingly chosen. Simultaneous left ventricular function assessment allows infarction to be distinguished from signal attenuation due to obesity or breast tissue (commonly seen in the inferior wall). Here, the presence of normal regional wall contraction makes full thickness myocardial infarction unlikely. An abnormal SPECT scan is shown in Figure 4.33.

Cardiac MRI

This rapidly emerging technique has the potential to provide all the information and more than both stress echo and SPECT combined. Left ventricular wall thickening and motion can be accurately measured at rest and under stress with a greater precision than can be achieved with echo. This is principally due to better endocardial and epicardial definition. Myocardial perfusion at rest and under stress can be assessed following the intravenous injection of gadolinium. Myocardium with reduced perfusion appears dark in contrast to surrounding normal myocardium where the signal is enhanced by gadolinium (Fig. 4.26B). This takes less time than is required for a SPECT scan and can be combined with delayed imaging to visualize 'delayed enhancement' of infarcted tissue (Fig. 4.34). Here, images are taken 15 minutes after an intravenous injection of gadolinium. At this point, gadolinium concentrates in scar and necrotic tissue and results in an increased signal from both acutely and chronically infarcted myocardium. The technique has high resolution, and can define the transmural extent of infarction for the first time in vivo (Fig. 4.34).

Imaging of the proximal coronary arteries is now becoming possible with 'navigator' techniques to allow for cyclical cardiac and respiratory motion.

Summary

Stress echo, nuclear cardiology and cardiac MRI can all provide complementary information to exercise testing and angiography. Each modality has

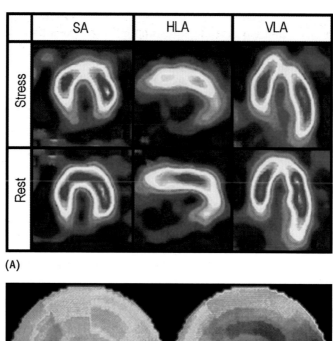

(A)

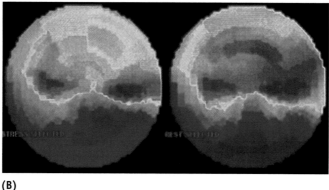

(B)

Fig. 4.33 SPECT scan demonstrating prognostically significant three vessel disease (A). The short axis (SA) images show no perfusion at both stress and rest inferiorly (the lower part of the complete 'doughnut' is missing compared to normal). This is due to full thickness inferior myocardial infarction (right coronary artery territory) and is also apparent in the horizontal long axis (HLA) views. Anteriorly, the signal is reduced under stress but normalizes at rest in keeping with 'reversible' ischaemia in the left anterior descending (LAD) territory. This is seen in short axis and horizontal long axis. The vertical long axis (VLA) view shows that the lateral wall signal is subtly reduced under stress compared to rest, consistent with reversible ischaemia in the circumflex territory. The polar plots (B) show an alternative representation of this data in short axis only with apical regions centrally and basal regions shown peripherally.

different roles in answering particular questions and currently none are perfect (Table 4.3).

Which technique is chosen will depend on local expertise and availability, as well as the particular question being asked. The complex nature of these tests and their interpretation make it unlikely that they will replace exercise testing for baseline assessment. The necessity to catheterize the coronary arteries for coronary intervention will ensure that coronary angiography continues but with developments in non invasive imaging, this may reduce to a test performed only when coronary intervention has been shown to be likely.

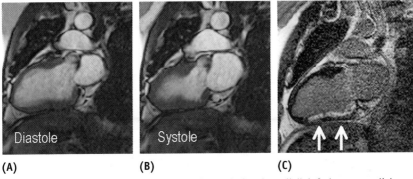

(A)   (B)   (C)

Fig. 4.34 Cardiac MRI showing partial thickness (subendocardial) inferior myocardial infarction. Diastolic (A) and systolic (B) frames show that wall motion and thickening are reduced inferiorly. The delayed enhancement image (C) shows a rim of enhancing subendocardial tissue but a significant amount of inferior myocardium epicardially, which does not enhance implying viability (arrows). Significant viability is considered present if less than half of the thickness of the left ventricle wall in a given segment shows delayed enhancement.

Table 4.3 Ability of different imaging modalities to detect important abnormalities in coronary artery disease

Technique	Perfusion	Wall motion/ thickening	Hibernation	Transmural extent of infarction	Coronary stenoses
Stress echo	+	+++	++	+	−
SPECT	+++	+	+	+	−
MRI	++	+++	++	+++	+

FURTHER READING

Granger, R.G. & Allison, D.J. (Eds) (1986) *Diagnostic Radiology*. Edinburgh: Churchill Livingstone.

Rimmington H. & Chambers J. (1998). *Echocardiography: A Practical Guide for Reporting*. Lancaster: Parthenon.

Gerson, M.C. (Ed.) (1987) *Cardiac Nuclear Medicine*. New York: McGraw Hill.

Constantine, G., Shan, K., Flamm, S., Sivananthan M. (2003) The Developing Role of Magnetic Resonance Imaging in Clinical Cardiology. *Lancet* 363(9427): 2162.

Sivananthan, U.M. (ed) (2003) *Atlas and Manual of Cardiac MRI*. Oxford: Andromeda Interactive.

CHAPTER 5

Invasive investigations

As a result of advances in non-invasive cardiac investigations, cardiac catheterization is now required less frequently to establish a diagnosis in patients with heart disease. However, the proliferation of interventional techniques for the treatment of heart disease (including cardiac surgery, coronary angioplasty, percutaneous balloon valvuloplasty) has meant that cardiac catheterization is now being performed more frequently than ever to assess the patient's suitability for all forms of interventional treatment.

Invasive diagnostic techniques can be considered under the following headings:

- right heart catheterization
- left heart catheterization
- coronary angiography
- invasive electrophysiological studies.

CARDIAC CATHETERIZATION

Right heart catheterization

Under local anaesthesia, a catheter is introduced percutaneously into the femoral or basilic vein and advanced to the right atrium. It is manoeuvred under X-ray control through the tricuspid valve to the right ventricle, thence to the pulmonary artery and finally wedged in a distal pulmonary artery. The pulmonary arterial wedge (pulmonary capillary) tracing so obtained is an indirect measurement of pressure in the left atrium (Fig. 5.1).

If there is a septal defect, the catheter may be passed through this into the left side of the heart; if there is a persistent ductus arteriosus, this may be traversed.

The catheter can be used to record pressures in the different chambers of the heart and also to obtain blood samples from each vessel and chamber. Normal cardiovascular pressures are summarized in Table 5.1. Blood samples are usually taken for oxygen content or saturation. When a left-to-right shunt is present, the blood is found to be more oxygenated in the affected chamber and beyond than it is in the great veins:

- *Persistent ductus arteriosus.* The oxygen saturation in the left pulmonary artery exceeds that in the right ventricle

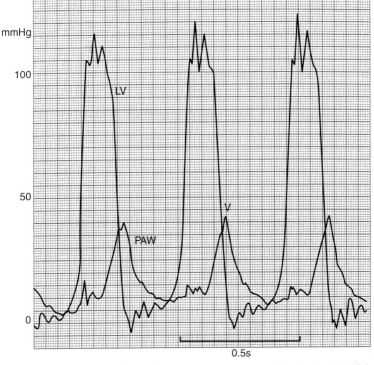

Fig. 5.1 Pulmonary artery wedge tracing. A pulmonary artery wedge tracing (PAW) is shown together with a left ventricular tracing (LV). There is a prominent V wave in the pulmonary wedge tracing due to mitral regurgitation.

Table 5.1 Normal cardiovascular pressures (mmHg)

	Mean	Range
Right atrium – mean	4	0–8
Right ventricle		
systolic	25	15–30
end diastolic	4	0–8
Pulmonary artery		
systolic	25	15–30
diastolic	10	5–15
mean	15	10–20
Pulmonary artery wedge – mean	10	5–14
Left atrium – mean	7	4–12
Left ventricle		
systolic	120	90–140
end diastolic	7	4–12
Aorta		
systolic	120	90–140
diastolic	70	60–90
mean	85	70–105

- *Ventricular septal defect.* The oxygen saturation in the right ventricle and pulmonary artery is greater than that in the right atrium
- *Atrial septal defect.* The oxygen saturation in the right atrium exceeds that in the superior and inferior venae cavae.

In modern clinical practice, left to right shunts, and all forms of valvular heart disease, are usually diagnosed by echocardiography without the need for invasive investigations to establish a diagnosis.

Cardiac output can also be measured during right heart catheterization using the Swan–Ganz catheter which has two separate lumens, one opening into the right atrium and the other to the pulmonary artery. This technique is based on the principle that the concentration of an injected substance is dependent on the volume injected and the volume of blood into which it is diluted. In this technique, cold saline of known volume and temperature is injected via the catheter into the right atrium. The temperature is then sampled in the pulmonary artery as the cold saline, diluted in the blood, passes the thermistor at the catheter tip. The transient fall in blood temperature is, therefore, indirectly related to the cardiac output, i.e. the greater the fall in temperature, the lower the cardiac output for a given volume of saline injected.

The Swan–Ganz catheter has an inflatable balloon close to its tip which allows the catheter to be 'floated' through the right side of the heart and into the pulmonary artery without the need for X-ray guidance. This catheter is still frequently used in intensive care units for monitoring of severely compromised patients. With the catheter tip in a pulmonary artery, both the pulmonary artery and the pulmonary capillary wedge pressures can be measured according to whether the balloon is inflated (pulmonary wedge pressure) or deflated (pulmonary artery pressure).

Left heart catheterization

Under local anaesthesia, a catheter is introduced into the femoral, brachial or radial artery and advanced retrogradely until it reaches the aortic valve. The catheter can then be manipulated across the valve and into the left ventricle. The catheter is used to measure pressures or to deliver contrast injections (angiography).

Pressure measurements

Pressure gradients across the aortic and mitral valves can be measured in suspected aortic and mitral stenosis respectively, but these diagnoses are now more commonly made by echocardiography.

- *Aortic stenosis* is assessed by the pressure difference between the left ventricle and the aorta. This can be distinguished from cases of subaortic stenosis or hypertrophic cardiomyopathy, in which the pressure drop lies within the cavity of the left ventricle.
- *Mitral stenosis* is assessed by the pressure difference between the pulmonary artery wedge and left ventricular pressures.
- measurement of the left ventricular end-diastolic pressure may be useful as an indicator of *left ventricular function.*

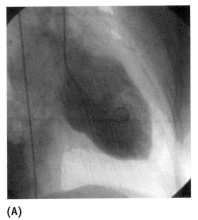 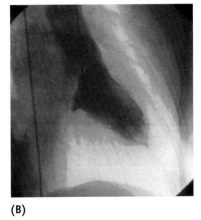

(A)   (B)

Fig. 5.2 Angiography demonstrating normal left ventricular function in a patient with competent mitral valve. (A) shows a frame taken at the end of diastole when the left ventricle is full of contrast. (B) shows a frame at the end of a systole when the ventricle has contracted and ejected blood into the aorta.

VENTRICULOGRAPHY AND AORTOGRAPHY

The rapid injection of 30–40 ml of contrast medium by a power injector can be used to demonstrate the anatomy of the chambers of the heart and to look for evidence of valvular regurgitation. The images can be stored either on cine film at 25 to 50 frames per second, on analogue video cassette, or digitally. Injection into the left ventricle (left ventricular angiography) is used to assess left ventricular function (Fig. 5.2) and also to look for mitral regurgitation (Fig. 5.3). If the mitral valve is competent, there should not be any contrast leakage from the left ventricle into the left atrium. Similarly, injection of contrast into the ascending aorta will demonstrate whether or not there is significant aortic regurgitation.

CORONARY ANGIOGRAPHY

This is by far the most commonly performed invasive cardiac investigation in Western countries. It is used both to establish whether or not a patient has significant coronary artery disease and to determine their suitability for interventional treatment including percutaneous transluminal coronary angioplasty and coronary artery bypass surgery. The procedure is carried out under local anaesthesia and usually as a day case. After administering a local anaesthetic, fine plastic catheters (approximately 2 mm in diameter) are introduced. Access to the arterial system may be via the femoral, brachial or radial artery. The most commonly used catheters are the Judkins shapes which are designed to be used from the femoral artery. Different catheters are generally used to cannulate the left and right coronary arteries (Fig. 5.4), although it is often possible to cannulate both coronary vessels using a single catheter from the brachial approach. Multiple views are taken of both coronary arteries from different angles to ensure that all proximal segments of the arteries are adequately visualized. For each view, 5–10 ml of contrast medium is injected by hand and the films are recorded on to cine film, video

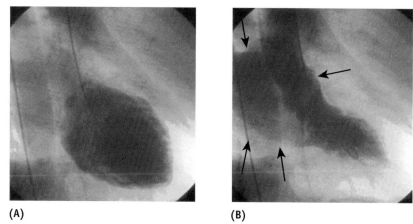

(A)   **(B)**

Fig. 5.3 Left ventricular angiography in a patient with mitral valve regurgitation.
(A = end diastole, B = end systole.) Note the large amount of contrast medium which
refluxes into the left atrium particularly during systole (arrowed). This should be compared
with the normal angiogram in a patient with a competent mitral valve (Fig 52A and B).

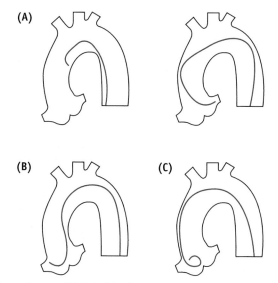

Fig. 5.4 Cardiac catheters. (A) A Judkins left coronary catheter advanced around
the aortic arch to engage the left coronary artery. (B) Judkins right coronary catheter.
(C) Pigtail catheter in aortic root.

cassette or digital storage system. Examples of abnormalities seen at
angiography are shown in Figures 5.5, 5.6 and 5.7.

Selective angiography is also the investigation of choice when re-examining
patients who have recurrent symptoms following coronary artery bypass surgery. Specially shaped catheters are used to obtain views of the aortocoronary
vein grafts and also of the left internal mammary artery if this has been used
as a conduit at the time of surgery.

All invasive procedures carry some risk for the patient but the risk of
diagnostic coronary angiography with currently available equipment (soft-
tipped catheters, non-ionic contrast media) should be very low. Most series

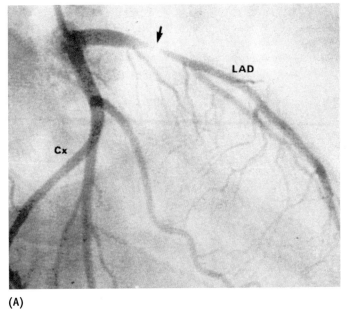

(A)

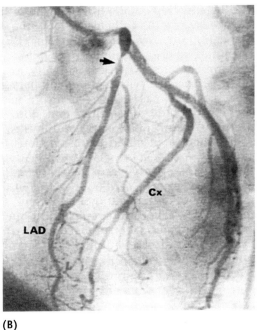

(B)

Fig. 5.5 Coronary angiography. Contrast medium has been injected into the left coronary artery. (A) Right anterior oblique projection. (B) Left anterior oblique projection. The left coronary artery divides into left anterior descending (LAD) and circumflex (Cx) branches. A stenosis in the proximal LAD is arrowed.

report mortality rates of less than 1 per 2000, with a risk of non-fatal stroke or myocardial infarction of 1 in 1000. Local femoral artery complications, such as haematoma or arterial dissection, are more common but are not usually severe.

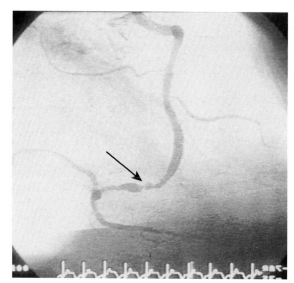

Fig. 5.6 Angiogram of a right coronary artery demonstrating a ruptured atheromatous plaque (arrowed).

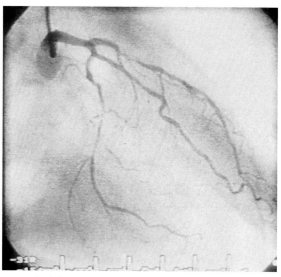

Fig. 5.7 Angiogram of a left coronary artery showing diffuse disease with multiple areas of narrowing (stenoses).

INVASIVE ELECTROPHYSIOLOGICAL STUDIES

It is possible to position electrodes in various parts of the heart, having introduced them percutaneously through a peripheral vein (or rarely an artery). Thus, electrodes may be placed in juxtaposition to several sites in the atria and ventricles, and also adjacent to the bundle of His (Fig. 5.8). The sequence of activation of the heart may then be determined, and specific sites found where conduction is accelerated (as in the Wolff–Parkinson–White syndrome) or delayed (as in heart block).

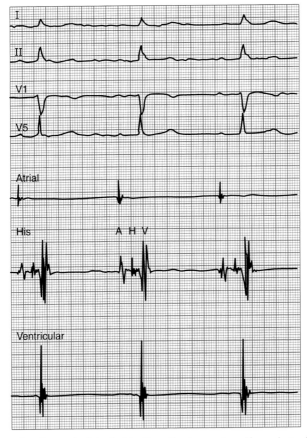

Fig. 5.8 Invasive electrophysiological testing. The traces show (from above downwards) four surface electrocardiogram (ECG) channels, atrial, His bundle and ventricular intracardiac electrograms. The His bundle recording shows three wave forms, A, H and V corresponding to atrial, His and ventricular excitation respectively.

Furthermore, by introducing stimuli at an appropriate time and place, an arrhythmia may be triggered in susceptible patients, and the effect on it of various pharmacological and electrical measures assessed. This technique is particularly valuable in:

- *arrhythmia diagnosis*, e.g. distinguishing the mechanisms of supraventricular tachycardias
- identification of the origin of a ventricular arrhythmia or of the site of a bypass tract in Wolff–Parkinson–White syndrome
- assessing the efficacy of antiarrhythmic therapy. This is of particular value in patients with malignant ventricular arrhythmias. If a drug is successful in preventing arrhythmia induction, this indicates that it is also likely to be successful in preventing spontaneous occurrences of the arrhythmia
- *ablation* of accessory pathways or of the atrioventricular node using radio-frequency current (see Ch. 9).

CHAPTER 6

Diseases of the coronary arteries – causes, pathology and prevention

THE CORONARY CIRCULATION

There are two major coronary arteries – right and left (Fig. 6.1). The right coronary artery arises from the right coronary sinus of Valsalva and runs down in the groove between the right atrium and the right ventricle. In most hearts, its branches supply the sinus node, the atrioventricular node and bundle, the right ventricle and the inferior part of the left ventricle. The left coronary artery, which arises from the left coronary sinus of Valsalva, soon divides into two large branches: the anterior descending branch which runs down between the two ventricles anteriorly, and the left circumflex branch which passes around in the groove between the left atrium and the left ventricle. The anterior descending artery supplies the interventricular septum and the anterior wall of the left ventricle. The circumflex supplies the lateral and posterior aspects of the left ventricle. The major vessels traverse the external surface of the myocardium, sending branches perpendicularly into the muscle mass. There are normally many small anastomoses between the coronary arteries, but these are of no functional importance. When an area of the heart becomes ischaemic, the anastomoses enlarge and then provide a collateral blood supply to the affected muscle which is often vital for its survival.

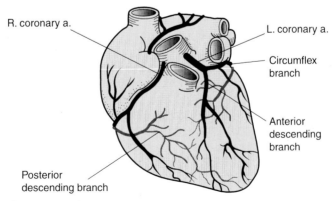

R. coronary a.

L. coronary a.

Circumflex branch

Anterior descending branch

Posterior descending branch

Fig. 6.1   The anatomy of the coronary arteries.

The arteries divide to form arterioles and capillaries similar to those elsewhere in the body, and the venules and veins join to form larger venous channels. Virtually all the blood from the left coronary artery eventually drains into the coronary sinus; that from the right coronary artery drains mainly into the anterior cardiac veins. From these veins the blood passes into the right atrium.

The blood flow in the coronary arteries resembles that in other regions in being dependent on the blood pressure and on the vascular resistance of the arteries and arterioles. A distinctive feature of the coronary circulation is that the arteries are compressed by the contracting myocardium during systole so that the resistance to flow at that time is sharply increased. Consequently, coronary blood flow occurs mainly during diastole. Flow is largely determined by the calibre of the small coronary arteries. Certainly, the aortic diastolic pressure is also a determinant of coronary flow, but, according to Poiseuille's equation, flow is dependent directly on pressure differences but related to the fourth power of the radius. Therefore, a doubling of aortic diastolic pressure doubles coronary flow, whereas a doubling of the radius of the coronary arteries leads to a 16-fold increase in flow. In health, variations in coronary blood flow are mainly due to changes in impedance in the small coronary arteries; these dilate in response to metabolic signals from the myocardium, but they are also under the influence of neurohumoral agents. A further influence is the flow-related release of nitric oxide. Variations in tone also occur in the large coronary arteries but these affect blood flow only if these vessels are narrowed by disease or if they are extreme (spasm).

In the normal resting heart, almost all the oxygen is extracted during its passage through the capillaries; coronary sinus blood is therefore almost completely desaturated. Unlike other organs, the heart cannot call upon a venous oxygen reserve when faced by increased demands, and is largely dependent upon the ability of the coronary arteries to increase their diameter.

CORONARY ARTERY DISEASE

Coronary artery disease is the commonest cause of heart disease and the most important single cause of death in the affluent countries of the world. In the overwhelming majority of cases, disease of the coronary arteries is due to atherosclerosis.

However, the coronary arteries may also be involved in other disorders:

- congenital abnormalities such as arteriovenous fistulae and anomalous origin from the pulmonary artery
- coronary embolism associated with thrombosis arising in the left atrium or ventricle, or from mitral or aortic valve prostheses, or from infective endocarditis
- syphilitic aortitis involving the coronary ostia
- occlusion of a coronary artery due to dissecting aneurysm
- polyarteritis and other connective tissue diseases
- coronary artery spasm which may affect both diseased and otherwise normal vessels.

Definitions

Atherosclerosis has been defined (by a World Health Organization study group) as 'a variable combination of changes of the intima of arteries (as distinguished from arterioles) consisting of a focal accumulation of lipids, complex carbohydrates, blood and blood products, fibrous tissue and calcium deposits, and associated with medial changes'. It is synonymous with *atheroma* but not with *arteriosclerosis*, which is a less specific term used to describe hardening of arteries and arterioles.

Coronary artery disease is the term used to describe coronary arteries that are affected by a pathological process. Coronary artery disease usually exists for many years before a disorder of myocardial function develops. It is, therefore, not synonymous with coronary (or ischaemic) heart disease.

Ischaemic heart disease is disease of the heart muscle resulting from ischaemia. Although myocardial ischaemia also occurs in such conditions as aortic stenosis, the term 'ischaemic heart disease' is generally applied only to cases of atherosclerotic origin.

Coronary heart disease and *atherosclerotic heart disease* are synonymous with ischaemic heart disease.

Coronary thrombosis refers to occlusion of a coronary artery by thrombus. This may or may not lead to myocardial infarction.

Coronary occlusion is the term used to describe occlusion of the coronary artery by any cause. Again, this may or may not cause myocardial infarction.

Myocardial infarction is necrosis of a portion of heart muscle as a result of inadequate blood supply.

Silent ischaemia is ischaemia in the absence of symptoms. The term is applied particularly to episodes of ST elevation or depression unaccompanied by pain.

Vasospastic angina *(Prinzmetal's angina)*

This term is used to describe a syndrome of which the essential features are angina pectoris due to an increase in coronary vasomotor tone and ST elevation in the electrocardiogram (ECG). The angina is attributable not to an increase in myocardial oxygen demand, as it is in classic angina, but to a transient reduction in coronary blood flow. The disorder may occur either in otherwise apparently normal coronary arteries or in atherosclerotic vessels. In the former case, the increase in tone must be extreme (spasm), but in severely stenotic arteries, even physiological changes in tone can produce a critical reduction in blood flow. The mechanism for coronary spasm is unknown, but it may be provoked by certain drugs, notably ergometrine.

The clinical picture is typically one of anginal pain occurring at rest, particularly in the early morning. The attacks are usually self-limiting, but the pain may be severe; they very seldom lead on to myocardial infarction. Nitrates and calcium antagonists are effective both in the treatment of individual episodes and when used prophylactically.

Coronary atherosclerosis

Pathology of coronary atherosclerosis and its complications

The atherosclerotic process probably starts with the 'fatty streak'. Fatty streaks are a common finding in the intima of young people; macroscopically, they

Issues Summary   11/10/2013 10:27
University of Bedfordshire

Id :: 1310815

Item : 3403063354 , Cardiology / Desmond G
Julian, J. Campbell Cowan, James M.
McLenachan ; with contributions from Wil
25/10/13
Item : 3402734415 , Handbook of diabetes /
Gareth Williams, John C. Pickup
18/10/13

Total Number of Issued Items 2

Renewals: library.beds.ac.uk

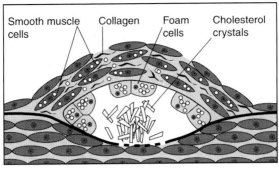

Fig. 6.2 A diagrammatic representation of an atheromatous plaque showing outer cap containing collagen and smooth muscle cells, and inner core showing foam cells and extracellular cholesterol crystals. (With permission from Thompson G.R. [1989] *A Handbook of Hyperlipidaemia*. Current Science.)

appear as yellow patches within the arterial wall. They are mainly composed of lipid-laden foam cells which are derived from macrophages and, to a lesser extent, from smooth muscle cells. Depending upon their location and the presence of the relevant risk factors, the fatty streak may progress to the characteristic lesion of atherosclerosis – the fibrolipid plaque (Fig. 6.2). The major components of the plaque are lipid and arterial smooth muscle cells and their products, such as fibrous proteins and complex carbohydrates. Plaques vary from one another in their composition. At one extreme are fatty plaques, containing a large pool of cholesterol and its esters, separated from the lumen by a thin fibrous cap. At the other extreme are solid plaques, consisting of smooth muscle cells and connective tissue. Calcification may be superimposed. These deposits are focal and are most commonly located at the bends and bifurcations of arteries.

The atheromatous plaque, which is produced by this process, may itself narrow the lumen of the artery. The fibrous cap is prone to fracture, allowing the necrotic core to ulcerate and trigger off platelet aggregation and fibrin deposition. This is a repetitive process and leads to further narrowing, which may proceed to complete occlusion.

Necropsies on patients who have experienced *angina pectoris* usually reveal widespread but patchy coronary atherosclerosis and myocardial fibrosis. Evidence of old coronary occlusion and myocardial infarction is common. The basic pathological cause for the angina is the coronary arterial narrowing which has reduced the lumen of at least one of the three main coronary arteries by 75%. In most cases, two or all three of these arteries are affected.

Sudden death is often attributed to coronary artery disease when widespread coronary atherosclerosis is present. Recent coronary occlusion or myocardial infarction can be demonstrated in only a minority of cases but plaque rupture and non-occlusive thrombus are common. In most instances, it is probable that acute myocardial ischaemia has provoked fatal ventricular fibrillation.

The essential pathological feature of *acute myocardial infarction* is myocardial necrosis. This is usually, but not always, the consequence of total occlusion of a coronary artery. Plaque rupture is commonly found at necropsy;

plaques that rupture are typically rich in lipid and have only a thin cap. There is often evidence of an inflammatory state with many macrophages and T lymphocytes within the plaque. Disruption of the cap allows blood to enter the lipid pool; collagen, crystalline cholesterol and oxidized low-density lipoproteins trigger the formation of a platelet-rich thrombus within the intima. A fibrin-rich thrombus may become superimposed and project into the lumen. It may further expand as many red cells infiltrate the network of fibrin to cause total occlusion. The thrombus will usually lyse spontaneously in the days after infarction but the process can be greatly accelerated by thrombolytic drugs.

If death occurs soon after the onset of myocardial infarction, there may be no gross changes in the myocardium, but enzyme-staining reactions and electron microscopy will reveal evidence of damage. Later, the infarct ed area appears pale and is surrounded by a reddish area due to hyperaemia. Microscopically, the muscle cells lose their nuclei and, subsequently, necrotic changes take place in adjacent connective tissue and blood vessel walls. Leucocytic infiltration occurs at the edges of the infarct. The removal of necrotic muscle starts about the third day and continues for about 2 weeks. At the same time, granulation tissue containing blood vessels and fibroblasts invades the necrotic area. Finally, the infarct zone is replaced by scar tissue over a period lasting between 2 and 8 weeks. If the infarction involves the endocardial surface, a mural thrombus may develop; if it affects the epicardium, there may be pericarditis.

The location and size of a myocardial infarct depend upon the artery that is occluded and the collateral blood supply. In some cases, the infarct extends from the endocardium to the epicardium (transmural infarction); in others, only the subendocardial territory is involved. If the left anterior descending artery is occluded, the infarction involves the anterior wall of the left ventricle and may involve the septum. If the left circumflex is occluded, the infarction affects the lateral or posterior walls of the left ventricle. If the right coronary artery is occluded, the infarction chiefly affects the inferior (diaphragmatic) surface of the left ventricle but also the septum and right ventricle. Coronary artery occlusion may not lead to myocardial infarction if the area supplied by the occluded artery has an adequate collateral supply from adjacent arteries.

The infarcted tissue may thin and stretch in the days after infarction, particularly if this has been anterior. It is due to a combination of stretching of the tissues and the sliding of muscle bundles over each other. This process, known as infarct expansion, has adverse effects on left ventricular shape and contractile ability and is probably an important component of subsequent cardiac failure. It may be preventable if the load on the left ventricle is minimized in the early post-infarction period, as by the use of angiotensin-converting enzyme inhibitors.

The pathogenesis of atherosclerosis
Atherosclerosis results from interactions between the arterial wall and the constituents of the blood. A number of elements play important roles:

- endothelium
- monocytes/macrophages

- smooth muscle cells
- platelets
- blood lipids.

The *endothelium* is composed of a single layer of cells that acts as a barrier, albeit a highly selective one, between the components of the blood and the arterial wall. Endothelial cells are also metabolically active, generate vasoactive substances, and present a non-thrombogenic surface (because they can form prostacyclin and because they have a coating of heparan sulphate). They can produce growth factors (mitogens) such as platelet-derived growth factor (PDGF), and nitric oxide that causes relaxation of the underlying smooth muscle. The loss of integrity of the endothelium is of critical impotance in the development of atherosclerosis. Very often the endothelium is denuded over plaques. Even when it is not, there is endothelial dysfunction.

Macrophages, which are derived from circulating monocytes, secrete seveal biologically important substances, including a number of growth factors and toxic oxygen metabolites. They also have receptors for oxidized low-density lipoprotein (LDL), which they ingest and degrade. They are the major source of foam cells in the fatty streak and the fibrolipid plaque, and play a key role in connective tissue proliferation.

Smooth muscle cells, derived originally from the media, change their characteristics when they migrate to the intima. Instead of being primarily contractile, they take on many secretory functions. They also become resposive to growth factors and are then able to proliferate. They are an essential component of advanced atherosclerotic lesions, in which they accumulate lipid and form foam cells.

Platelets are crucially involved in the complication of thrombosis but also play a major role in the development of atherosclerosis. When activated, they release vasoconstrictor substances and growth factors which can stimulate virtually all the cell types found in the tissues.

Lipids are important components of most plaques, and affect the function of the endothelium, smooth muscle cells and macrophages. They contribute to the formation of foam cells, but there is also a considerable amount of free cholesterol in the tissues of many lesions. Much of the lipid that is taken up is in chemically altered form, having been modified by oxidation or acetylation. Modified LDL is a powerful chemoattractant for monocytes, and macrophages take up LDL avidly in the modified but not in the unmodified form.

'Response to injury' hypothesis

There is still much to be learned about the genesis of atherosclerosis, but current thinking is best integrated under the *'response to injury'* hypothesis. This proposes that the initial lesion is one in which the endothelium is 'injured' in some way, although the term 'injury' is used to cover functional disorders as well as physical disruption. Chronic hyperlipidaemia, with an increase in circulating LDL, leads to changes in the function of monocytes and platelets, as well as in the endothelial cells. The monocytes adhere to the endothelium, and are attracted to migrate into the subendothelial layer, where they become macrophages and take up lipid. These macrophages may secrete free oxygen radicals that further damage the endothelium; they also secrete growth factors that stimulate the migration and proliferation of smooth muscle cells. Damage to the intima may lead to exposure of platelets to the underlying connective tissue and foam cells, with consequent adherence, aggregation and thrombus formation. Mural thrombi may become incorporated into the plaque and contribute to progression of the atherosclerotic process.

Incidence and prevalence of ischaemic heart disease

The incidence of ischaemic heart disease varies greatly between countries and within them, but in all, the mortality from this cause rises rapidly with age. Relatively few females, however, suffer from coronary disease under the age of 45; indeed under the age of 65, more than three times as many men die from coronary disease as do women. Nonetheless, coronary disease is the most common single cause of death in women of that age. In the older age groups the incidence is approximately equal in the two sexes.

Myocardial infarction was seldom recorded as a cause of death until the 1920s, but subsequently the number of deaths attributed to coronary heart disease rose rapidly in Western countries, particularly after the Second World War. It peaked in the USA and Australia in the 1960s; subsequently the mortality in these countries has virtually halved. Mortality from the disease rose until the 1970s in the UK, since when there has been a fall of about 40%. Within the UK, at least twice as many people die from coronary heart disease in parts of south-west Scotland as in south-east England. UK residents of South Asian extraction have substantially higher rates than the UK population as a whole. There is a much lower incidence of coronary heart disease in the countries bordering the Mediterranean Sea than in Northern Europe, and there has been a striking rise in coronary heart disease deaths in Eastern Europe and the developing countries of Asia in recent years.

The reasons for the differences in incidence and the remarkably changing mortality rates are not well understood, but probably relate mainly to diet and smoking behaviour.

Risk factors for ischaemic heart disease and their control

Epidemiological studies and clinical trials have provided valuable information about the risk factors associated with the development of coronary disease and the ways in which the risk of the disease can be reduced. The best identified risk factors are cigarette smoking, high lipid levels and hypetension but several others have been implicated. These include physical inactivity, obesity, diabetes, insulin resistance, genetic inheritance, and homocysteinaemia. These risks are multiplicative so that the possession of several factors greatly increases the chance of developing coronary heart disease.

Lipid disorders

There is much circumstantial evidence to incriminate lipid abnormalities in the genesis of atheroma. Thus, there is a strong and graded relationship between plasma cholesterol and the risk of subsequent coronary heart disease. Furthermore, clinical trials have demonstrated that the reduction of cholesterol by the use of lipid-lowering regimens reduces the risk of myocardial infarction and death from coronary heart disease.

There are several lipid fractions which have different relationships to coronary heart disease. About two-thirds of plasma cholesterol is transported as LDL and it is this that has been most strongly correlated with subsequent disease. By contrast, high-density lipoprotein (HDL) appears to be protective, because it transports lipid out of the arterial wall. The higher the plasma HDL concentration, the lower the risk of disease. There is less certainty about the role of triglycerides, although they appear to increase risk further when the LDL concentration is raised and/or the HDL level is low.

In countries, such as the USA and the UK, in which the average plasma cholesterol level of the community is relatively high, there is a much higher incidence of coronary artery disease than in countries (such as Japan and China) in which hypercholesterolaemia is rare. The cause of the high cholesterol levels is not yet fully established, although it seems likely that it is related in part to dietary factors. A high content of saturated fat (mainly of animal origin) in the diet is particularly suspect but a relative deficiency of polyunsaturated fats may also be important. In some countries, such as France, coronary heart disease is relatively rare in spite of lipid levels that are not greatly different from those in the UK. It is probable that a high intake of fruit and vegetables is protective because of their antioxidant effects.

Certain metabolic and endocrine disorders that disturb lipid metabolism are associated with a high incidence of coronary disease. These include hypothyroidism and diabetes mellitus. Women who have had bilateral oöphorectomy are liable to develop hypercholesterolaemia and premature coronary disease.

PRACTICE GUIDELINES

The *detection* of hyperlipidaemia depends upon blood sampling. Cholesterol estimates can be undertaken in the non-fasting state, but some other lipid measurements, such as triglyceride, require that the subject is fasting. Single measurements may be misleading both because of inaccuracy of the method and because of variability in the cholesterol level from time to time. Therefore, if a high level is suspected, a repeat measurement should be obtained and, particularly if drug treatment is contemplated, a full lipid profile (to include HDL) obtained.

The significance of a particular cholesterol level depends upon many factors, such as age, sex and the presence of other risk factors such as cigarette smoking and hypertension. Thus a cholesterol level of 6.0 mmol/L without other risk factors is associated with a good prognosis, while a much lower value is associated with a high risk of disease if the subject smokes and has a high blood pressure. The risk is particularly high in those with manifest coronary disease and the indications for lipid lowering are very strong in this context. Thus, the decision of how to treat an individual does not depend on the lipid level alone, but upon the presence of other risk factors. In those with coronary heart disease and those with multiple risk factors even in its apparent absence, an attempt should be made to reduce total cholesterol concentration to well below 5.0 mmol/L and low density lipoprotein to 3 mmol/L.

Blood lipids should be measured in anyone with known ischaemic heart disease, diabetes or hypertension requiring drug treatment, or with a family history of hyperlipidaemia or coronary disease at a relatively young age (e.g. under the age of 55).

Treatment of hyperlipidaemia should start with dietary measures. Weight reduction alone substantially reduces hypertriglyceridaemia; alcohol restriction reinforces this. For hypercholesterolaemia, total fat should be reduced to 25–30% of food energy, polyunsaturated fatty acids, especially linoleic acid, providing 7–10%.

Several types of drug are used to correct hyperlipidaemia:

- *HMG CoA reductase inhibitors* ('statins') block cholesterol synthesis in the liver by inhibiting the enzyme 3-hydroxy-3-methy-glutaryl coenzyme A reductase. They reduce plasma cholesterol by 25% or more. Large clinical trials have confirmed not only their effectiveness in reducing mortality and morbidity rates from coronary heart disease, but the absence of serious side-effects. The most impressive results are seen in those who have angina or have had a myocardial infarction and in those with hypertension and diabetes. There is little to choose between the various agents available which include simvastatin, pravastatin, atorvastatin, and fluvastatin. They are all capable of producing rhabdomyolysis that can, in a small number of cases, lead to renal failure. It is important to measure creatine phosphokinase in any patient with muscle pains on these drugs.
- *Bile acid sequestrants* are anion exchange resins, which are not absorbed. Cholestyramine 8–12 g twice daily is effective in hypercholesterolaemia, but is unpleasant to take, and may cause dyspepsia and constipation. A large trial with this drug showed a reduction in myocardial infarction but no effect on total mortality.
- *Nicotinic acid* reduces triglycerides and, to a lesser extent, cholesterol. The most troublesome side-effect is flushing, which can be diminished by aspirin. Treatment should start with 100 mg three times daily, and rise slowly to 1–2 g three times daily.
- *Fibrates* reduce triglycerides and, to a lesser extent, cholesterol. Trials with fibrates have shown a reduction in coronary events, including myocardial infarction and death, but not in overall death rate.

Dietary fat and ischaemic heart disease

Major differences in lipid levels in different communities can be largely accounted for by diet. The LDL cholesterol level in the blood is determined chiefly by the intake of saturated fat, which is converted into cholesterol by the liver. There is relatively little cholesterol in the diet, so that the control of saturated fat is more important than limiting cholesterol intake. Polyunsaturates lower LDL cholesterol; monounsaturates also do so if they are substituted for saturates. The ratio of polyunsaturated fat to saturated fat in the diet is known as the P/S ratio; there are wide variations between P/S ratios in different countries, being high (about 1.0) in Japan and about 0.37 in the UK. Most of the saturated fat is derived from dairy products and fatty meat; a substantial impact on the P/S ratio can be made by substituting skimmed or semi-skimmed milk for the full fat form, a polyunsaturated margarine for butter, olive or polyunsaturated oil for saturated oils, and lean meat, chicken or fish for fatty meat. There is evidence that fish oils (omega-3 fatty acids) have a protective effect.

Other dietary factors

Epidemiological studies show that those who eat five or more helpings of fruit and vegetables a day have a lower prevalence of coronary heart disease. It is not clear whether this is due to the presence of high levels of the antioxidant vitamins A, C and E; it is therefore recommended that, rather than vitamin supplements, the public should be advised to consume more fruit and vegetables.

Hypertension

The higher the blood pressure, whether systolic or diastolic, the greater is the risk of developing ischaemic heart disease. Hypertension may contribute to its development in two ways: by accelerating the development of arterial disease and by increasing the work load of the left ventricle. Evidence from clinical trials suggests that antihypertensive agents lower coronary mortality only moderately – less than one might have anticipated. This may be because the trials have been short-lived, or because the agents used have had adverse effects that counteracted the benefit of lowering blood pressure.

Obesity

This is common in patients with ischaemic heart disease, but is often associated with other risk factors such as diabetes, hyperlipidaemia and hypertension. It is probably an independent risk factor, particularly in women. A high waist-to-hip ratio (common in South Asian men) has been linked to coronary disease. Weight loss is to be encouraged as a way of diminishing risk.

Family history

Coronary artery disease often occurs in several members of the same family. While this may indicate a genetic factor, a shared environment (e.g. diet and smoking) may partially explain it, but it is likely that both genetic and environmental factors are involved. The inherited tendency is usually mediated through hyperlipidaemia or hypertension. Although nothing can be done to correct the family history, it is important to recognize that those with familial disorders are very susceptible to environmental influences. The other risk factors should be attended to particularly diligently.

Cigarette smoking

Heavy consumption of cigarettes is associated with a high incidence of myocardial infarction and sudden death. The association is particularly striking in the younger age groups, but applies at all ages. Giving up smoking reduces the risk, but the full effect may take some years to achieve. The avoidance of smoking is perhaps the most important single preventive measure in Western countries.

Physical activity

Physical exercise appears to have a protective effect. Its mechanism is not clear, but it may increase HDL levels, reduce blood clotting and, perhaps, encourage the enlargement of the coronary arteries and their anastomoses. Everyone who can do so should exercise regularly. Simple forms of physical activity such as brisk walking, cycling and swimming are adequate if performed for at least 30 min three times a week. The middle-aged, if unfit, should take up exercise gradually and should avoid the most vigorous competitive games such as squash.

Mental stress
It is widely believed that stress contributes to the development of coronary disease. This may well be so, but convincing evidence is not, as yet, available, perhaps because it is a very difficult area to study. There is no doubt, however, that stress can aggravate the symptoms of those with heart disease.

Diabetes
Ischaemic heart disease develops more frequently and at an earlier age in those with diabetes.

Insulin resistance
Many individuals with ischaemic heart disease who are not frankly diabetic are insulin resistant, i.e. they require a higher insulin level than others to maintain a normal blood glucose level. Obesity and physical inactivity seem to be important factors in its occurrence.

Haemostatic factors
Individuals with high levels of factor VII activity and fibrinogen have an enhanced risk of coronary events.

Alcohol
Alcohol in moderation (e.g. 1–2 glasses of wine a day) is associated with a reduced incidence of ischaemic heart disease, but heavier drinking leads to hypertension and an increased risk.

PUBLIC HEALTH APPROACHES TO PREVENTION OF ISCHAEMIC HEART DISEASE

Changes in lifestyle are clearly important in the prevention of coronary disease, and these to a large extent are the responsibility of the individual. However, health professionals and the Government also play an important role.

Two strategies have been suggested to prevent coronary disease: a 'high-risk' strategy, involving the identification and treatment of those at high risk, e.g. hyperlipidaemic individuals, or a 'population' strategy, aimed at reducing risk factors in the community at large. The two approaches are not incompatible and both should be pursued, because whilst the high-risk patients are those most likely to benefit, they are relatively few in number and constitute only a small proportion of those who develop coronary disease.

Those at high risk can be identified on the basis of a family history of hyperlipidaemia or of coronary disease at a young age, or by a combination of risk factors such as hypertension, smoking and diabetes. Such individuals should have their lipids checked; they require skilled advice on the control of their risk factors. The population at large needs advice about a healthy diet and not smoking, the need for exercise and for having their blood pressure taken at least every 5 years. Both doctors and the Government need to be involved in providing such information; national food and taxation policies can strongly influence behaviour.

FURTHER READING

Wood, D., De Backer, G., Faergeman, O. et al (1998) Prevention of coronary heart disease in clinical practice. *European Heart Journal* **19**:1434–1503.

Diseases of the coronary arteries – causes, pathology and prevention

Clinical presentations of coronary disease

Coronary artery disease may present in any of the following ways:

- stable angina
- unstable angina/non-Q wave myocardial infarction/non-ST segment elevation myocardial infarction (NSTEMI)
- ST segment elevation myocardial infarction
- heart failure (see Ch. 9)
- sudden death
- as an incidental finding (asymptomatic).

Coronary disease presenting as an incidental finding in young people is rare. This may occur if a patient has a resting electrocardiogram (ECG) for some other reason and the ECG shows evidence of previous myocardial infarction. Alternatively, an exercise ECG carried out for employment or insurance reasons may show evidence of myocardial ischaemia. In general, patients identified in this way should be fully investigated and treated in the same way as patients with stable angina. The reason for this is that the individual patient's prognosis is related closely to the extent of their coronary disease and to their left ventricular function; symptoms are a poor guide to prognosis.

STABLE ANGINA

Definition

Angina pectoris is a discomfort in the chest and adjacent areas due to a transiently inadequate blood supply to the heart. As originally described by Heberden, it was only a symptom complex; there was no implied association with the heart. Today, the term is still used to describe a symptom, but its relationship to myocardial ischaemia is an essential component of the definition. There are many causes but coronary atherosclerosis is much the commonest. Almost invariably, at least one of the major coronary arteries has a reduction in luminal diameter of 70% or more; frequently two or three major arteries are involved. In most patients, there is a clear relationship to exercise, but the threshold for this may vary.

Characteristics of angina pectoris

The four major characteristics of anginal pain are its:

- location
- character
- relation to exercise
- duration.

Location of angina pectoris

Angina pectoris is most often felt behind the middle or upper third of the sternum. Even when the discomfort may be more obvious in another area, the sternal region is usually involved to some extent. Angina may also be felt in the lower sternal or xiphisternal region, over both sides of the chest, more commonly the left, in the neck and lower jaw and in both arms, again particularly the left. It may affect only the upper arm, but often reaches the elbow, the wrist or the fingers. In some patients, the elbow region escapes and the patient is aware of discomfort in the upper arm and a tingling feeling in the fingers. Rarely, it may radiate through to the left scapular region. It is very unusual for the pain to be located predominantly under the left nipple and it is virtually never confined to this area.

Character of angina pectoris

Angina pectoris is most frequently likened to a pressing feeling, a tight band, or a heavy weight. Many patients deny actual pain and refer only to a sense of discomfort. It is not usually severe but can cause much anxiety and distress. It is not stabbing in quality, but the terms 'sharp' (meaning intense rather than knife-like) and 'burning' are sometimes used. The sensations in other areas are often different in character. In the neck, it is frequently described as 'choking'; in the lower jaw it may be 'like toothache'. The feeling in the arms is usually one of numbness, heaviness or tingling.

Relationship of angina pectoris to exercise and other provoking factors

Angina pectoris is usually provoked by exertion, nearly always that of walking, particularly uphill. The amount of exercise required to produce angina varies from time to time in any individual, but it is more readily provoked after a heavy meal or in cold weather. There is also a diurnal variation. Patients often describe angina provoked by minimal exertion (such as washing or dressing) after rising from bed in the morning but are able to undertake much more strenuous activities later in the day without symptoms. This reflects changes in coronary vasomotor tone or 'conditioning' of the myocardium. Emotion is also an important provoking factor; angina may be readily induced by anger and irritation. Angina often develops during sexual intercourse. Some patients experience nocturnal angina, which wakes them up. In some cases this may be due to dreams, but it is probable that increased coronary artery tone, which is maximal in the early morning, is often responsible.

Angina pectoris may be provoked by several different types of tachycardia, particularly paroxysmal tachycardia associated with very rapid ventricular rates. Anaemia also contributes to its development, although it is unusual for it to do so in the absence of coronary atherosclerosis.

Duration of the angina attack

Most attacks last 1–3 min. Their duration is seldom less than 30 s or more than 15 min, although a vague sensation of discomfort may persist after the pain has stopped.

Other symptoms and signs of angina pectoris

Some patients complain of breathlessness accompanying the anginal pain. Other symptoms include flatulence, feelings of faintness and acute anxiety. Tachycardia and a rise in blood pressure may be noted during an attack but there are usually no abnormal signs.

The electrocardiogram

Between attacks of angina pectoris, the ECG is usually normal. There may, however, be evidence of old myocardial infarction, or non-specific changes such as flattening or inversion of T waves, bundle branch block or left ventricular hypertrophy. If the patient is seen during an attack, there are usually clear abnormalities which take the form of a horizontal or downward sloping depression of the ST segment (Fig. 7.1). Similar changes may be provoked by an exercise test (see below).

Diagnosis

By definition, angina is a symptom complex with a pathophysiological basis of myocardial ischaemia. The diagnosis must, therefore, depend on the history, combined with evidence of inadequate coronary blood flow.

There is usually no problem in determining the location of the pain and the factors that provoke it, but patients often find it difficult to find the words to describe the sensation they experience and estimates of the duration of the attack are often inaccurate. Most weight must therefore be placed on the first two elements. If the pain is located solely in the left submammary region, or if it lasts for only a few seconds, it is almost certainly not ischaemic. Angina is seldom associated with tenderness of the chest wall, although it may occasionally be so. It is usually, but not always, relieved by glyceryl trinitrate. Angina pectoris is unlikely if walking is not a provoking factor, but some patients take so little exercise that the symptom arises only with emotion or at night.

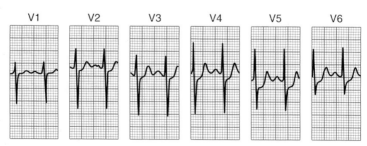

Fig. 7.1 ST depression during myocardial ischaemia. The chest leads are shown during an episode of angina. Extensive ST depression is evident, most marked in leads V5 and V6.

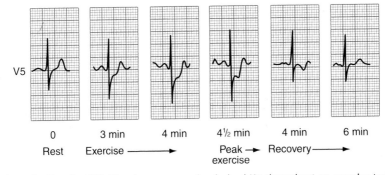

Fig. 7.2 Exercise EGC. The changes occurring in lead V5 throughout an exercise test are illustrated. During exercise there is a progressive depression of the ST segment, which returns to normal in the subsequent recovery period.

Physical examination is of comparatively little value except for the exclusion of such causes as aortic stenosis and cardiomyopathy. However, because angina pectoris is often associated with hypertension, with diabetes and with aortic valve disease, the characteristic findings of these conditions may be observed.

Evidence of myocardial ischaemia is provided by the presence of characteristic ST segment changes during an attack. As spontaneous attacks are seldom witnessed, it is usually necessary to carry out an exercise test. The patient may be made to exercise on a bicycle ergometer or a treadmill, preferably until chest discomfort is provoked. Standard and chest lead ECGs should be obtained during exercise and during the first 10 min of rest (Fig. 7.2). A positive exercise test is one that shows horizontal or downward sloping ST depression of 1.5 mm or more. ST segments that slope upwards from the J point should not be regarded as evidence of ischaemia as they are often seen in normal individuals with tachycardia.

Even after careful history taking and ECG examination, the diagnosis may remain uncertain. Stress echo or SPECT scanning (Ch. 4) may be helpful, but it is often necessary to carry out coronary angiography to confirm or refute the diagnosis of coronary artery disease (see Ch. 5).

Differential diagnosis

Although the diagnosis of angina can usually be established on the basis of the history and ECG, there are a number of other conditions that have to be considered in the differential diagnosis. Perhaps the most common difficulty arises with musculoskeletal pains in the chest wall. Frequently no cause is found for such pains which are often associated with tenderness and usually located on one side of the chest rather than centrally. These pains are most likely to be provoked by such actions as lifting and pulling, which produce tension of the muscles attached to the ribs. Amongst identifiable musculoskeletal conditions may be included Tietze's syndrome (in which there is an inflammation of one or more costochondral junctions), a slipping rib cartilage, fractured ribs, or metastatic lesions in ribs. In these conditions, unlike angina, there is tenderness and the symptoms may be aggravated by inspiration. The pain of cervical spondylosis is sometimes most severe in the upper chest region and accompanied by discomfort in the shoulders and arms.

Stabbing pains under the left breast and persistent aches in the same region are common and are most unlikely to be due to ischaemic heart disease. It is often not possible to establish their cause, but these symptoms are very common in anxious individuals.

Disorders of the gastrointestinal tract may be difficult to differentiate from angina pectoris. Oesophageal reflux, often associated with hiatus hernia, gives rise to a central chest pain, but this seldom radiates to the arms, is of a more burning or bursting character, and is more readily provoked by stooping or lying flat, although it may be produced by exercise. The pain of peptic ulcer is usually situated in the epigastric region, and is associated with tenderness. It is related to food rather than to exertion and is usually relieved by alkalis or milk and not by glyceryl trinitrate. Cholecystitis and cholelithiasis may give rise to pain in the lower sternal region, but there is usually tenderness either in the epigastrium or in the right subcostal area; there is frequently associated nausea, and the pain is not related to exertion. It is important to recognize that these gastrointestinal conditions, particularly hiatus hernia and cholecystitis, are common in patients with ischaemic heart disease, and the presence of one of these disorders does not preclude the coexistence of angina pectoris.

Prognosis

Most patients who develop angina pectoris live a normal or nearly normal life for many years. Symptoms are liable to vary from time to time, becoming worse in winter and improving the subsequent summer. Symptoms are poorly related to prognosis. Instead, prognosis is related to the extent of coronary artery disease and to the degree of left ventricular dysfunction. Single vessel disease in a patient with good left ventricular function carries a good prognosis while diffuse disease of all three major coronary vessels and poor left ventricular function are associated with a poor prognosis.

Treatment

The general management of angina pectoris is of great importance. The anxiety that the diagnosis arouses may cause incapacity, and it is important to emphasize the relatively good prognosis. Intense cold, walking into a wind or unnecessarily uphill should be avoided if they provoke the pain, as should taking large meals. Patients quickly learn to avoid activities that are likely to provoke episodes of angina. Usually, patients can continue their occupations. Driving is permitted for patients with stable angina but the diagnosis of angina may have serious consequences for 'vocational' drivers (i.e. heavy goods vehicle drivers and coach drivers) as well as for airline pilots. Physical exercise is to be encouraged provided it does not induce discomfort, as it increases the threhold at which angina develops, but sudden strenuous effort should not be undertaken.

Risk factor modification

All modifiable risk factors should be addressed in the patient with angina. Cigarette smoking should be strongly discouraged and guidance given about weight reduction. The blood pressure should be recorded and, if necessary, treated. Blood cholesterol should be measured; the threshold for starting treatment with an HMG CoA reductase inhibitor (such as simvastatin or pravastatin) has been controversial but there is growing evidence that all patients with proven coronary artery disease should be treated with one of these drugs. This treatment is likely to be for life.

Drug treatment of angina

Aspirin

All patients with coronary artery disease, unless there are strong contraindications, should be commenced on treatment with aspirin for life. The dose should be 75 or 150 mg once daily. The ideal dose is not known but there is no evidence of any additional benefit from doses exceeding 150 mg once daily.

Nitrates

Nitrates have been in use in the management of angina for more than 100 years, but they remain the first-line treatment.

The major pharmacological effect of nitrates is the relaxation of smooth muscle, which seems to result from an increase in intracellular cyclic guanosine monophosphate (cGMP) levels. Dilatation occurs in the coronary arteries, the peripheral arteries and the veins. Coronary artery dilatation leads directly to an increase in coronary blood flow, arterial dilatation leads to a fall in afterload, and a reduction in venous tone causes pooling, with a diminished venous return and preload. The relative importance of these different effects varies from one patient to another. Thus, the coronary vasodilator action is of particular value when an increase in coronary artery tone is an important component of angina, whereas it may have little influence in an artery with a fixed stenosis. In the latter situation, it is probably the venodilator action that is most relevant.

Most nitrates undergo extensive first-pass metabolism in the liver; this may be overcome by administering large doses, but the effects are rather unpredictable. Alternatives are to use isosorbide mononitrate which does not undergo first-pass metabolism, or to bypass the gut by sublingual, buccal or transdermal administration.

Nitrates have relatively minor side-effects, but headache is very common. This tends to diminish with continued use, but some patients find it even more distressing than the angina. Nitrates (particularly glyceryl trinitrate) may cause hypotension and syncope; patients should be advised to take at least their first dose sitting down.

A problem with continuous nitrate therapy is the development of tolerance. This can be avoided by a regimen that ensures a period in the day with little or no nitrate in the blood.

Glyceryl trinitrate (nitroglycerin, trinitrin) is standard therapy in angina pectoris. It is given sublingually either in tablet form or as an aerosol spray. The dose is usually 0.2–0.5 mg. It will stop an attack of angina in about 2 min, but is particularly effective if given prophylactically. Patients should, therefore, be encouraged to take a tablet or use the spray when they anticipate an attack; they should also be advised that the drug is not addictive, as many fear that they will become drug dependent.

Long-acting oral nitrates are effective if given in sufficient dosage, but headache is a common problem, and the regimen should ensure a nitrate-free period. Sustained-release once-daily preparations of isosorbide mononitrate (as 25, 50 or 60 mg preparations) appear to be more effective than smaller doses given at frequent intervals and do ensure a nitrate-free interval. The same considerations apply to transdermal patches.

Beta-adrenoceptor blocking drugs

These are now given routinely to most patients with angina unless there are contraindications to their use. They block the action of catecholamines to increase heart rate, blood pressure and cardiac contractility and thereby limit the myocardial oxygen needs during exercise. Beta-blockers have been shown to reduce the frequency of angina, to reduce the consumption of glyceryl trinitrate, to prolong exercise time during treadmill testing and to reduce ECG evidence of myocardial ischaemia at a given workload. Beta-blockers may exacerbate congestive cardiac failure and airways obstruction and should be avoided in patients with asthma, and introduced very cautiously in patients with heart failure (see Ch. 8). When given to patients free of heart failure or a history of asthma, the main side-effects of beta-blockers are fatigue and cold extremities, both of which disappear on stopping the drug.

In general, the choice of a particular beta-blocker is not of importance, but compliance is more likely to be achieved if a preparation that requires only once or twice daily administration (such as atenolol or bisoprolol) is used.

Calcium antagonists

Currently, available calcium antagonists fall into two main groups, the dihydropyridines and the phenylalkylamines. The phenylalkylamines (verapamil and diltiazem) have potent depressant actions on the myocardium and the conducting system. They slow the heart rate both at rest and during exercise and are useful antianginal agents when beta-blockers are contraindicated. These drugs can be combined with beta-blockers but this combination may lead to excessive bradycardia or to heart block. A usual dose is 60 mg three times daily for diltiazem and 80 mg three times daily for verapamil, although long-acting once-daily preparations of both drugs are available. Side-effects with diltiazem are rare and the only commonly reported problem with verapamil is constipation.

The dihydropyridine calcium antagonists (nifedipine, nicardipine and amlodipine) have little effect on the myocardium and conducting tissue; their main action is to dilate the peripheral arteries and to reduce the workload on the heart. Used alone, they often cause a reflex tachycardia which can be avoided by concomitant use of a beta-blocker. Side-effects are common and include headache, facial flushing and ankle swelling. The usual dosage for nifedipine is 30–60 mg daily in divided doses or as a single slow-release preparation. The dose for nicardipine is 5–30 mg three times daily and for amlodipine is 5–10 mg once daily.

Calcium antagonists can worsen cardiac performance in those with poor left ventricular function, and generally should be avoided in patients with cardiac failure.

Nicorandil

Nicorandil is a potassium channel activator and also has nitrate-like coronary vasodilator effects. It has been shown to reduce symptoms and to reduce events (cardiac death, myocardial infarction and admission to hospital with unstable angina) in patients with chronic stable angina. It is given orally in a dose of 10 mg bd, increasing to 20 mg bd if required.

Revascularization treatments for patients with angina

Patients with angina should be considered for some form of revascularization. This may take the form of coronary angioplasty (percutaneous coronary intervention or PCI) or coronary artery bypass grafting (CABG). In the past, these treatments were considered only in patients who failed medical therapy (i.e. patients with ongoing angina despite medical treatment). However, it has now been established that an individual patient's prognosis is more closely related to left ventricular function and to the extent of coronary artery disease than to symptoms and that revascularization can improve prognosis in certain patient groups; it follows, therefore, that all patients should have some form of assessment regarding their suitability, and appropriateness, for revascularization. This assessment should include some form of testing for ischaemia (e.g. exercise ECG) and will often include coronary angiography.

Percutaneous coronary intervention (PCI)

PCI is carried out on a conscious patient under local anaesthetic. Access to the coronary vessels is gained via the femoral, radial or brachial artery. A balloon catheter is then passed over a guidewire and into the stenosed segment of the artery. The balloon is then inflated, causing disruption of the stenosis. This is shown schematically in Figure 7.3. This produces a substantial increase in the diameter of the artery (Fig. 7.4); however, the injured artery tends to renarrow ('restenose') in 25–40% of cases within 6 months, with a return of angina. In current clinical practice, therefore, most patients are treated with coronary artery 'stents' (Fig. 7.5). These are metal (usually steel) devices that are crimped onto the outside on an angioplasty balloon. The balloon-mounted stent is then passed to the narrowed segment of the artery and the balloon is inflated, usually to a pressure of 10–14 atmospheres for 30–60 s. This expands and deploys the stent. The balloon is then deflated and removed, leaving the stent as a permanent internal scaffolding within the artery. Restenosis can still occur, but the rates are around 10% and are substantially lower than in PCI without stenting.

The advent of coronary artery stents has greatly expanded the indications for PCI. Lesions that were previously considered unsuitable for PCI, or had a very high restenosis risk, can often now be stented. These include:

- long coronary lesions (> 20 mm) (Fig. 7.6)
- total coronary occlusions (Fig. 7.7)

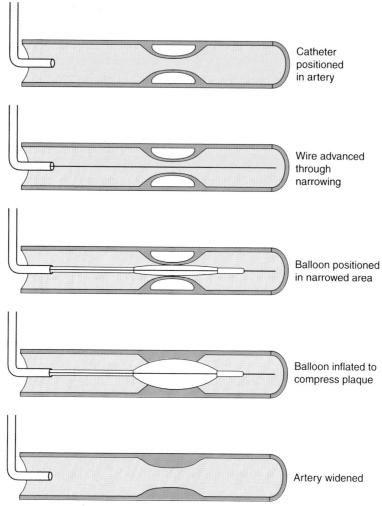

Catheter
positioned
in artery

Wire advanced
through
narrowing

Balloon positioned
in narrowed area

Balloon inflated to
compress plaque

Artery widened

Fig. 7.3 Percutaneous transluminal coronary angioplasty. (With permission from Julian D.G. & Marley C. [1991] *Coronary Heart Disease: The Facts*. Oxford: Oxford University Press.)

- bifurcation lesions
- vein graft stenoses (Fig. 7.8)
- lesions of the left mainstem.

Adjunctive medication in PCI

Once a stent has been deployed in a coronary vessel, there is then a period of 'endothelialisation' during which the endothelial cells of the vessel wall proliferate and cover all the struts of the stent. This period takes 2–4 weeks. At the end of this period, the coronary stent is effectively incorporated into the wall of the artery with no bare metal exposed to the circulating blood. Within the first few weeks, however, there is a risk that the exposed stent will act as a focus for thrombus formation. If thrombus completely occludes the lumen (subacute stent thrombosis), then the patient may present acutely with recurrent pain, acute myocardial infarction, or sudden death. To reduce this risk, a number of antiplatelet drugs are given:

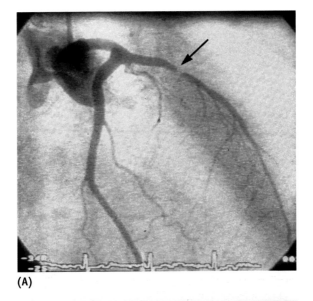

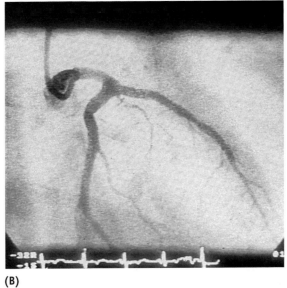

Fig. 7.4 A stenosis of the left anterior descending coronary artery (arrowed) before (A) and after (B) coronary angioplasty.

- *Aspirin 300 mg once daily.* This is given for 4 weeks to most stent patients. Thereafter, the dose can be reduced to 75 or 150 mg per day as long-term treatment.
- *Clopidogrel 75 mg once daily.* This is also given for a minimum of 4 weeks after the PCI procedure.
- *IIb/IIIa inhibitors.* These drugs act by blocking the GP IIb/IIIa receptor on the platelet and preventing the binding of fibrinogen. This in turn prevents platelet to platelet binding. There are three agents currently available (abciximab, tirofiban, eptifibatide). All are given intravenously. They reduce periprocedural complications such as myocardial infarction.

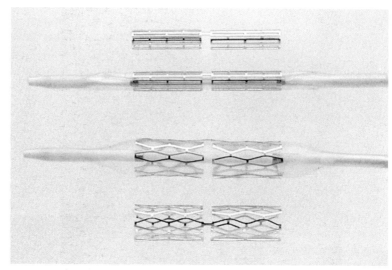

Fig. 7.5 Example of a coronary artery stent. From top to bottom: stent before insertion; stent crimped on a deflated angioplasty balloon; stent being expanded by inflation of the balloon; fully deployed stent.

Side-effects are rare and they can be used in all PCI procedures; in most centres, however, they are used mostly in higher risk PCI procedures (acute patients, bifurcation lesions, etc.)

Other angioplasty techniques have not been shown to reduce late restenosis but may be useful in certain situations. These include the following:

- *Rotational atherectomy.* This device comprises an olive-shaped burr with multiple tiny diamonds embedded in the burr. This is rotated at high speed, resulting in emulsification of the atheroma. This device appears to be useful in patients with diffuse coronary atheroma and in ostial lesions.
- *Directional atherectomy.* As its name implies, this device has a cutter that can remove and retrieve atheromatous lesions. This technique may be useful in eccentric stenoses.
- *Laser angioplasty.* Laser energy is transmitted through multiple optic fibres to cut through stenotic or occluded coronary lesions.

However, two new techniques have shown great promise in terms of reducing restenosis:

- *Brachytherapy.* Following a normal angioplasty or stent procedure, a radioactive ribbon is advanced into the artery and the treated arterial segment is then irradiated with either a beta or a gamma emitting radiation source. Brachytherapy has been shown to reduce restenosis and is generally reserved for patients in whom the lesion has already restenosed once. It delays endothelialization of the stent and leaves the patient at risk of late thrombosis for much longer than after a simple stent procedure.
- *Drug-eluting stents.* These are stents that are coated in a drug or drugs designed to prevent, or at least reduce, restenosis. The early results have been very encouraging with restenosis rates in the actively treated groups around 20–30% of those seen in the control groups. The two stents

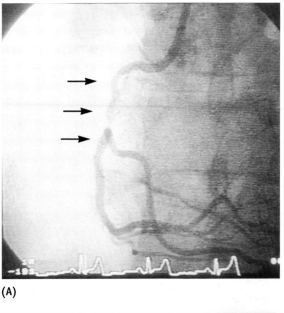

(A)

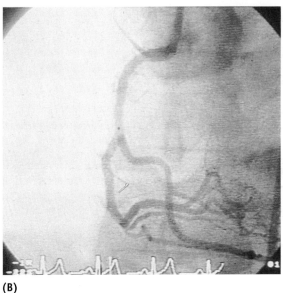

(B)

Fig. 7.6 Angiographic appearance (A) before and (B) after stenting of a long stenosis of a right coronary artery (arrows).

currently available in the UK use antiproliferative agents (sirolimus and paclitaxel) and it seems likely than more drug-eluting stents, perhaps with multiple agents, will follow.

Coronary artery bypass surgery

The narrowed segments of coronary arteries can be bypassed using a length of saphenous vein taken from the leg. One end of the vein is attached to the ascending aorta and the other to the affected artery beyond the most distal

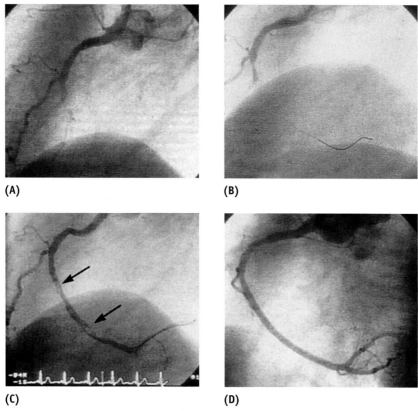

(A) **(B)**

(C) **(D)**

Fig. 7.7 Reopening of a totally occluded right coronary artery. (A) Occlusion of a right coronary artery; (B) a guidewire has been passed through the occluded segment and into the distal right coronary artery; (C) after multiple balloon dilatations, the artery is now patent although there are areas of arterial dissection (arrowed); (D) two arterial stents have been positioned in the right coronary artery establishing a smooth outline with good flow.

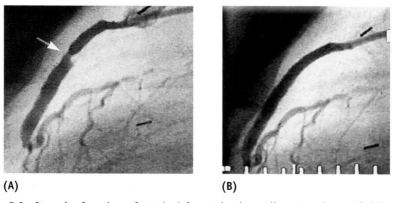

(A) **(B)**

Fig. 7.8 Stenosis of a vein graft to the left anterior descending artery (arrowed) (A) before and (B) after coronary stenting.

obstruction as demonstrated by coronary arteriography (Fig. 7.9). Surgeons are increasingly trying to use lengths of artery instead of vein. The most commonly used artery for this purpose is the left internal mammary artery.

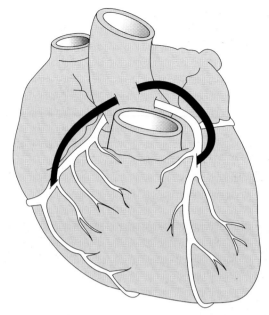

Fig. 7.9 Two saphenous vein bypass grafts, from the aorta to the anterior descending and right coronary arteries, respectively. (With permission from Julian D.G. & Marley C. [1991] *Coronary Heart Disease: The Facts*. Oxford: Oxford University Press.)

In this case, the proximal end of the vessel is not detached from the left subclavian artery; the artery is, however, mobilized, its major side branches are tied off and the distal end is anastomosed to the coronary artery (most commonly the left anterior descending artery). Other arteries can be used in this way, including the right internal mammary artery and the gastroepiploic artery. Recently, free arterial grafts (such as an excised radial artery) have also been utilized. This allows some patients to undergo 'total arterial revascularization' in which only arterial conduits are used. The long-term success, however, of arterial grafts other than the mammary arteries, has not yet been demonstrated.

Grafts may, if necessary, be inserted into all the three major arteries, and into their larger branches. Provided left ventricular function is not severely impaired, the mortality rate of the operation is less than 1% in most centres. A small proportion of grafts close shortly after insertion. Approximately 50% will remain patent for at least 5 years with much higher patency rates (of around 90%) if an arterial conduit has been used. It has been found that antiplatelet therapy (e.g. aspirin 150 mg once daily) is helpful in maintaining patency, and lipid-lowering drugs such as simvastatin, pravastatin or atorvastatin should be given to all patients.

The results of surgery are usually very satisfactory, at least for 5–10 years. Angina is abolished in at least 50% of cases, and greatly improved in a further 30%. As well as relieving angina, coronary artery surgery benefits the prognosis of patients with disease of the left main coronary artery, and also those who have disease of the three major vessels, together with left ventricular dysfunction. Late deterioration may be due to graft closure, or to progression of disease in the ungrafted vessels.

Surgery is indicated for those whose angina is not adequately relieved by full medical treatment, but it should also be considered as a measure to improve prognosis, even in the absence of symptoms, in certain groups of patient (see below).

Most centres carry out coronary artery bypass grafting under cardiopulmonary bypass after a sternotomy with full exposure of the heart and great vessels. Recent interest has focused on coronary artery bypass surgery without the need for cardiopulmonary bypass or sternotomy (so-called minimally invasive approaches). The safety of these techniques when compared with conventional coronary artery bypass grafting has yet to be established but this is certain to be a major interest in cardiac surgery over the next 10 years.

Choice of treatment for the individual patient with angina

In the patient with stable angina, treatment should include aspirin and a beta-blocker together with identification and treatment of any modifiable risk factors such as hypercholesterolaemia or hypertension. In practice, most patients are treated with a statin and with an angiotensin-converting enzyme (ACE) inhibitor. Although there are no large-scale mortality studies looking at the effects of drug treatment on prognosis in angina, beta-blockers have been shown to reduce mortality if given early during the course of myocardial infarction. In the absence of other data, therefore, it seems logical to treat patients with angina with a beta-blocker, as they are at risk of myocardial infarction at some time. If the patient's symptoms are not controlled, a long-acting nitrate, nicorandil and/or a calcium antagonist can be added.

The decision as to when to undertake invasive investigations with a view to either percutaneous transluminal coronary angioplasty (PTCA) or coronary artery bypass surgery has been controversial and varies widely from country to country and from region to region. In general, angiography should be undertaken if a patient's symptoms are not controlled on medical therapy or if an exercise test shows evidence of ischaemia at a low workload. This implies that most patients with angina should have an exercise ECG, not only to confirm the diagnosis of angina, but to help stratify the individual patient's risk of major adverse events such as myocardial infarction and death. This is necessary because the relationship between symptomatic status and the extent of coronary disease at angiography is often poor. In certain groups of patients, such as those with stenosis of the left main stem or stenoses of all three major coronary vessels and reduced left ventricular function, coronary bypass surgery has been shown to improve both symptoms and prognosis. It follows that patients with a strongly positive exercise test should be considered for angiography even if their symptoms are mild or absent. The decision as to whether or not an individual patient should undergo angiography will be influenced by other factors such as the patient's age and the presence of other medical conditions that might increase the risk of any interventional treatment.

If revascularization is warranted, this may take the form of either PCI or surgery. In general, PCI (usually with coronary artery stenting) is preferred for patients with one- or two-vessel disease, and coronary artery bypass surgery is preferred for those with triple vessel disease, left main stem disease or diffusely diseased arteries. There are, however, no hard and fast rules and clinical practice will vary depending on local expertise. Several studies have compared the outcome of coronary surgery and PCI in patients with multi-vessel disease; no significant differences have been demonstrated in major events such as death and myocardial infarction. If the initial treatment is PCI, however, the patient should accept that reintervention (in the form of further PCI or surgery) is more likely than if the initial treatment is surgical.

UNSTABLE ANGINA, NON-Q WAVE MYOCARDIAL INFARCTION AND NON-ST SEGMENT ELEVATION MYOCARDIAL INFARCTION

These three terms are now often used interchangably. Another commonly used term, 'acute coronary syndrome', covers all of these conditions, together with acute ST segment myocardial infarction.

The term 'unstable angina' is a clinical definition and refers to:

- recent onset angina
- angina occurring with increasing frequency
- angina occurring with less exertion or at rest
- angina not rapidly relieved by GTN.

Until recently, it was believed that unstable angina was not associated with myocardial necrosis. Within the last few years, however, more sensitive assays of myocardial damage have become available, including the measurement of troponin T and troponin I in peripheral blood samples. Troponin levels are generally raised in patients with unstable angina even when the more traditional cardiac enzyme levels (CK or CK-MB) are normal. This has resulted in an expansion of the definition of acute myocardial infarction. Many patients who were previously labelled as having had unstable angina are now considered to have had a myocardial infarction based on raised troponin levels. In this chapter, the term unstable angina will be used to include non-Q wave MI and non-ST segment elevation MI. This is reasonable because the diagnosis on admission is one of 'unstable angina' or 'acute coronary syndrome'; the confirmation of any myocardial infarction is not generally possible until blood test results become available 12–24 h after admission.

Prevalence and pathogenesis of unstable angina

It is reasonable to group these conditions together since their pathology and treatment is the same. The pathogenesis relates to plaque rupture and thrombus formation. The reasons for the infarction not progressing to a full thickness or Q wave myocardial infarction may relate to incomplete or intermittent occlusion of the infarct-related vessel, to the presence of collateral channels or to the small size of the affected vessel.

In the UK, non-ST segment elevation MI is becoming more common and ST segment elevation MI less common. The reasons for this are not clear. In a recent UK study, it was estimated that there were 115 000 hospital admissions per annum with unstable angina. The same study also drew attention to the high risk of recurrent events in these patients. Although immediate in-hospital mortality was relatively low, more than 25% of patients had either died, sustained a major myocardial infarction or been readmitted to hospital with a further episode of unstable angina within the subsequent 6 months. Older patients, patients with previous myocardial infarction and patients with ST segment depression on the resting ECG were at highest risk.

Clinical presentation and diagnosis of unstable angina

The diagnosis of unstable angina is based on the clinical history, the ECG findings and the blood enzyme levels.

Clinical history

The patient may be admitted following a first episode of angina or because of an increase in the frequency or severity of pain in someone with pre-existing angina. The patient will usually describe an episode of chest pain which is similar to the description of chronic stable angina but which lasts longer (10 min to several hours) and is usually not related to exercise. The pain may be intermittent and may be partially relieved by GTN.

ECG changes

The ECG may show ST segment depression or T wave inversion. ST segment depression carries a higher risk of further events than does T wave inversion. The leads in which the changes are seen give some indication as to the area of myocardium affected and the likely 'culprit' artery but this should serve as a rough guide only and 'surprises' are common:

Leads II, III, aVf	inferior surface	? RCA lesion
Leads V1–V4	anteroseptal surface	? LAD lesion
Leads V4–V6	anterolateral surface	? Circ. lesion

Serial ECG tracings should be recorded since the ECG is most useful when there are sequential or progressive changes over a period of hours or days. For example, an ECG which is initially normal but later shows T wave inversion in leads V1 to V6 is strongly suggestive of an acute coronary syndrome secondary to an unstable lesion of the left anterior descending artery. An ECG during pain is particularly useful to diagnose or exclude coronary disease as a cause of chest pain.

Enzyme levels

The CK and CK-MB levels may be mildly raised to 2–3 times the upper limit of normal; they may, however, be within the normal range and have been superceded by the use of assays for troponin T and troponin I which are much more sensitive indicators of myocardial damage. These are fairly specific but can be raised in patients with heart failure or patients with arrhythmias, even in the absence of coronary disease. In most cases, however, a significant elevation in the troponin level is diagnostic even in the setting of a normal resting ECG.

Treatment

Medical treatment of unstable angina

General

These patients should be admitted to hospital, preferably to a coronary care unit equipped with full resuscitation facilities and facilities for continuous ECG monitoring. Appropriate pain relief (with intravenous diamorphine) should be given. Since the pathogenesis relates to plaque rupture, platelet aggregation and thrombus formation, it follows that the cornerstone of medical treatment will be anticoagulant and antiplatelet therapy.

Aspirin

Soluble aspirin 75 or 150 mg daily should be given. Aspirin inhibits cyclo-oxygenase, reduces synthesis of thromboxane A2 and reduces platelet adhesiveness. In clinical trials, aspirin has been shown to reduce myocardial infarction and death in this group of patients.

Clopidogrel

Clopidogrel is given orally in a dose of 75 mg daily. It is usually given in combination with aspirin to all patients with unstable angina and has been shown to reduce major events including death, Q wave myocardial infarction and recurrent ischaemia. It is usually given for 1 year after the acute event.

Heparin

Until recently, patients with unstable angina were treated with unfractionated heparin. This was given by continuous intravenous infusion. Because of its variable action, regular blood monitoring (once or twice per day) was required to ensure that the patient was appropriately anticoagulated. Currently, heparin treatment is given as low molecular weight heparin. There are two preparations available – dalteparin (Fragmin) and enoxaparin (Clexane). They are probably more efficacious than unfractionated heparin but their main advantages are that they are given by subcutaneous injection rather than by continuous intravenous infusion and that they do not require regular monitoring of blood clotting. The dose regimens used in unstable angina are:

Dalteparin: 120 units/kg twice daily by s.c. injection
Enoxaparin: 1 mg/kg twice daily by s.c. injection

Glycoprotein IIb/IIIa receptor antagonists

These drugs prevent platelet deposition and aggregation. There are three agent available, all given intravenously. Abciximab is an antibody and is expensive to produce. Most of the studies of abciximab have centred on its use in patients undergoing PCI. The other agents, tirofiban and eptifibatide are peptides and are less expensive to manufacture. Most of the studies of these agents have centred on their role as part of the medical management of unstable angina, where they are normally given by intravenous infusion for 48–72 h. They are effective in preventing infarction, ongoing ischaemia, etc., but a recent meta-analysis suggests that the benefit of these drugs is only maintained if the patient subsequently undergoes revascularization either by PCI or CABG (see below).

Beta-blockers

Patients with unstable angina should be treated with an oral beta-blocker provided thay have no contraindications (asthma, severe peripheral vascular disease, acute heart failure, etc.). Atenolol 25–50 mg bd, bisoprolol 5 mg once daily or metoprolol 25–50 mg three times daily are all appropriate.

Calcium antagonists

These are not front-line drugs in unstable angina but, as in stable angina, a rate-limiting calcium antagonist (diltiazem or verapamil) can be used if the patient has contraindications to beta-blockade.

Nitrates

If the patient has ongoing or recurrent ischaemic pain, particularly if accompanied by ST segment depression, then intravenous nitrates can be given starting at 1 mg per hour and increasing as required.

Coronary intervention in unstable angina

Most patients with unstable angina, non-Q MI and non-ST segment elevation MI should be considered for coronary revascularization, either by PCI or by CABG. This has been a controversial area in the past. Early studies in this group suggested either no overall benefit, or harm, from interventional treatment. However, many of these studies were carried out prior to the advent of coronary stents and IIb/IIIa inhibitors, both of which make angioplasty (PCI) safer. Furthermore, these early studies were complicated by a high rate of patient crossover from conservative to interventional treatment which makes interpretation difficult.

Three recent studies have clearly established the benefits of early revascularization in this patient group. In general, therefore, most patients with unstable angina should be stabilized on medical treatment and should then be considered for coronary angiography with a view to coronary revascularization by either PCI or CABG.

If doubt exists about the diagnosis (e.g. troponin negative patient with no ECG changes), then exercise testing may be useful. If the patient has already demonstrated dynamic ECG changes, then exercise testing is unlikely to be helpful and may be harmful.

ST SEGMENT ELEVATION MYOCARDIAL INFARCTION

Myocardial infarction is the term applied to myocardial necrosis secondary to an acute interruption of the coronary blood supply. The pathological changes underlying myocardial infarction are described in detail in Chapter 6. Rupture of an atheromatous plaque leads to deposition of intracoronary thrombus, which leads in turn to coronary occlusion. The term myocardial infarction refers to the consequent necrosis of myocardium. The morbidity and mortality of infarction arise from the resultant arrhythmias and loss of pump function.

The management of myocardial infarction has been transformed in the past two decades. Whereas in the past, management was largely reactive, treating complications as they arose, recent advances have led to a proactive approach, addressing the underlying pathological processes. This proactive approach to myocardial infarction is one of the success stories of modern cardiology. Large clinical trials have shown that the use of aspirin and thrombolytic therapy can reduce the mortality rate from acute infarction by almost 50%. Furthermore, in the recovery phase after infarction, intervention with beta-blockers and ACE inhibitors offer further substantial reductions in mortality.

It is reasonable to anticipate, therefore, that with current therapies the long-term mortality rate after infarction can be reduced by over 50%.

Clinical presentation

Clinical features

The common presenting symptom of myocardial infarction is severe chest pain. This is predominantly in the sternal region, but may radiate to both sides of the chest, to the jaw, to the shoulders and to one or both arms. It is usually described as tight, pressing, heavy or constricting. Sometimes the patient may deny 'pain' and describe a discomfort, not amounting to pain, in the centre of the chest. Although it can be brief, the pain usually lasts for more than half an hour and may continue for several hours. Unlike the pain of angina, it is seldom associated with exertion and is not relieved by rest or glyceryl trinitrate. The pain may be maximal at the onset, but often increases in intensity for a period of minutes or hours and then remains constant until it gradually recedes. Frequently, the patient gives a history of the recent onset of angina or the exacerbation of pre-existing angina in the preceding days or weeks.

The pain may be overshadowed by other symptoms, such as breathlessness or syncope. Occasionally, it is obscured because the infarction develops during anaesthesia or at the time of a cerebrovascular accident. Rarely, infarction may be truly pain-free.

Once the pain has been controlled, the patient may remain free of symptoms and make an uninterrupted recovery. However, complications develop in a substantial proportion of cases. The most important of these are:

- arrhythmias
- cardiogenic shock
- left ventricular failure.

These complications, which will be considered in detail later, are the common causes of death and are responsible for many of the abnormal physical signs that may be observed.

Physical signs

During the earliest stages of the attack, patients are obviously distressed and may be sweaty and cold. The general appearance improves when the pain is controlled and often, within a few hours, the patient looks well.

The pulse may be normal in volume and rate, but in severe attacks it is small and fast. Tachyarrhythmias or bradycardia are also common.

The blood pressure usually falls progressively over a period of hours and days, reaching its minimum some time during the first week, and returning towards normal slowly over the next 2–3 weeks. There may, however, be a sharp fall in blood pressure at the onset of the infarction, which may progress to the severe hypotension of cardiogenic shock, or may resolve. Transient hypertension, perhaps resulting from intense pain, is sometimes observed.

The jugular venous pressure is usually normal or slightly elevated early in the course of acute myocardial infarction; it is seldom markedly elevated due to right-sided heart failure.

The apex beat, which is often difficult to feel, may be displaced outwards. Between the apex and the left sternal edge, a systolic pulsation may be detectable, due to a protrusion of the infarcted anterior wall of the heart.

The first and second heart sounds are often soft. A fourth (or atrial) sound can be heard in most cases; a third heart sound is common when there is heart failure or shock.

A soft pansystolic murmur at the apex is not uncommon and is caused by mitral regurgitation either as a result of papillary muscle malfunction or secondary to dilatation of the left ventricle. Rarely, a loud systolic murmur may develop at the left sternal edge, due to a rupture of the ventricular septum, or at the apex, due to rupture of a papillary muscle. A transient pericardial rub occurs in some patients, usually on the second or third day.

Pulmonary crepitations may be present: they are a poor prognostic indicator if widespread and numerous because of pulmonary oedema.

Most of the abnormal physical signs described disappear within a few days of the onset of infarction, except in the most severely affected patients.

A fever, seldom exceeding 38°C, usually commences within the first 24 h and subsides in under a week.

There is often a slight leucocytosis and an increase in the erythrocyte sedimentation rate (ESR). The pyrexia, leucocytosis and raised ESR represent a reaction to myocardial necrosis.

Diagnosis

This is based on:

- clinical history (see above)
- ECG changes
- raised enzyme measurements.

ECG changes

The ECG is virtually always transiently or permanently abnormal after acute myocardial infarction. Because the ECG diagnosis of infarction depends upon the observation of a sequence of changes with time, serial records are vital. Many coronary care units will have the facilities for continuous 12 lead ECG monitoring.

The characteristic abnormalities (Fig. 7.10) are:

- ST segment elevation
- Q wave formation
- T wave inversion.

Although the precise mechanisms responsible for these ECG changes are not yet determined, it is probable that the Q wave changes are the result of

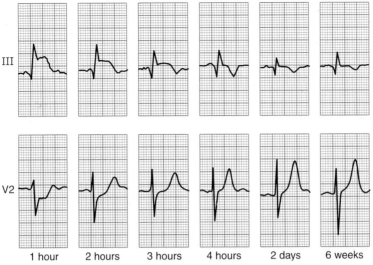

| | 1 hour | 2 hours | 3 hours | 4 hours | 2 days | 6 weeks |

Fig. 7.10 Progression of ECG changes in myocardial infarction. The progression of ECG changes during and after an inferior infarct is shown. Lead III (upper series) faces the area of infarction. V2 (lower series) demonstrates reciprocal changes. The time of each ECG from onset of symptoms is shown. The patient received thrombolytic therapy on initial presentation at 1 h. In lead III, early ST elevation rapidly resolves, to be succeeded by a biphasic T wave and subsequently by T wave inversion. A Q wave develops over several hours. In the remote lead, V2, there is initial ST depression. This resolves with the disappearance of ST elevation in lead III.

muscle death, that the ST abnormalities are due to muscle injury, and that the T wave abnormalities are due to ischaemia.

Classically, the earliest change in acute myocardial infarction is ST elevation. This occurs within minutes of arterial occlusion and represents transmural ischaemia in the territory of the infarct. Q waves, by contrast, arise due to myocardial necrosis and take some hours to develop fully (Fig. 7.10). The ST segment progressively returns to normal to be succeeded by T inversion in the first 24–48 h after infarction. Persistent ST segment elevation suggests the possibility of a ventricular aneurysm. Over a time course of weeks and months, the T wave generally becomes less inverted and may even normalize. This is in contrast to Q waves, which usually persist indefinitely. Since Q waves are a marker of previous infarction, distinguishing pathological from physiological Q waves is of some importance. Normally, Q waves in leads facing the left ventricle do not exceed 2 mm in depth or 0.03 s in width. Q waves and QS waves are normal in aVR, and are commonly found in V1 and V2. Deep Q waves are often also seen normally in lead III. The Q wave in lead III should be considered definitely abnormal only if it exceeds 0.03 s in duration, and if it is accompanied by Q waves in either lead II or aVF. The 'normal' Q wave in lead III usually diminishes or disappears on deep inspiration, whereas the 'pathological' Q wave persists.

The time sequence of ECG changes in acute infarction is of importance in relation to thrombolysis. Firstly, patients seen in the earliest phase of infarction may not have developed Q waves. It is entirely appropriate in such cases to base the decision to commence thrombolytic therapy on the presence of ST elevation alone. Secondly, the rapidity of resolution of ST elevation provides a rough guide to the success of reperfusion: ST segments show rapid resolution in patients achieving successful reperfusion, compared with a more gradual resolution in those failing to reperfuse. As a rough guide, if ST segments have resolved by 50% or more within 90 min of the commencement of thrombolytic therapy, this indicates successful reperfusion. Finally, with the advent of reperfusion therapy, a greater proportion of infarcts may be 'arrested' in the course of development before the development of Q waves and fall into the category of 'T wave infarcts'. T wave infarcts are in general smaller than those resulting in the development of Q waves.

Left bundle branch block may also obscure the changes of infarction because in this disorder, the septum is depolarized from right to left; this produces an initial R wave in left ventricular leads, preventing the appearance of a Q wave. The diagnosis can sometimes be made from ST and T wave changes.

Distribution of ECG changes in infarction
The leads in which the infarct patterns are seen depend upon its location:

- Anteroseptal infarction produces changes in one or more of the leads V1 to V4 (Fig. 7.11).
- Anterolateral infarction produces changes from V4 to V6, and lead I and aVL.
- Anterior infarction is indicated by more widespread changes including most of the leads from V1 to V6, as well as lead I and aVL.
- Inferior (or diaphragmatic) infarction is registered by changes in leads II, III and aVF (Fig. 7.12).
- Strictly posterior myocardial infarction does not produce Q waves in the standard 12 leads. However, the loss of electrical activity from the posterior part of the left ventricle, leads to a tall R in V1, because the forces depolarizing the right ventricle are unopposed (Fig. 7.13).
- Right ventricular infarction (which is almost always associated with inferior infarction) produces transient ST elevation in V4R.
- Further leads may be required for infarcts in unusual sites, V7 and V8 being helpful in lateral infarcts, and leads in the second or third intercostal spaces for high anterior and lateral infarcts.

Raised enzyme measurements
Certain enzymes, present in high concentration in cardiac tissue, are released by necrosis of the myocardium. Their activity in the serum, therefore, rises and falls after myocardial infarction. The amount of enzyme released roughly parallels the severity of myocardial damage. The time-course of the release of the cardiac enzymes is summarized in Figure 7.14. Enzymes include:

- *Troponin T and troponin I.* These are very sensitive tests which detect small amounts of myocardial necrosis. They can be used for the confirmation of myocardial infarction in patients with ST segment elevation myocardial infarction but are more commonly used in the diagnosis of non-ST segment elevation myocardial infarction where the enzyme assays

(A)

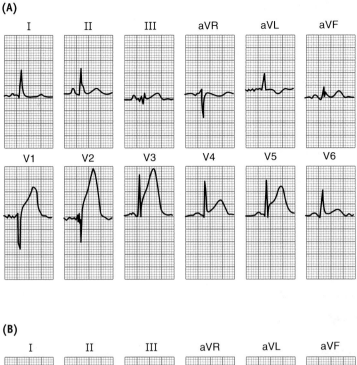

(B)

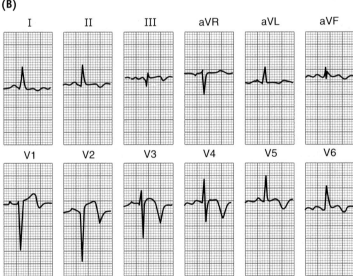

Fig. 7.11 Anteroseptal myocardial infarction. (A) 12-lead ECG recorded within one hour of onset of symptoms. Hyperacute changes are evident with marked ST elevation across the anterior chest lead. Tall peaked T waves are present in lead V2 and V3. (B) 12 h later the acute ST changes have largely resolved, and have been succeeded by T wave inversion. A deep Q wave is present in lead V2.

described below (CK and CK-MB) are often negative but the highly sensitive troponin assays are usually positive.

- *Creatine kinase (CK).* Creatine kinase, which occurs in heart, skeletal muscle and brain, rises within 6 h of the onset of infarction, reaching a peak in 18–24 h. It may become normal after 72 h. Apart from myocardial

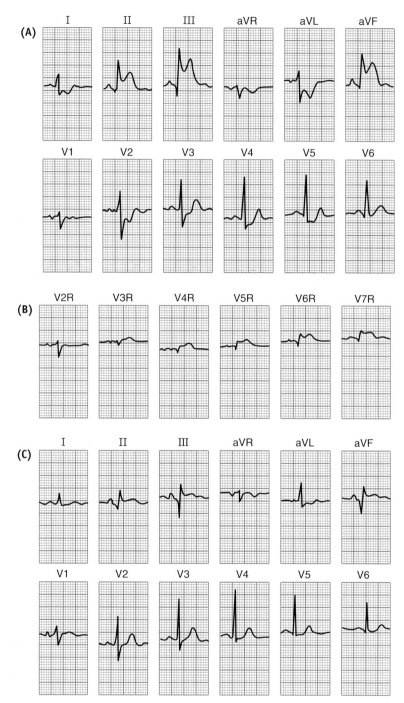

Fig. 7.12 Inferior myocardial infarction. (A) Conventional 12-lead ECG recorded 1 h after the onset of symptoms showing ST elevation in leads II, III and aVF. There is reciprocal ST depression across the anterior chest leads, extending into leads I and aVL. (B) Right-sided chest leads recorded simultaneously. ST-elevation is apparent in leads V3R to V7R, indicating right ventricular infarction. (C) Conventional 12-lead ECG recorded 12 h later. The acute ST segment changes have largely resolved. There are now deep Q waves in leads II, III and aVF.

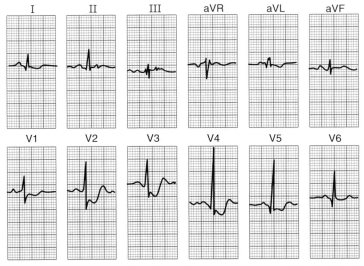

Fig. 7.13 Posterior myocardial infarction. Tall R waves are present in leads V1 and V2 accompanied by deep ST depression. These are reciprocal changes arising from a posterior infarction.

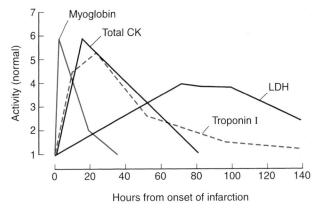

Fig. 7.14 Changes in serum enzyme activity following myocardial infarction are shown, demonstrating the differing rate of rise, peak level and direction of election for a number of enzyme reactors. (Adapted, with permission from Antman, E.M. [1994] General hospital management. In: Julian, D.L. and Brunwald, E. (eds) *Management of Acute Myocardial Infarction*, p. 63. London: W.B. Saunders.)

infarction, abnormally high levels occur in muscle diseases, in cerebrovascular damage, after muscular exercise and with intramuscular injections.

* *The MB isoenzyme of CK* is virtually specific for cardiac muscle and is now widely used in the diagnosis of myocardial infarction. The assay is of particular value in patients who have sustained skeletal muscle damage as an additional or alternative cause of a rise in CK concentration, for example patients who have received a d.c. shock, intramuscular injections or external cardiac massage.
* *Serum glutamic-oxalo-acetic transaminase (SGOT)* (also called aspartate transaminase) is found particularly in the heart, skeletal muscle, brain, liver

and kidney. After infarction, the SGOT level rises in about 12 h and reaches its peak in 24–36 h, returning to normal from the third to the fifth day.

- *Serum lactate dehydrogenase (LDH)* is found in the heart, but also in red cells. It rises relatively late after infarction, reaches its peak 24–48 h afterwards, and may remain abnormal for 1–3 weeks. Unfortunately, even slight haemolysis raises its level. Isoenzymes are more specific.

Differential diagnosis of acute ST segment elevation myocardial infarction

In most cases, the diagnosis is suspected from the character, location and duration of the chest pain. The persistence of the pain beyond 15 min, its lack of relationship to exercise and the failure of glyceryl trinitrate to relieve it usually serve to differentiate it from angina pectoris. The development of abnormal physical signs and, more particularly, the appearance of arrhythmias, shock and failure also suggest that infarction has occurred. Fever, leucocytosis and raised ESR indicate necrosis rather than ischaemia. The definitive diagnosis depends upon the recognition of the ECG changes, supported by abnormal serum enzyme levels. Infarction is virtually certain if Q waves appear during the course of the illness, or if sequential ST and T wave changes are accompanied by transient but significant elevations of serum enzyme levels. Difficulties in diagnosis arise when the ECG or enzyme level changes are equivocal, or if serial ECG records or enzyme estimations are not made at appropriate times.

The differentiation of myocardial infarction from massive pulmonary embolism may be difficult, but the chest pain of myocardial infarction is usually more severe and the breathlessness less marked. In pulmonary embolism, the ECG may be normal, or there may be characteristic abnormalities and although there may be changes in LDH and SGOT, the more specific enzymes (CK, CK-MB and troponin) are usually not raised while the D-dimer level is raised. In cases of doubt, spiral CT scanning or radioisotope scanning of the chest are helpful. Pulmonary infarction can be recognized by the location and pleural character of the pain and the radiographic appearances.

Acute pericarditis may produce symptoms and signs similar to those of an acute myocardial infarction. In many cases, the pericarditis is preceded by an upper respiratory infection and cough. The chest pain is more aching or stabbing in character, and is made worse by deep inspiration, movement or lying flat. Pyrexia often precedes the pain, whereas the temperature rise of myocardial infarction usually takes at least 12 h to develop. Although pericarditis may produce ST elevation and T wave inversion, the ST elevation is concave upwards and is widespread rather than focal. Abnormal Q waves do not occur and enzyme changes occur only if there is accompanying myocarditis.

Dissecting aneurysm can cause severe central chest pain similar to that of acute myocardial infarction. The pain usually has a tearing quality, and tends to move into the upper dorsal spinal region and into the abdomen. The ECG does not show the changes of myocardial infarction, except when the dissection involves the origin of a coronary artery. In cases of doubt, some form of imaging (trans-oesophageal echocardiography, CT scanning or magnetic resonance imaging) of the thoracic aorta should be arranged urgently.

Treatment of acute infarction

- Immediate treatment
- Aspirin
- Reperfusion therapy
  - thrombolysis
  - angioplasty (PCI)
- Beta-blockers
- Anticoagulants
- Other drugs.

Immediate treatment

The management of the early phase of myocardial infarction is critical; resuscitation from cardiac arrest is most often required at this time and interventions to limit infarct size should be administered as soon as possible. It is, therefore, of great importance that resuscitation and other relevant facilities should be available outside hospital. Depending upon local circumstances, these can be provided by suitably trained and equipped doctors or by paramedical personnel.

Usually, the most urgent measure is the relief of pain. When this is severe, opiates such as intravenous morphine sulphate (10 mg) or diamorphine (5 mg) are required and may have to be repeated. Unfortunately, these drugs may produce bradycardia, hypotension and respiratory depression, and it is advisable to combine them with atropine (0.6 mg) if there is bradycardia. Nausea and vomiting may occur and may require the administration of an intravenous antiemetic such as cyclizine (50 mg).

It is usual to admit all patients with suspected acute myocardial infarction to hospital, usually to a coronary care unit (CCU). The purpose of this is to ensure that emergency treatment (defibrillation, resuscitation, temporary pacing, etc.) is available, if required, during the first few unpredictable hours. The patient must be confined to bed immediately, but the degree of restriction depends upon the severity of the infarction. If this has been mild and there is no evidence of cardiogenic shock or cardiac failure, patients should be allowed to feed themselves, use a commode, and gently exercise their legs from the outset. Within 1–2 days it may be possible for them to sit out of bed. Mobilization thereafter is rapid and the majority of patients should be ready for discharge within 5–7 days. In patients with extensive infarcts or experiencing complications due to heart failure or arrhythmias, mobilization and discharge are necessarily slower.

One of the greatest dangers after a myocardial infarction is the development of unwarranted anxiety. This can be prevented by encouragement and explanation from the onset; the patient must understand that there is a good chance of recovery and return to near normal activity. At every stage an optimistic attitude should prevail, and it should be apparent that the physician expects the patient to recover.

Aspirin

Aspirin reduces the mortality rate of acute myocardial infarction by approximately 20%. Its benefits are additive to those of thrombolytic therapy (see below). A 300 mg tablet of soluble aspirin should be given as early as possible in acute infarction, which may mean before admission or in the emergency receiving room, rather than delaying treatment until the patient has arrived on the coronary care unit.

All patients in whom myocardial infarction is a possibility should be considered for aspirin therapy. Unlike thrombolytic therapy, distinguishing cases of myocardial infarction from those with unstable angina is not crucial, as aspirin therapy is appropriate for both. Moreover, contraindications to aspirin are encountered less often than contraindications to thrombolytic agents. In general, a history of peptic ulceration in the past should not be regarded as a contraindication to aspirin. Cases in which a contraindication to aspirin should be regarded as sufficiently strong to forego a 20% mortality rate reduction in acute infarction are rare.

Reperfusion therapy

Once the patient with acute myocardial infarction has been resuscitated, their pain and anxiety relieved by appropriate analgesia and aspirin administered, the next step is to try to restore patency of the occluded coronary artery. The earlier this can be achieved, the better. If the vessel is successfully reopened within 1 h, mortality is reduced by 50% and the amount of myocardium lost may be very small. Reperfusion can be achieved by pharmacological means (thrombolysis) or by physical means (coronary angioplasty).

Pharmacological reperfusion – thrombolysis

Thrombolysis, the use of drugs to break down the thrombus in the artery, has been shown to reduce mortality by around 20%. Streptokinase was the first agent to be widely used. It is given in a dose of 1.5 million units intravenously over 1 h. Streptokinase is a protein and can stimulate antibody production. The presence of preformed antibody can occasionally lead to allergic reactions and may block the effects of a second dose of streptokinase. For this reason, repeated administration of streptokinase is best avoided.

The next agent to pass into widespread use was tissue plasminogen activator (t-PA). This acts by promoting the conversion of plasminogen to plasmin which then breaks down preformed thrombus. It is usually given as a 15 mg intravenous bolus followed by a 30 min infusion of 0.75 mg/kg and then a 60 min infusion of 0.5 mg/kg. This is the so-called 'accelerated' or 'front-loaded' t-PA regimen. Heparin is given for 24 h with t-PA but is not required with streptokinase. More recently, a number of newer plasminogen activators have been developed; these include reteplase (r-PA), tenecteplase (TNK) and lanectaplase (n-PA). All three have longer half-lives than t-PA and are administered as a single or double bolus.

Indications for thrombolysis. Patients with suspected myocardial infarction who have ST segment elevation on the resting ECG should be considered for thrombolytic therapy. As in the case of aspirin, the reduction in mortality rate achieved with thrombolytic therapy has been of the order of 20%.

However, unlike aspirin, the treatment carries significant risks, and careful consideration needs to be given to the risks and benefits in each individual patient. This will involve consideration of the extent and site of infarction, the time delay from the onset of symptoms and any possible contraindications to thrombolysis.

In general, the larger the infarct the greater is the potential benefit of thrombolytic therapy. Anterior infarcts are generally bigger than inferior ones and are associated with a higher mortality rate. Patients with anterior infarction, therefore, gain more in absolute terms from thrombolysis than those with inferior infarction.

Patients with new-onset left bundle branch block on the ECG (LBBB) should also be given thrombolytic therapy. The association of benefits of thrombolysis with LBBB may at first seem surprising. However, in patients presenting with a history consistent with infarction, the presence of LBBB suggests extensive infarction and defines a group who stand to gain substantially from thrombolysis.

By contrast, patients with ST depression or T wave inversion do not benefit from thrombolytic therapy. These patients represent a heterogeneous group, some with unstable angina and others with smaller infarctions, in whom the risks of thrombolytic therapy outweigh the benefits.

Timing of thrombolytic therapy. The benefits of thrombolysis diminish rapidly with time and the goal should be to administer therapy as early as possible. Candidates for thrombolysis should either be 'fast-tracked' from the receiving room to the CCU or should have thrombolytic therapy commenced in the receiving room. In rural communities with a substantial delay to hospital admission, out-of-hospital thrombolysis should be considered as an alternative.

The time window during which the benefits of thrombolysis exceed the risks is defined imprecisely. For the majority of infarcts, thrombolysis should be considered in patients presenting within 6 h of the onset of symptoms. Treatment between 6 and 12 h is still likely to benefit high-risk groups, such as patients with large anterior infarcts. Treatment beyond 12 h is unlikely to be beneficial.

Complications of thrombolytic therapy. Not surprisingly, bleeding is the major complication of thrombolytic therapy. Of potential bleeding sites, by far the most significant is intracerebral haemorrhage. This occurs with a frequency of approximately 1 in every 200 patients receiving thrombolytic therapy and is very frequently fatal. Consequently, a history of previous intracerebral or subarachnoid haemorrhage should be regarded as an absolute contraindication to thrombolytic therapy. A history of recent head injury or cerebrovascular accident (whether embolic or haemorrhagic) should similarly be regarded as a major contraindication. Recent severe gastrointestinal bleeding must also be regarded as a major contraindication. Other contraindications are relative. The significance of these relative contraindications must be considered in relation to the potential benefit of treatment.

The hazards of thrombolytic therapy tend to be greater in the elderly. However, the elderly are also at increased risk of dying as a result of infarction and, in general, the benefits of thrombolytic treatment out-weigh the risks.

Physical reperfusion (Coronary angioplasty and stenting)

Several studies have demonstrated that urgent coronary angioplasty (PCI) reduces mortality from acute myocardial infarction. Furthermore, very few patients have contraindications to coronary angioplasty. Patients with a history of recent stroke, recent gastrointestinal bleeding and recent surgery can usually all undergo angioplasty if necessary. Like thrombolysis, the benefits are greatest if the procedure is carried out early, preferably within 3–4 h of the onset of symptoms.

Thrombolysis or PCI?

Who should receive thrombolysis and who should undergo PCI? This is a contentious issue. One of the difficult issues is the interpretation of clinical trial results. Many recent clinical trials of acute myocardial infarction have shown mortality rates of around 5–6%. Registry data, however, suggest a 'real-life' mortality of around 20%. The reason for this is that younger and fitter patients tend to be included in clinical trials. It is difficult, therefore, to apply the results of these trials to the older, sicker patients with extensive comorbidity who are seen in everyday practice. In the UK, most patients presenting with acute myocardial infarction are admitted to district hospitals without facilities for urgent PCI. Even when patients are admitted to centres with interventional facilities, primary PCI (i.e. angioplasty as the first choice treatment of acute myocardial infarction patients) is reserved for those patients with a contraindication to thrombolysis (recent stroke, recent surgery, active bleeding, etc.). The vast majority of acute myocardial infarction patients in the UK, therefore, are treated with thrombolysis. In the USA, and in many Western European countries, the proportion treated by primary PCI is much higher.

When a patient is given a thrombolytic agent but then shows little resolution of the ST segment elevation, it is said that they have 'failed to reperfuse'; the treatment options at this stage include conservative management, repeat thrombolysis (with the same or a different agent), and referral for urgent angioplasty (so-called 'salvage' or 'rescue' angioplasty). Clinical trials are ongoing to tell us which of these strategies is the most effective. A special case should be made for those patients with cardiogenic shock; these patients have a mortality risk of more than 50% and should all be considered for emergency PCI.

Beta-blockade

Long-term beta-blockade has been shown to reduce mortality by 25% following myocardial infarction. Provided there are no contraindications (acute left ventricular failure, asthma, complete heart block, etc.), oral beta-blockers should be given to all patients with acute myocardial infarction. Suitable dose regimens would include atenolol 25–50 mg twice daily, bisoprolol 5 mg once daily or metoprolol 25–50 mg two to three times daily. Early intravenous beta-blockade confers some marginal advantages in acute infarction. There is a small reduction in mortality, which reflects a decreased incidence of death due to left ventricular rupture. However, early intravenous beta-blockade has not gained wide acceptance in UK coronary care units. The reasons for this are unclear but may reflect a cautious approach based on the experience that treatment may exacerbate heart failure and bradycardia in some patients.

Anticoagulant therapy

The routine use of anticoagulant therapy with subcutaneous heparin has not been found to confer any advantage when applied globally to all patients with myocardial infarction. There remain, however, a number of situations where heparin is given:

- to prevent reocclusion following t-PA, intravenous heparin is given for 24 h
- to prevent deep venous thrombosis in patients with complicated infarction or other reasons for immobility
- to prevent thromboembolism in patients with atrial fibrillation or extensive infarction with early aneurysm formation.

Other drugs

Most patients with acute myocardardial infarction are treated with an ACE inhibitor but these drugs are generally started 1 or 2 days after admission. The same is true of the statin drugs for lowering cholesterol. The value of various other drugs, which include lidocaine (lignocaine), nitrates and magnesium, in acute infarction has been addressed in other large studies. It has been concluded that a global approach to the administration of these drugs confers no overall benefit. This is not to deny a continuing value of these therapies in specific situations, such as the use of lidocaine (lignocaine) to treat arrhythmias or the use of nitrates to treat continuing angina.

Prognosis

In about one-quarter of all episodes of acute myocardial infarction, death occurs suddenly within minutes of the onset. Such cases are seldom seen by a physician. The remainder of this discussion is concerned with the prognosis of those who survive this immediate period.

The overall natural mortality rate, excluding the very early deaths, is approximately 15–30%. The risk of death depends upon many factors, including the age of the patient, previous myocardial infarction and the presence of other diseases, as well as the extent of the infarction.

The mortality rate of the acute attack rises sharply with age. Today the death rate is probably less than 5% in those under 50 years of age, but may rise to 20–30% in the elderly. Mortality is higher in women than in men, but this is largely accounted for by the fact that infarction occurs relatively uncommonly in the younger female. The mortality rate is greater in recurrent compared with first infarction, particularly when there has been preceding cardiac failure.

The risk of dying is highest in the first few hours and decreases rapidly thereafter. Some 60% or more of all deaths within 4 weeks occur within the first 2 days. During this time, prognostication is difficult because dangerous arrhythmias may develop unpredictably. At the end of 48 h, the assessment of the prognosis for the rest of the 4-week period is reasonably accurate if the blood pressure, the signs of cardiac failure and the occurrence of serious arrhythmias are taken into account. Cardiogenic shock carries a mortality rate of 50–70%. Persistent tachycardia, continuing gallop rhythm and the development of right-sided heart failure are unfavourable features. Ventricular tachycardia, bundle branch block and atrial fibrillation are associated with a high mortality rate. Death may occur unexpectedly, late in the course of acute myocardial infarction, from further myocardial infarction, ventricular rupture or pulmonary embolism.

Complications of acute myocardial infarction and their management

Disturbances of rate, rhythm and conduction

These occur in 95% of patients with acute myocardial infarction. In about half of these, they are severe enough to be of clinical importance.

Ventricular arrhythmias

Ventricular ectopic beats are almost invariable in the early phase of infarction. They are generally of no consequence, but those of the R-on-T variety (Fig. 7.15) are of significance as they may be a prelude to ventricular fibrillation.

Ventricular tachycardia is more sinister both because of the haemodynamic compromise it may cause in its own right and because of the possible progression to ventricular fibrillation. Ventricular tachycardia complicating acute infarction is generally polymorphic and nonsustained, in contrast to ventricular tachycardias arising late after infarction, which are frequently sustained and monomorphic.

The general rule for the treatment of both ventricular ectopics and non-sustained ventricular tachycardia is to avoid treatment unless the arrhythmia is causing haemodynamic compromise. A slow ventricular rhythm (often around 60–120 bpm) is common after thrombolysis and is often a sign of successful thrombolysis ('reperfusion arrhythmia'). Treatment is generally not required. Hypokalaemia and hypomagnesaemia should be corrected. If treatment is necessary, then intravenous lidocaine (lignocaine) is the treatment of choice.

Ventricular fibrillation is the most important single cause of death in acute myocardial infarction and occurs in 8–10% of hospitalized patients. In about half of these cases, there has been no preceding shock or cardiac failure and the ventricular fibrillation is 'primary'. In the remainder, it can be regarded as being secondary to these complications.

Ventricular fibrillation is best treated by immediate DC shock of 200 J (see Ch. 9). If a defibrillator is not immediately available, external

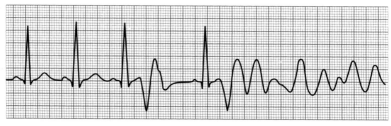

Fig. 7.15 Ventricular ectopic beats interrupting the T wave of preceding beats (R-on-T phenomenon). The second such beat initiates ventricular fibrillation.

resuscitation must be initiated and continued until the apparatus arrives. The prognosis of patients with ventricular fibrillation depends on their condition before the onset of this arrhythmia. If free of shock or cardiac failure, and if d.c. shock is immediately available, 90% have a chance of being alive 1 month later. If either of these complications has been present, survival falls to around 25%.

Atrial arrhythmias

Atrial fibrillation and atrial flutter are relatively common following myocardial infarction. They generally indicate a substantial infarction causing significant ventricular dysfunction and as such are an adverse prognostic indicator.

Any underlying failure should be treated. Episodes of atrial fibrillation can be treated with either digoxin or amiodarone. Digoxin is a more conventional treatment, but its benefits are confined to limiting AV node conduction and hence ventricular response rate with no direct antifibrillatory action. Amiodarone offers the advantage of a class III antiarrhythmic action (see Ch. 9), with a direct antifibrillatory effect and so offers the haemodynamic advantage of restoration of sinus rhythm. On rare occasions it may be necessary to restore sinus rhythm quickly with a synchronized d.c. shock.

Bradyarrhythmias

Sinus bradycardia is common in the early phase of acute myocardial infarction, particularly in inferior and posterior infarcts. In some patients, the bradycardia may be due partly to a vagal response to severe pain. Adequate pain relief may help to relieve the bradycardia. When sinus bradycardia does not result in haemodynamic compromise, no specific treatment is necessary. In cases of hypotension, intravenous atropine should be administered.

Junctional bradycardia is a frequent accompaniment of reperfusion and indeed can be used as a marker of successful reperfusion. Specific treatment is seldom necessary.

Heart block is a relatively common complication of inferior myocardial infarction, reflecting the fact that the right coronary artery provides the arterial supply to the AV node. All degrees of block may occur from PR prolongation to complete heart block, and transition between the phases of block is generally gradual. Second-degree block is common and is generally of Wenckebach (Mobitz I) type (see Ch. 9), with a gradually prolonged PR interval before the non-conducted P wave.

Pacing is rarely required in inferior infarction. Even if complete heart block ensues, there is generally a satisfactory escape focus ensuring the maintenance of an adequate heart rate. Pacing is indicated only in patients showing haemodynamic compromise. Complete heart block complicating inferior infarction generally resolves within a few days and permanent pacing is seldom necessary.

Complete heart block complicating anterior infarction is rare, but has a very different significance. It implies very extensive infarction, which of itself carries a poor prognosis. The site of block is more distal in the conduction system. As a consequence, block may occur suddenly or may be preceded by evidence of bundle branch block or Mobitz II second-degree block (see Ch. 9), but not by PR prolongation. As a further consequence the escape rhythm is unstable and has a wide QRS complex; temporary pacing is likely to be necessary. Permanent pacing may also be required, although whether this leads to any improvement in mortality in this very high risk group is unclear.

Bundle branch block

Block occuring lower in the conduction system will give the appearance of bundle branch block. This may involve any of the three subdivisions of the His–Purkinje system, the right bundle and either the anterior or the posterior division of the left bundle. If two fascicles are involved, this results in bifascicular block. All combinations are possible:

- Left anterior and posterior fascicles (causing complete left bundle branch block).
- Right bundle and left anterior fascicle (causing right bundle branch block and left axis deviation).
- Right bundle and left posterior fascicle (causing right bundle branch block and right axis deviation). This combination is rare.

When, in addition to the changes of bifascicular block, the PR interval is prolonged, this may indicate delay in conduction in the sole remaining fascicle. This is termed trifascicular block.

The development of changes of bundle branch block are indicative of a poor prognosis, which primarily reflects the extent of infarction rather than susceptibility to bradyarrhythmias. The role of pacing (temporary or permanent) is controversial.

Heart failure and cardiogenic shock
Left ventricular failure

This is seldom present at the onset, but develops within 48 h in perhaps one-third of patients with acute myocardial infarction. It can be suspected from tachycardia, a third heart sound, widespread pulmonary crepitations and pulmonary venous congestion or oedema on the chest radiograph. Catheterization, using a Swan–Ganz or similar catheter, will show a pulmonary wedge pressure in excess of 20 mmHg.

Cardiogenic shock

The patient at the onset of infarction is often pale, distressed and hypotensive. This situation, which is often transient, may be attributed to pain and should not be described as cardiogenic shock. This term should be restricted to those patients who have the clinical picture of hypotension, with cold cyanosed extremities, sweating and mental torpor, which lasts at least half an hour, or who deteriorate rapidly until the blood pressure can no longer be recorded. There is a low cardiac output and a peripheral resistance insufficient to compensate for this, together with oliguria, hypoxia and acidosis. Arrhythmias and cardiac failure are frequently associated and the mortality rate is more than 50% irrespective of treatment. Shock is largely the result of severe myocardial damage with more than 40% of the ventricular wall being infarcted.

The most important single factor is the extent of myocardial damage sustained in the current and previous myocardial infarctions. Others, which are more amenable to correction, are:

- arrhythmias and conduction disorders
- hypovolaemia, sometimes the consequence of previous treatment with diuretics or antihypertensive drugs
- right ventricular infarction, which may produce a clinical picture of high venous pressure, with low systemic arterial and pulmonary wedge pressures
- previous treatment with beta-adrenoceptor drugs
- lesions which are surgically correctable such as a ventricular septal defect or a papillary muscle rupture leading to severe mitral regurgitation.

The intra-aortic balloon pump can produce temporary clinical improvement, but this is not maintained unless some major factor can be corrected, e.g. the surgical closure of a ventricular septal defect or the early reopening of an occluded vessel at angioplasty. In general, most patients with cardiogenic shock following thrombolysis should be transferred to an interventional centre for attempted angioplasty because their prognosis with conservative treatment is so poor.

Right ventricular failure

It is important to distinguish right ventricular failure from other causes of heart failure following myocardial infarction as recognition can lead to appropriate corrective measures. Right ventricular infarction is usually seen as a complication of inferior and true posterior infarcts. The jugular venous pulse is characteristically raised, although the other classical features of right heart failure (ankle oedema and hepatomegaly) usually take several days to develop and are uncommon in the acute phase of infarction. The ECG can be used to provide confirmation of right ventricular infarction. To do this, the right chest leads should be recorded, transposing the normal left precordial leads to the right precordium. Most patients with right ventricular infarction have ST elevation in lead V4R (right precordial lead in V4 position).

Hypovolaemia and right ventricular dysfunction can be difficult to detect clinically and can appear like cardiogenic shock. Unlike cardiogenic shock, hypovolaemia and right ventricular dysfunction have a good prognosis provided they are recognized and treated appropriately. Treatment comprises plasma expansion by administration of intravenous fluids to increase right-sided filling pressures. If there is any doubt about whether a patient has true cardiogenic shock, defined as hypotension secondary to pump failure in the presence of an adequate filling pressure, or right heart failure, then the patient should be considered for Swan–Ganz catheterization. In this procedure, a balloon catheter is passed from a peripheral vein through the right atrium and right ventricle and into a pulmonary artery. When the balloon is inflated in the pulmonary artery, the pressure measured at the tip of the catheter, the 'pulmonary artery wedge pressure' is an indirect measurement of the left atrial filling pressure.

Using this technique, three major patient groups can be identified:

- Those with a high cardiac index (>2.2l/min/m^2) and a high pulmonary wedge pressure (>25 mmHg). These patients have pulmonary oedema but will usually respond to intravenous diuretics and oxygen.

- Those with a high cardiac index and a low pulmonary wedge pressure. This is typical of patients with hypovolaemia or right ventricular dysfunction. These patients will usually respond to volume replacement with intravenous fluids.
- Those with a low cardiac index and a high pulmonary artery wedge pressure. (cardiac output $<2.21/min/m^2$ and pulmonary artery wedge pressure >18 mmHg). These patients have cardiogenic shock. Clinically they have pulmonary oedema and systemic hypotension. The mortality rate in this group is very high. If there are no correctable factors (see above), an attempt should be made to improve left ventricular function by reducing afterload (with vasodilators) and increasing contractility with inotropic drugs such as intravenous dobutamine. Intra-aortic balloon pumping and salvage angioplasty (PCI) should also be considered.

It is important neither to overload the circulation nor to lower the filling pressure of the left ventricle excessively. One should aim to keep the pulmonary artery wedge pressure between 15 and 20 mmHg.

Mechanical complications of infarction

A number of mechanical complications may occur giving rise to heart failure or cardiogenic shock. Their recognition is important as the conditions are potentially treatable.

Ventricular septal defect

This occurs in approximately 1 in every 200 patients with acute infarction. It results in the development of severe heart failure, and frequently leads to cardiogenic shock. Characteristically, the patient suddenly deteriorates accompanied by the development of a pansystolic murmur, maximal at the left sternal edge. The differential diagnosis is papillary muscle rupture (see below). The two conditions can generally be distinguished by transthoracic echo. Alternatively, right heart catheterization can be undertaken to demonstrate a step-up in oxygen saturation at the right ventricular level. Untreated, the complication is almost invariably fatal. Urgent surgical repair is generally indicated, although surgical mortality is high.

Papillary muscle rupture

Papillary muscle rupture is another cause of acute haemodynamic deterioration after infarction, and is similarly accompanied by the development of a new pansystolic murmur. Echocardiography reveals the regurgitant jet across the mitral valve. Unlike ventricular septal defect, which generally complicates large infarcts, papillary muscle rupture may complicate relatively small infarcts. The treatment is surgical repair.

It is important to distinguish papillary muscle rupture from other causes of mitral regurgitation following myocardial infarction. Extensive left ventricular damage frequently results in functional mitral regurgitation. Treatment is the management of accompanying heart failure.

Cardiac rupture

Rupture through the wall of the left ventricle is responsible for about 10% of all deaths and particularly affects elderly and hypertensive patients. It is most likely to occur during the first few days and most commonly presents with the clinical features of cardiac arrest, but with continuing electrical activity in the electrocardiogram (electromechanical dissociation).

While rupture generally leads to immediate death, occasionally subacute rupture can occur, which may be amenable to surgical repair. Some cases of subacute rupture later give rise to the features of a pseudoaneurysm. In this condition organizing thrombus seals an area of left ventricular rupture, preventing the development of a haemopericardium. With time, the area of thrombus and the overlying pericardium may form a pseudoaneurysm, communicating with the left ventricular cavity.

Recurrent ischaemia and infarction
Following infarction, patients are vulnerable to recurrent ischaemia and extension of the original infarct. In addition, patients who have undergone successful reperfusion are vulnerable to reocclusion. In practice, it may be difficult to distinguish between infarct extension and reinfarction, and the two are best considered under the single term of recurrent infarction. Diagnosis is based on the development of additional ECG changes or a second peak in the level of cardiac enzymes.

Postinfarction angina is an indication for early coronary angiography with a view to coronary angioplasty or bypass surgery as appropriate. Patients developing further ST elevation should be considered for repeat thrombolysis or urgent angioplasty.

Miscellaneous complications of myocardial infarction
- Pulmonary embolism and infarction
- Systemic arterial embolism
- Cerebrovascular accident
- Pericarditis.

Pulmonary embolism and infarction
Twenty or more years ago, pulmonary embolism caused death in about 3% of all patients admitted to hospital with acute myocardial infarction. It has become relatively rare, presumably because patients are now mobilized much earlier than they were. It is usually preceded by deep vein thrombosis in the legs, but this may not be clinically evident. Pulmonary embolism should be suspected if hypotension or right heart failure develop some days after the onset of myocardial infarction, and also when there is a pleuritic type of chest pain with or without haemoptysis.

Systemic arterial embolism
Embolism may occur from mural thrombi situated in the left ventricle or left atrium. Hemiplegia is a common result, but there may be occlusion of any artery.

Cerebrovascular accidents
Cerebrovascular accidents may precede, accompany or follow acute myocardial infarction. As mentioned, cerebral embolism is one cause, but cerebral infarction may develop, as may cerebral haemorrhage, particularly when thrombolytic drugs are used.

Pericarditis

The main differential of recurrent chest pain in the first few days after infarction lies between recurrent ischaemia/infarction and pericarditis. The diagnosis is generally a clinical one, based on the nature of the patient's discomfort. Characteristically, pericarditic pain varies with inspiration and with body posture – worse on inspiration and alleviated by sitting up and leaning forward.

Treatment of pericarditic discomfort consists of aspirin. Non-steroidal antiinflammatory agents and steroids are best avoided because of the concern that they may contribute to adverse ventricular remodelling and infarct expansion (see below). Caution is also advisable in the use of anticoagulants at this time because of the risk of haemorrhagic pericarditis.

Late complications of infarction

There are two main late consequences of myocardial infarction: impaired pump function and arrhythmias.

Infarct expansion

Ventricular impairment following myocardial infarction is due only in part to the myocardial necrosis that occurs at the time of the infarct. In the ensuing weeks and months ventricular remodelling occurs, which may lead to further deterioration in ventricular function. This secondary deterioration in ventricular function arises from expansion and thinning of the infarct-zone (Fig. 7.16). This infarct expansion results in an increase in ventricular volume, which in turn causes an increase in wall tension. As a result, a vicious circle may be established resulting in progressive ventricular dilatation.

ACE inhibitors reduce infarct expansion and help to prevent adverse ventricular remodelling. As a consequence, ACE inhibitors now have a major role in the management of patients after infarction (see below). Patients at increased risk of adverse remodelling include those with large infarcts, anterior infarcts and infarcts that have failed to reperfuse. ACE inhibitors are particularly important in these patient groups.

Ventricular aneurysm formation

Ventricular aneurysm formation represents the most extreme form of infarct remodelling; the area of paradoxically moving non-contractile myocardium

Infarct expansion

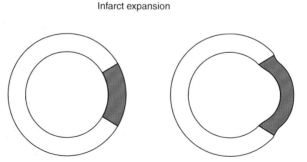

Fig. 7.16 Infarction thinning and elongation of the infarcted myocardium results in infarct expansion. This infarct expansion has an additional adverse effect on cardiac pump function.

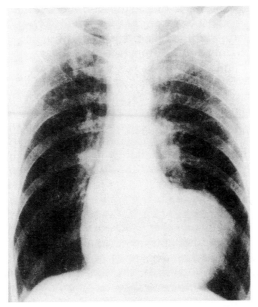

Fig. 7.17 Left ventricular aneurysm. An abnormal, rounded protrusion of the left heart border is apparent.

leads to extra work for the remaining heart muscle. In some cases this contributes to cardiac failure together with a risk of embolism from mural thrombi. There is also an increased risk of serious ventricular arrhythmias. The presence of an aneurysm is suggested by a systolic pulsation of the anterior chest wall lasting more than 3 weeks after the infarction. Other evidence includes persistent QS waves and ST elevation in the affected leads, an abnormal rounded protrusion from the left ventricular wall on the chest X-ray (Fig. 7.17). These features are often not present. The aneurysm may be demonstrated by echocardiography, radionuclide studies and left ventriculography. If it is causing heart failure or serious arrhythmias, surgical removal of the aneurysm may be necessary. Anticoagulants reduce the risk of thromboembolism.

Late arrhythmias
The electrical changes occurring as a consequence of infarction lead to electrical instability and, in a small proportion of patients, to a long-term susceptibility to serious ventricular arrhythmias. In the majority of cases these arise from areas of electrically viable myocardium, separated by areas of fibrosis, which result in delayed conduction and create the re-entry circuits that give rise to ventricular tachycardia and ventricular fibrillation. Whereas ventricular tachycardia and fibrillation occurring within the first 24–48 h of infarction are due to the electrical instability of acute infarction, and do not imply a long-term electrical instability, sustained ventricular arrhythmias occurring after this time are indicative of long-term electrical instability and a risk of sudden death. Such patients should be considered for electrophysiological investigations, antiarrhythmic drug therapy or an implantable defibrillator (see Ch. 9).

Risk stratification at hospital discharge

In patients who have survived acute myocardial infarction, the outlook is better than is often appreciated. The prognosis is best in those who are free of hypertension, angina and cardiac failure. Overall, between 80 and 90% of patients survive at least 1 year, approximately 75% survive 5 years, 50% 10 years and 25% 20 years. The risk of further infarction and sudden death persists but diminishes as time elapses.

Attempts should be made before discharge to identify patients at higher than average risk of recurrent infarction or death. Long-term prognosis is determined by three factors:

• left ventricular function
• the extent of residual coronary disease
• susceptibility to serious ventricular arrhythmias.

Some attempt, therefore, should be made to assess these potential problems in all patients who have sustained a myocardial infarction.

Assessment of ventricular function

Left ventricular function is the single strongest determinant of long-term outcome. This is most easily assessed by measuring left ventricular ejection fraction. This can be achieved by either echocardiography or radionuclide imaging. The relation between ejection fraction and prognosis is non-linear, mortality increasing markedly for values of ejection fraction below 30%.

Assessment of ischaemia

Estimating the risk of further infarction and appropriate intervention to reduce risk would be highly desirable objectives. There is, however, little clinical trial evidence defining an optimal approach to this problem, and clinical practice varies.

Coronary angiography offers the advantage of an accurate measure of the extent of residual coronary disease, but does not provide information on the functional severity of lesions. In many healthcare systems, offering coronary angiography to all patients recovering from infarction is not a feasible practical proposition.

Exercise testing is more generally applicable and enables a low-risk group not requiring further investigation to be identified. Exercise testing can be performed either before discharge using a relatively modest exercise protocol or after discharge using conventional submaximal testing. The former has the advantage of identifying high-risk individuals before discharge, while the latter offers the advantage of providing more complete diagnostic information. Once again, preference for pre- or post-discharge testing will depend on local circumstances. If a patient has a positive exercise ECG at a low workload, then they should be considered for coronary angiography. If the treadmill test shows a good effort capacity with no or minimal evidence of reversible ischaemia, then angiography may not be necessary.

Exercise testing following myocardial infarction fulfills a further most important objective: increasing patient confidence in their ability to resume a reasonably normal lifestyle and hence playing an important role in rehabilitation (see below).

Assessment of electrical instability

A number of non-invasive investigations have been shown to identify patients at risk of serious ventricular arrhythmias and sudden death following myocardial infarction. These include Holter monitoring, high-resolution electrocardiography, assessment of heart rate variability and measures of autonomic dysfunction. However, the tests have a relatively low positive predictive value. Moreover, at this time no simple drug treatment has been identified to improve prognosis. On this basis, screening methods for arrhythmia risk are still best considered a research tool rather than part of routine clinical practice. Patients with very poor left ventricular function, however, may be at such high risk of arrhythmic death to justify use of an implantable cardioverter defibrillator (Ch. 9).

Drug treatment at discharge

A number of drug therapies have been shown to improve long-term prognosis after infarction and every patient postinfarction should be considered for these therapies. The therapies concerned are:

- beta-blockers
- ACE inhibitors
- cholesterol-lowering agents ('statins')
- aspirin.

Beta-blockers

Long-term beta-blockade has been shown to reduce the mortality rate by about 25%. The benefit arises largely from a reduction in the number of patients dying suddenly. The potential benefits are greatest in those at greatest risk, particularly patients with more severely impaired ventricular function. Previously, beta-blockers were contraindicated in patients with heart failure; they are still not given to patients with acute heart failure, but have now been shown to improve prognosis in established heart failure and should be given to these patients. They are started at very low dosage and the dose is then slowly titrated upwards (see Ch. 8).

ACE inhibitors

ACE inhibitors have also been shown to reduce long-term mortality following myocardial infarction. A global approach of treating all patients, starting therapy in the acute phase of infarction on the day of admission, has been shown to provide a small but statistically significant overall mortality benefit. Thus most patients with established coronary artery disease are treated with an ACE inhibitor although the patients who stand to benefit most are the following groups:

- patients manifesting clinical or radiological evidence of heart failure
- patients with a moderate or large anterior infarct
- patients with significant left ventricular impairment as reflected by an ejection fraction of less than 40% or significant regional wall motion abnormalities on echocardiography.

Cholesterol-lowering agents ('statins')

Hypercholesterolaemia is a risk factor for further infarction, and lowering of cholesterol levels has been shown to reduce recurrent coronary events after infarction. Patients with infarction have already identified themselves as at risk from coronary disease and an aggressive approach to cholesterol lowering is therefore justified. The threshold cholesterol level for considering the addition of cholesterol-lowering drug therapy is uncertain. Benefits of statin therapy have been demonstrated in a population of post-infarct patients, irrespective of cholesterol levels at presentation, suggesting that whatever the initial cholesterol level, the patient will benefit from having it lowered further. In practice, therefore, most patients who have sustained a myocardial infarction will be treated with a statin, usually for life.

Checking cholesterol levels in patients after infarction is problematic. In the first 24 h after infarction, values are representative of the patient's normal cholesterol level. Following this, cholesterol levels fall for several weeks and may give a falsely low estimate in comparison with long-term values. Ideally, therefore, samples for cholesterol estimation should be drawn within the first 24 h of infarction or else delayed until subsequent outpatient follow-up.

Aspirin

Aspirin is of proven benefit in the acute and subacute phases after myocardial infarction. In common with other patients with established coronary disease, it is conventional to continue with long-term aspirin therapy unless the drug is contraindicated or the patient experiences significant side-effects relating to its use.

CARDIAC REHABILITATION

Patients who survive a myocardial infarction are often anxious about their future and have many questions. Cardiac rehabilitation programmes, involving appropriately trained nurses and physiotherapists, have a very important role to play in restoring the confidence and sense of well-being of the patient, and returning them to a normal and active life. The patient usually attends two or three out-patient sessions a week for a period of 3–6 months. A graduated exercise programme, tailored to the individual patient, is accompanied by counselling on lifestyle, and advice on preventive measures.

This is often the setting in which various lifestyle issues are discussed. These include the following:

Exercise

Even before attending rehabilitation classes, the patient should be encouraged to take short walks (15–30 min) each day and to gradually increase the length of the walk. Early angina occurring soon after discharge from hospital is unusual and merits urgent investigation. Regular exercise should be encouraged as part of lifestyle modification. Ideally, patients should exercise for at least 30 min two to three times per week. They should be encouraged to exercise to around 75% of their maximum heart rate (maximum = 220 minus the patient's age). If the patient is taking a beta-blocker, this will not be achievable and they should aim for a heart rate of around 100–110 beats per min.

Smoking

Patients must stop smoking completely. The patient must understand that continuing to smoke after a first myocardial infarction greatly increases the risk of further infarction, and of death.

Alcohol

Moderate alcohol consumption is allowable (up to around 28 units per week for men and 21 units for women). If weight loss is important, then alcohol, and especially beer drinking should be discouraged or restricted because of the high calorie content of alcoholic drinks.

Diet

Patients who are overweight should be encouraged to lose weight. Extreme diets (e.g. zero saturated fat diets) should not be encouraged; instead, patients should be advised to eat a balanced diet including reasonable quantities of cereals, vegetables and fruit. Most patients will be on treatment with an HMG CoA reductase inhibitor (statin) regardless of their initial cholesterol level.

Return to work

Most patients should aim to return to work 2 months after a myocardial infarction. If the job involves heavy manual labour, the patient should, if possible, seek a lighter job. For a small number of occupations (e.g. airline pilot), return to work may not be possible. For others (e.g. coach or lorry drivers), return to work is possible provided certain criteria are satisfied. For professional drivers, the British licensing authority requires that the driver is free from angina and able to complete three stages (9 min) of the standard Bruce treadmill test protocol without major evidence of reversible ischaemia.

Sex

Patients may be reluctant to discuss sexual problems. Sexual intercourse should probably be avoided for 1 month after a myocardial infarction. Thereafter, a gradual return to normal sexual relations should be encouraged. Impotence following myocardial infarction may be related to medication (especially beta-blockers) or to psychological factors. It is important that patients do not use sildenafil (Viagra) if they are using nitrate preparations for angina because of the known drug interaction.

Travel

Patients should be advised against travelling abroad for 2 months after a myocardial infarction. Thereafter, they can travel abroad on holiday but should be aware of the need for appropriate medical insurance cover and the need to 'declare' their medical history to the insurance company. They should also be aware that travel to areas with poorly developed cardiac services (e.g. central Africa) carries some risk.

FURTHER READING

Braunwald, E. (2001) *Heart Disease. A Textbook of Cardiovascular Medicine*, 6th edn. Philadelphia: W.B. Saunders.

CHAPTER 8

Heart failure

Failure in anything implies expectations unfulfilled, and one's definition of heart failure depends upon what one expects of the heart. No single definition suffices because the clinical and physiological criteria necessarily differ.

The clinician regards the patient as having heart failure when there are symptoms or physical signs attributable to inadequate cardiac performance. The physiologist regards the heart as failing when the contractility of the ventricles or the cardiac output falls outside the statistically defined normal range. There is no clear distinction between normality and abnormality; values in the 'abnormal' range may be found in normal hearts in the face of extreme demand, and 'normal' values may be encountered in diseased hearts when the demands are slight.

Cardiac failure, as it is understood in clinical practice, denotes the presence of one of the complexes of symptoms and signs associated with the 'congestion' of tissues and organs or attributable to the inadequate perfusion of tissues and organs:

- *Pulmonary venous congestion* results from disordered function of the left ventricle or left atrium.
- *Systemic venous congestion* is similarly due to disorders of the right ventricle and atrium, but is often the end-result of left-sided heart failure. The clinical features derive, in the main, from engorgement of the systemic veins and capillaries.
- The heart has also failed when it cannot maintain an adequate blood pressure in spite of a peripheral vascular resistance that is normal or high but, by convention, this type of cardiac failure is referred to as acute circulatory failure or *cardiogenic shock* rather than heart failure.

THE PATHOPHYSIOLOGY OF HEART FAILURE

The causes of heart failure

The heart fails either because it is subjected to an overwhelming load, or because the heart muscle is disordered:

- *A volume load* is imposed by disorders which demand that the ventricle expels more blood per minute than is normal. Examples include thyrotoxicosis and anaemia, in which the total cardiac output is increased; and mitral regurgitation and aortic regurgitation, in which the left ventricle has to expel not only the normal forward flow into the aorta but also the large volume of regurgitated blood as well.

- *A pressure load* is imposed by disorders which increase resistance to outflow from the ventricles (typified by systemic hypertension due to increased impedance of the peripheral arterioles, and by aortic stenosis in which there is narrowing of the outflow orifice of the left ventricle).

- *Disorders of myocardial function* result not only from diminished contractility but also from loss of contractile tissue, as occurs in myocardial infarction. This is the commonest cause of heart failure. An additional factor in this condition is a paradoxical movement of infarcted muscle which further increases the work of the remaining myocardium.

In many cases, a combination of mechanisms contribute to failure. For example in patients with rheumatic heart disease, myocardial damage, valve narrowing and regurgitation may all be contributory.

Cardiac and circulatory responses in heart failure

The heart at first responds to pressure and volume overloads in much the same way as it does to normal increases in demand, such as those imposed by exercise. As the disorder progresses, more cardiac and circulatory adjustments take place which, for a time, may maintain an adequate circulation but many of the so called 'compensatory' mechanisms are inappropriate. During evolution the circulatory system has had to evolve methods of combating blood loss and trauma rather than, for example, myocardial infarction, and the responses invoked are relevant to the former stresses rather than the latter. Indeed, the clinical manifestations of heart failure are largely the effects of 'compensatory' mechanisms which eventually embarrass the circulation.

Dilatation of the heart – increase in end-diastolic volume

In response to a volume load, the heart dilates, i.e. the ventricular volume is increased. Up to a point, dilatation is a normal and efficient response but it is abnormal when it cannot be wholly ascribed to the volume load. Pathological dilatation of this kind occurs when there is myocardial disease, when, because of decreased contractility, the ventricle must be stretched to a greater extent for a given stroke volume. Even in those cases in which dilatation may at first be regarded as a physiological response, it eventually becomes disadvantageous because, as the ventricle increases in size, greater tension is required in the myocardium to expel a given volume of blood. This is in accordance with the *Law of Laplace* which indicates that the tension in the myocardium (T) is proportional to the intraventricular pressure (P) multiplied by the radius (R) of the ventricular chamber ($T \propto PR$). The greater tension results in increased oxygen requirements.

This sequence is a major contributory factor in the deterioration in ventricular function following myocardial infarction. Following infarction, 'remodelling' of the ventricle occurs involving expansion and thinning of the infarct zone (p. 128). This *infarct expansion* causes an increase in the end-diastolic volume. In some patients this may help to compensate for the impaired contraction and to restore stroke volume to normal, but in others the resultant increase in wall tension causes progressive expansion, establishing a vicious circle of increasing wall tension and further expansion. In extreme cases this can lead to aneurysm formation.

Hypertrophy of the heart

When the ventricle has to face a chronic increase of pressure load, such as that imposed by arterial hypertension, aortic stenosis or pulmonary hypertension, the myocardium hypertrophies, i.e. it increases in weight as a result of an enlargement of individual muscle fibres. The process affects only those chambers upon which there are increased demands. The mechanism responsible for the development of cardiac hypertrophy is uncertain but it seems likely that it is a response to increased stretching or tension in muscle fibres which result from a raised diastolic volume or pressure. Hypertrophy may be regarded as a normal compensatory mechanism which permits the heart to cope with the increased demands, but becomes self-defeating when it is excessive. The thickening of the fibres increases the distance by which oxygen has to diffuse from the capillaries; eventually this leads to impaired oxygenation of the centre of the fibre. It is probable that this hypoxia is an important factor in the fibrosis which frequently develops in hypertrophied muscle.

Cellular changes in heart failure

Changes occurring within the myocyte in heart failure have been intensively studied. Changes include:

- *Abnormal calcium metabolism.* Heart failure results in changes in excitation contraction coupling. The ability of the sarcoplasmic reticulum to reaccumulate calcium is significantly reduced, together with the ability of the cell to eliminate calcium by the sodium–calcium exchange mechanism. As a consequence, contraction and relaxation may be prolonged.
- *Changes in myocardial gene expression.* Haemodynamic overload of the ventricles has effects on contractile protein gene expression which may result in additional adverse effects on cardiac function.
- In some types of heart failure, a process of *cell self-destruction* may be initiated, resulting in further loss of myocytes and progressive impairment of ventricular function. The process of 'programmed cell death' is termed *apoptosis.*

The cardiac output in heart failure

By definition, cardiac failure is present when the cardiac output is insufficient for the needs of the body, but some patients with an output in the normal range manifest the clinical features of cardiac failure, whereas other patients with low outputs are free of symptoms and signs. However, in cardiac failure, even if the cardiac output is normal at rest, it usually responds inadequately to exercise. In conditions such as beri-beri and thyro-toxicosis, in which the cardiac output is abnormally high, it is still insufficient for the exceptional metabolic demands.

Neuroendocrine response to heart failure

Cardiac failure activates several components of the neuroendocrine system, which play an important intermediary role in its clinical manifestations (Fig. 8.1):

- *Sympathetic nervous system.* Activation of the sympathetic nervous system results in an increase in myocardial contractility, heart rate, and vasoconstriction of arteries and veins. Although this may be beneficial in maintaining blood pressure, it is adverse in so far as it increases preload, afterload, and myocardial oxygen requirement. There is also an increased plasma noradrenaline (norepinephrine), but myocardial catecholamines are reduced.
- *Renin–angiotensin–aldosterone systems.* Both the fall in cardiac output itself and the increase in sympathetic tone reduce effective blood flow to the kidney and, consequently, increase renin secretion. Salt restriction and diuretic therapy also augment this. As a result, there is a rise in angiotensin II levels, which leads directly to vasoconstriction and indirectly, by stimulating aldosterone secretion, to sodium retention and the expansion of blood volume. This is advantageous in so far as increasing preload helps to maintain stroke volume by the Starling mechanism, but it does so at the expense of circulatory congestion.
- *Arginine vasopressin (antidiuretic hormone).* The reduced effective blood volume of heart failure stimulates the release of arginine vasopressin, leading to water retention. This is a feature of late, rather than early, cardiac failure.

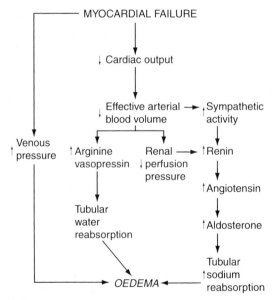

Fig. 8.1 Some of the neuroendocrine and renal responses to cardiac failure.

- *Atrial natriuretic peptide (ANP)*. Distension of the atria leads to the release of this peptide which has natriuretic and vasodilator properties. Levels of ANP are elevated in patients with heart failure and correlate with functional class. In addition, ANP has been suggested as a screening test to aid in the diagnosis of heart failure.
- Heart failure results in local vasoconstriction. This is partly a result of a reduced responsiveness to local vasodilators (*endothelial derived relaxing factor*) and to increased levels of the local vasoconstrictor, *endothelin*. A role for endothelin antagonists in the treatment of heart failure has been suggested.

Regional circulations in cardiac failure

There is a redistribution of blood flow to different organs and tissues in cardiac failure, as there is on exercise. This redistribution is mediated through vasoconstriction in certain areas, notably the renal arterioles. The renal blood flow falls disproportionately, and may be reduced to one-quarter of normal. There is little reduction in the coronary or cerebral blood flow, but there is vasoconstriction of the skin and splanchnic vessels.

Salt and water retention

An almost invariable feature of cardiac failure is the retention of sodium and water. This leads to a substantial increase in extracellular and plasma volume and plays a large part in the production of the clinical features of cardiac failure. Glomerular filtration is reduced in cardiac failure, although to a lesser extent than is renal blood flow. Diminished glomerular filtration may play some part in sodium retention, but it is probably not an important factor except when the failure is severe. There is also evidence that tubular reabsorption of sodium is increased in cardiac failure. There is no doubt that, in certain patients, there is increased aldosterone secretion, and that this hormone, by its action on the distal tubule, promotes the reabsorption of sodium whilst increasing the excretion of potassium and hydrogen. However, evidence of hyperaldosteronism is confined to advanced failure; aldosterone antagonists are relatively ineffective in the treatment of sodium retention in early failure.

As mentioned, water retention in heart failure is usually secondary to sodium retention. In some patients with advanced cardiac failure, however, there is a disproportionate retention of water. In these patients, the kidneys can no longer excrete solute-free water and the serum sodium concentration falls as a result of dilution ('dilutional hyponatraemia').

Raised venous pressure in cardiac failure

When the left ventricle fails the pulmonary venous pressure rises, and when the right ventricle fails the pressure rises in the systemic veins. This can be largely explained by the inability of the failing ventricle to discharge the blood presented to it effectively. The increased blood volume resulting from sodium and water retention contributes to the venous return and is thus a factor in producing the raised venous pressure, as is venoconstriction.

The effect of left ventricular failure on the lungs

As explained above, when the left ventricle fails, the diastolic pressure in the left ventricle rises and with it the left atrial pressure. Since the pulmonary veins and capillaries are in continuity with the left atrium, the pressures in these vessels rise concomitantly. In mild left ventricular failure, the pressures in the left atrium and pulmonary veins are within normal limits at rest but rise on exercise. As failure advances, the left atrial pressure progressively increases from its normal level of 5–10 mmHg to one of 25–30 mmHg. The hydrostatic pressure in the capillaries is then close to that needed to overcome the osmotic pressure exerted by the plasma proteins and may lead to an exudation of fluid from the capillaries into the alveolar walls and alveoli. If the pressure in the atrium rises rapidly, there may be a sudden exudation of fluid into the alveoli. If this process takes place slowly, exudation may proceed gradually with a slow build up of tissue tension occurring in the alveolar wall. This restricts further exudation of fluid and limits the risk to the alveoli. In response to this process, some fibrosis may take place in the alveolar wall. The pulmonary congestion caused by the high pulmonary venous pressure and by the changes in the alveolar walls makes the lung more rigid (less compliant). As a result of this, more work must be done by the respiratory muscles to move a given volume of air.

Arrhythmias in heart failure

Patients with heart failure have a high incidence of sudden death. The majority of deaths are thought to be due to ventricular tachycardia or ventricular fibrillation.

A number of factors contribute to the occurrence of ventricular tachyarrhythmias in patients with heart failure. These include:

- high circulating catecholamine levels
- electrolyte disturbance, particularly diuretic-induced hypokalaemia
- proarrhythmic effects of inotropic drugs
- stretch on the myocardium may result in arrhythmias through the process of 'contraction–excitation feedback'.

Arrhythmia prevention in patients with heart failure is a particular problem. The efficacy of antiarrhythmic drugs is reduced and there is, moreover, an increased incidence of proarrhythmic side-effects. In addition, most antiarrhythmic drugs have negative inotropic effects.

CLINICAL SYNDROMES OF HEART FAILURE

Left heart failure

Aetiology

The features of left heart failure develop when there is a major obstruction to outflow from the left atrium (e.g. mitral stenosis) or when the left ventricle can no longer cope with the demands upon it. The common causes of left ventricular failure are:

- myocardial infarction
- systemic hypertension
- valvular heart disease
- cardiomyopathy.

Clinical features

The *clinical features* of left-sided cardiac failure are largely the consequence of pulmonary congestion. The symptoms are:

- dyspnoea on exertion
- orthopnoea and paroxysmal nocturnal dyspnoea
- acute pulmonary oedema.

The *physical signs* of left ventricular failure may include:

- pulmonary crepitations
- third heart sound
- pleural effusion
- pulsus alternans – alternate large and low volume pulse – this is an indication of severe left ventricular failure.

Investigations

- The *chest radiograph* may show features of pulmonary venous congestion, particularly of the upper lobe, interstitial oedema and alveolar oedema.
- The *electrocardiogram (ECG)* may be of value although it does not provide direct evidence of left heart failure. For example, it is unusual for hypertension or aortic valve disease to lead to the symptoms of left heart failure without producing ECG evidence of left ventricular hypertrophy first. Again, it is unusual for coronary artery disease to lead to left heart failure if the ECG is normal. This is not, however, true of mitral regurgitation.
- *Echocardiography* plays a particularly important role in the investigation of patients with heart failure. Typically, left ventricular end-diastolic dimensions are increased and decreased systolic function is apparent. Echocardiography is also important in the exclusion of other potentially treatable causes of heart failure such as aortic stenosis or mitral regurgitation.
- *Atrial natriuretic peptide (ANP)* levels and the closely related *brain natriuretic peptide (BNP)* are elevated in patients with heart failure. Although these tests are not currently widely available, they have been suggested as a useful diagnostic marker for heart failure.

Differential diagnosis

The diagnosis of left heart failure is usually not difficult when there is progressive dyspnoea coupled with clinical evidence of advanced left-sided heart disease. However, this evidence may not always be unequivocal and there may be difficulty in distinguishing the symptoms of heart failure from those of pulmonary disease. The dyspnoea of left heart failure is more likely to be provoked by lying down flat. Patients with dyspnoea due to pulmonary disease usually have a history of asthmatic attacks or of chronic cough and sputum.

Paroxysmal nocturnal dyspnoea and acute pulmonary oedema may be difficult to differentiate from acute respiratory attacks. The latter are commonly associated with bronchospasm and purulent sputum. In contrast, the patient with acute pulmonary oedema is usually free of pulmonary infection, has fine crepitations rather than rhonchi and is liable to cough up pink frothy sputum. Furthermore, examination usually reveals the signs of left-sided heart disease. Correct diagnosis is of great importance because the therapy of the two conditions is different. For example, morphine may be lethal in respiratory failure, but invaluable in acute pulmonary oedema. Similarly, high concentrations of oxygen are useful in acute pulmonary oedema but may be dangerous in respiratory failure. The chest radiograph is also helpful in showing signs of oedema or infection. In cases of doubt, estimation of the arterial CO_2 tension is of value because this is usually low in acute pulmonary oedema and high in respiratory failure.

Right heart failure

Aetiology
Failure of the right side of the heart occurs when the right ventricle can no longer cope with the demands upon it, or when there is tricuspid stenosis. Common causes of right ventricular failure include:

- left ventricular failure with its consequent effects upon the pulmonary circulation
- right ventricular infarction (see p. 125)
- pulmonary disease, particularly chronic bronchitis and emphysema
- pulmonary hypertension (see p. 333)
- pulmonary valve disease
- tricuspid regurgitation.

Clinical features
The characteristic features of right heart failure are:

- *Elevated jugular venous pressure.* In the normal individual, the venous pressure in the internal jugular veins does not exceed 2 cm vertically above the sternal angle when the patient is reclining at 45°. In right heart failure this figure is exceeded. Even if normal at rest, it rises on exercise.
- *Hepatomegaly.* If chronic, this may result in cirrhosis.
- *Oedema.* This is of the dependent type and usually most evident in the pretibial and ankle regions.
- *Ascites.* This may occasionally occur in patients with severe right heart failure.
- *Tricuspid regurgitation.* This can occur in patients with severe or long-standing right heart failure, when right ventricular dilatation results in a functional incompetence of the tricuspid valve. A prominent V wave may be evident in the jugular venous pulse and a pulsatile liver edge may be palpable.

Differential diagnosis

In patients presenting with isolated signs of right heart failure, the possibility of pericardial constriction on tamponade should be considered as an alternative diagnosis.

Other clinical features of cardiac failure

There are a number of common but less specific features of cardiac failure:

- *Fatigue* is a frequent symptom which is difficult to evaluate.
- The nutrition of patients with cardiac failure is often good in the early stages, but *cachexia* sets in as disability increases.
- In the very advanced case, *cerebral symptoms* may develop with dulling of consciousness, confusion or changes in personality.
- Patients with cardiac failure are prone to develop *venous thrombosis and pulmonary emboli* are common.
- Mild jaundice, due to *hepatic congestion* or cirrhosis, is quite frequent in right-sided heart failure.
- *Proteinuria* due to renal congestion is often present.

GENERAL MANAGEMENT OF CARDIAC FAILURE

Ideally, the treatment of cardiac failure is the correction of the cause, but for a variety of reasons this may not be possible, at least initially. In some conditions, such as ischaemic heart disease and the cardiomyopathies, damage to the ventricular muscle may be irreversible and no currently available methods of treatment can correct the underlying muscle weakness. In other disorders, the radical treatment necessary for cure, such as major surgery, cannot be safely undertaken until cardiac failure has been corrected.

The principles of treating cardiac failure may be enumerated as follows:

- the correction or amelioration of the underlying disease
- the control of precipitating factors
- the reduction of demands on the heart by weight loss and the restriction of physical activity
- pharmacological therapy to modify the heart failure state and, particularly, to reverse the adverse consequences of neuroendocrine and renal responses to heart failure.

The objectives of therapy are twofold: to alleviate the symptoms caused by heart failure and to improve the prognosis.

The correction or amelioration of the underlying cause

When heart disease is due to such causes as thyrotoxicosis or hypertension, corrective treatment can be started immediately. In congenital and rheumatic heart disease, surgical management is usually required, but this may have to be deferred until the maximum benefit has been achieved from medical treatment.

In the case of ischaemic heart disease, the cause of heart failure is generally previous myocardial infarction rather than ongoing ischaemia. Coronary revascularization procedures cannot ameliorate the damage caused by previous infarction and for this reason play little part in the management of heart failure.

The control of complicating factors

Cardiac failure is often precipitated or exacerbated by factors superimposed on the underlying heart disease. Amongst these are:

- arrhythmias
- infections
- pulmonary embolism
- anaemia
- excessive sodium intake
- over-exertion.

The recognition of precipitating factors is of great importance in the management of heart failure, because the correction of these complicating conditions will often result in the abolition of symptoms.

Exercise

Rest reduces the demands on the heart and leads to a fall in venous pressure and a reduction in pulmonary congestion. It allows a relative increase in renal blood flow and often leads to a diuresis. However, bed rest also encourages the development of venous thrombosis and pulmonary embolism.

The degree of physical restriction necessary depends upon the severity of the cardiac failure. When there is severe pulmonary congestion or peripheral oedema, a period of complete rest may be required. At this time, the patient is usually most comfortable propped up by two or more pillows in bed or in an armchair. Complete bed rest is seldom necessary for more than a few days, after which a gradual increase in activity should be encouraged, depending upon the response.

In patients with lesser degrees of heart failure, regular exercise should be encouraged. This should not be exhaustive, but the patient should aim to undertake regular aerobic activities such as walking or swimming. Typical exercise would be to recommend 20 to 30 min walking three times per week. This helps to reverse the deconditioning of skeletal muscle, which contributes to the symptomatic limitation of patients with heart failure. Strenuous exercise and isometric exercises are best avoided.

Management of salt and water retention

Sodium and water retention are part of the neuroendocrine response to a fall in cardiac output in patients with heart failure (Fig. 8.1). Both may contribute to the patient's symptoms and hence both dietary sodium restriction and diuretics play an important role in the management of symptomatic heart failure.

Low salt diets effectively counteract cardiac failure. However, with the availability of potent diuretic drugs, no extreme limitation of sodium intake is usually necessary. Nevertheless, some restriction is desirable and inability to control cardiac failure is quite often due to the patient not reducing sodium intake sufficiently. All patients should be advised not to add salt at meals and to avoid obviously salty foods. Occasionally, a strict salt restriction must be applied. It is seldom necessary to practise water restriction, but in cases of dilutional hyponatraemia, a limitation of 1 litre per day may be helpful. These patients may be identified by a lack of response to conventional treatment for cardiac failure in association with a low serum sodium concentration.

PHARMACOLOGICAL THERAPY

The purposes of drug therapy in the management of heart failure are two-fold: the improvement of symptoms and improvement in prognosis. Some drugs act solely to improve symptoms whereas others improve both symptoms and prognosis (Table 8.1).

Diuretics

The loop diuretics: furosemide (frusemide), bumetanide
These drugs prevent reabsorption at multiple sites including the proximal and distal tubules and the ascending limb of the loop of Henle. They produce a profound diuresis with the excretion of large quantities of sodium and chloride. When given by mouth, action commences in about 1 h and is complete in 6–8 h. If given intravenously, the onset of action is almost immediate.

Thiazide diuretics
The many drugs in this group are essentially similar except in their potency and duration of action. Most of the thiazide diuretics act for 12–24 h whereas polythiazide and chlortalidone exert their effect for 48 h or more. They may have several sites of action, but the main mechanism is the inhibition of sodium reabsorption in the distal convoluted tubule.

These diuretics are less potent than the loop diuretics, but are rather more likely to produce hypokalaemia. If the serum potassium is low, supplements of slow release potassium chloride should be used.

Table 8.1 Pharmacological therapy for heart failure

Drug	Improvement in symptoms	Improvement in prognosis
Diuretics		
loop and thiazide	Yes	No
Spironolactone	Yes	Yes
Inhibition of the renin–angiotensin system		
ACE inhibitors	Yes	Yes
Angiotensin II blockers	Yes	Yes
Inotropes		
Digoxin	Yes	No
Beta-blockers	Yes	Yes

These drugs sometimes cause hyperglycaemia and hyperuricaemia, and may precipitate diabetes and clinical gout. Other occasional undesirable effects include agranulocytosis, thrombocytopenia, nausea, abdominal discomfort, impotence and skin rashes.

Thiazide and loop diuretic combinations

Combination of a thiazide and loop diuretic is of value in patients with refractory oedema. A particularly vigorous diuresis may ensue, and it is advisable to reduce the dose of both drugs to guard against intravascular volume depletion, severe hypokalaemia and deterioration in renal function. Close supervision of such combination therapy is essential.

Potassium-sparing diuretics

This group comprises two classes of agent:

- *Spironolactone.* This drug is an aldosterone antagonist, providing a weak diuresis with a potassium-sparing action.
- *Amiloride and triamterene.* These drugs inhibit sodium–potassium exchange in the distal tubule. They have a weak diuretic effect.

Potassium-sparing diuretics are relatively ineffective in the management of symptoms when used singly. Their chief symptomatic value in the treatment of heart failure is in combination with either a loop or a thiazide diuretic, to reduce the potassium losses associated with these agents.

Until recently, it had been assumed that spironolactone would be of little value in patients receiving angiotensin-converting enzyme (ACE) inhibitors, as ACE inhibition should theoretically suppress aldosterone levels. However, aldosterone levels remain high in heart failure despite ACE inhibitors, and spironolactone has been shown to confer an additional mortality benefit of approximately 30% in patients with severe heart failure.

Hyperkalaemia is a potential complication, particularly in patients with impaired renal function. Particular caution is necessary when adding potassium retaining diuretics to ACE inhibitor therapy. Spironolactone carries one very common and troublesome side-effect; it causes breast enlargement or pain in approximately 10% of men taking the drug.

Inhibitors of the renin–angiotensin system

Many of the neurohormonal changes which occur in heart failure are counterproductive and lead to worsening of the clinical syndrome of heart failure. The renin–angiotensin system is particularly important in this respect. Two types of pharmacological agent can be used to block the renin–angiotensin system:

- ACE inhibitors, which inhibit the conversion of angiotensin I to angiotensin II (Fig. 8.2).
- Angiotensin II receptor blocking agents provide an alternative approach to inhibition of the renin–angiotensin system. They block the vasoconstrictor and other actions of angiotensin II.

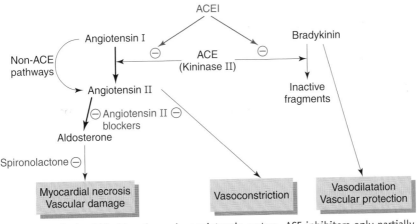

Fig. 8.2 Methods of blocking the renin–angiotensin system. ACE inhibitors only partially block conversion of angiotensin I to angiotensin II, because of the presence of ACE-independent pathways. ACE inhibitors have the additional effect of inhibiting the breakdown of bradykinin.

Although ACE inhibitors and angiotensin II blockers are clearly related in their mechanisms of action, they are not equivalent or interchangeable. ACE inhibitors do not fully prevent the formation of angiotensin II, because there are other pathways for its formation, which are ACE independent. For this reason, angiotensin II receptor blockers should theoretically provide a more complete inhibition of angiotensin II-mediated actions than ACE inhibitors. However, the effects of ACE inhibitors are not confined to inhibition of angiotensin II formation. ACE inhibitors also inhibit the breakdown of bradykinin. Bradykinin has a vasodilator action and may be responsible for some of the benefits observed with ACE inhibition. Angiotensin II receptor blocking agents do not share this effect of increasing bradykinin levels.

ACE inhibitors

ACE inhibitors are indicated both for the treatment of symptoms and to improve prognosis in patients with heart failure. There is a widespread consensus that ACE inhibitors are of value in improving symptoms of heart failure. In addition, a number of large well-controlled studies have shown that ACE inhibitors improve prognosis. In view of these benefits, ACE inhibitors should be prescribed, unless contraindicated, in patients with symptomatic heart failure and in all patients, irrespective of symptoms, with an ejection fraction of less than 40%.

Following myocardial infarction, ACE inhibitors are of particular value. They are indicated not only for the treatment of failure, but also for the prevention of adverse remodelling (see Ch. 7). A number of studies have shown that ACE inhibitors improve survival following infarction in a spectrum of patients, ranging from those who are asymptomatic but show significant ventricular dysfunction, to those who have clinical evidence of ventricular impairment.

ACE inhibitors are also of value in treating heart failure arising as a result of ventricular dilatation associated with either mitral or aortic regurgitation. The drugs are, however, contraindicated in patients with significant mitral or aortic stenosis.

ACE inhibitors are in general well tolerated. However, a number of problems may be encountered, including hypotension, renal impairment and cough:

- As many patients with congestive heart failure have low blood pressure, this restricts the use of these agents. The problem of *hypotension* is particularly marked after the first dose. First-dose hypotension can be minimized by reducing the dose of the ACE inhibitor on commencing therapy and omitting diuretics for 1–2 days beforehand.
- ACE inhibitors occasionally cause deterioration of *renal function*. They are contraindicated in patients with an initial creatinine level greater than 200 µmol/L. Renal function should be checked routinely 1–2 weeks after commencing therapy.
- *Cough* is a potentially troublesome side-effect, occurring in up to 10% of patients. The mechanism is unclear but may be due to inhibition of the metabolism of bradykinin in the lung. Switching to a different ACE inhibitor is rarely effective in alleviating the problem. Some patients will, however, respond to a reduction in dose.

Angiotensin II receptor blockers

Angiotensin receptor blockers represent another approach to inhibition of the renin-angiotensin system in patients with heart failure. The evidence for prognostic benefit is substantially greater for ACE inhibitors than angiotensin II antagonists and for this reason the two types of drug should not be regarded as interchangeable. In the management of heart failure, angiotensin II receptor blockers are generally regarded as second line drugs for those patients intolerant of ACE inhibitors, particularly those patients experiencing cough.

In patients intolerant of ACE inhibitors there is evidence that angiotensin receptor blocking drugs do improve prognosis. There may also be some benefit in adding an angiotensin receptor blocker to an ACE inhibitor, as the combination has been shown to have a symptomatic benefit, to reduce hospitalizations for heart failure, and to reduce cardiovascular mortality.

Other vasodilators

The widespread applicability and indications for ACE inhibitors have reduced the importance of other vasodilators in the management of heart failure.

Nitrate vasodilators remain of value in the management of acute left ventricular failure. Sublingual glyceryl trinitrate can be administered in the acute phase and can be followed by an intravenous infusion. Nitrates act predominantly as *venodilators*.

Hydralazine, by contrast, is predominantly an arterial dilator. The combination of hydralazine with a nitrate has been shown to improve both symptoms and prognosis in patients with heart failure. However, this use is largely historical and ACE inhibition has been shown to offer greater prognostic benefit. A nitrate–hydralazine combination may, however, still be of benefit in patients in whom ACE inhibitors are contraindicated.

Beta-blockers

It has been recognized for many years that the sympathetic system is activated in patients with heart failure. While sympathetic activation may initially be an adaptive response, it plays a mechanistic role in the progression of myocardial dysfunction. Excessive sympathetic stimulation may contribute to progression of heart failure in a number of ways, including additional energy requirements, ventricular hypertrophy and arrhythmias.

Superficially one might anticipate that beta-blockers would be contraindicated in heart failure. However, there is now very extensive clinical trial evidence proving their efficacy. Beta-blockers result in a reduction in mortality, of the order of 30%. The reduction in mortality relates substantially to a reduction in sudden deaths, but beta-blockers also benefit symptoms and have been shown to reduce hospitalizations for heart failure. Beta-blockers have been shown to benefit patients with class II and III heart failure and to benefit selected patients with class IV heart failure. In general, the more severe the degree of heart failure and the worse the prognosis of the patient, the greater the benefit to be gained from beta-blockade.

A number of features are important in the successful use of beta-blockers in heart failure:

- *Patient selection* is crucial. Beta-blockers should not be given in new onset or uncontrolled heart failure. Patients presenting with acute heart failure or with an exacerbation of chronic heart failure should be stabilized with diuretics and ACE inhibitors before initiating a beta-blocker. Bradycardia (heart rate < 60) and hypotension (systolic blood pressure < 100) are relative contraindications and require particularly careful monitoring on commencement of therapy.
- *Low dose initiation* of therapy is crucial. The usual starting doses, based on clinical trial experience, are given in Table 8.2.
- *Slow upward dose titration* with clinical monitoring. Titration should occur at intervals of not less than 2 weeks. Dizzyness, postural hypotension and worsening heart failure are all relatively common and may require dose reduction or cessation of beta-blocker therapy. Patients should be reviewed medically or by a nurse practitioner specializing in heart failure before upward dose titration. It is nonetheless important to try to achieve the target doses of beta-blockers used in the clinical trials of each agent (Table 8.2), if the substantial benefits seen in the trials are to be reproduced.

Great care is therefore necessary in determining which patients with heart failure should receive beta-blockers. Precise selection criteria are as yet unclear.

Inotropic agents

Digitalis glycosides
These were, for many years, regarded as standard therapy for cardiac failure. However, with the development of other effective treatments for heart failure, their role has become very substantially reduced.

Table 8.2 Beta-blocker dosage in heart failure

Agent	Initiating dose	Target dose
Bisoprolol	1.25 mg daily	10 mg daily
Metoprolol	12.5 mg daily	200 mg controlled release
Carvedilol	3.125 mg twice daily	25 mg twice daily

Mechanisms of action

The inotropic action of digitalis is mediated through the sodium/potassium-ATPase (sodium) pump, to which it binds. The inhibition of this pump leads to an accumulation of intra-cellular sodium; because of the sodium–calcium exchange system, this results in an increase in the amount of calcium available to activate contraction. Digitalis also has sympathomimetic and parasympathetic (vagal) effects. The latter is clinically important, in that it causes slowing of the sinus rate and delays.

Clinical trial evidence

The value of digoxin in the management of heart failure has long been controversial. Recent clinical trials have helped to clarify its role. Digoxin is of value in treating the symptoms of heart failure, but is neutral with respect to survival. This is in contrast to ACE inhibitors and beta-blockers, both of which improve survival.

For this reason, digoxin therapy should be regarded as second line, following the initiation of diuretics, ACE inhibitors and beta-blockers. The role of digoxin in patients already taking beta-blockers is particularly uncertain.

Indications

Digoxin is particularly indicated in patients with heart failure and atrial fibrillation, for its beneficial effects to reduce ventricular response rate (see p. 171). In this setting it is an appropriate first line agent.

Other inotropic agents

The long-term use of oral inotropic agents in the management of patients with heart failure has been largely discredited. The use of phosphodiesterase inhibitors, for example, is associated with an increased incidence of arrhythmias and increased mortality. Intravenous inotropic agents, however, still play an important role in the management of acute circulatory failure due to cardiogenic shock (see below).

VENTRICULAR RESYNCHRONIZATION THERAPY

There is growing evidence that some individuals with severe heart failure may be improved by biventricular pacing to provide ventricular resynchronization.

In many patients with severe heart failure, left ventricular contraction becomes incoordinate. Delay in the spread of the electrical impulse to different regions of the ventricle results in a dispersion of the onset of contraction. As a consequence, the regions of the ventricle activated earliest may be

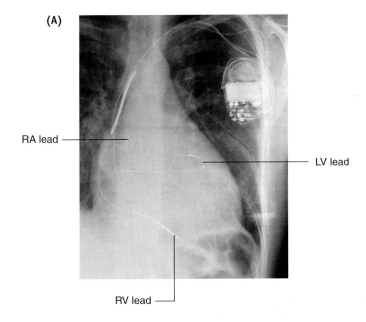

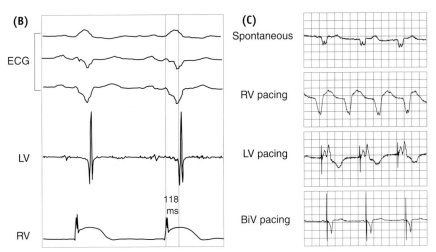

Fig. 8.3 Cardiac resynchronization therapy.

Resynchronisation pacing

A. Chest radiograph of a resynchronising pacemaker/implantable defibrillator. Three leads are placed in the heart – a right ventricular (RV) lead (with proximal and distal coils for shock delivery), a right atrial (RA) lead and a left ventricular (LV) lead positioned in a left ventricular branch vein of the coronary sinus.

B. Intracardiac electrograms recorded during *sinus* rhythm from the left ventricle and right ventricle. Recordings are at 50 mm/s. Three leads of the surface ECG are also shown. The RV electrogram lies early in the QRS and the LV electrogram late in the QRS. This corresponds to a delay of 118 ms between the two electrograms, showing that the left ventricle underlying the LV lead is activated late in *sinus* rhythm.

C. Surface ECG recorded during spontaneous rhythm, right ventricular pacing, left ventricular pacing and bi-ventricular pacing. Recordings are at 25 mm/s. Bi-ventricular pacing substantially reduces QRS width in comparison with either spontaneous rhythm or pacing either ventricle alone. The narrowing of the QRS results in a more synchronous ventricular activation.

relaxing by the time later regions have started to contract. This results in an additional inefficiency of pump function, responsible for an additional deterioration in ejection fraction and cardiac output.

Ventricular resynchronization pacing seeks to rectify this situation by pacing the right and left ventricles simultaneously, thereby reducing the time required for ventricular activation and improving the synchrony of contraction. One electrode is placed in the right ventricle, as for conventional pacing, and the other at a site of late activation in the left ventricle, most characteristically, the left free wall. Left ventricular pacing is achieved via the coronary sinus (Fig. 8.3). Simultaneous pacing at the two sites results in a narrowing of QRS width and an improvement in cardiac output.

Criteria of selection of patients likely to benefit most from ventricular resynchronization pacing include:

- severe heart failure, New York Heart Association class III or IV
- left bundle branch block
- QRS width greater than 120 ms
- evidence of incoordinate left ventricular contraction on echocardiography.

Ventricular resynchronization pacing has been convincingly shown to improve symptoms in patients with severe heart failure. Trials are currently in progress to determine whether it can also improve prognosis.

ARRHYTHMIA MANAGEMENT

About 50% of patients with heart failure die from progressive heart failure. The other 50% die suddenly as a result of ventricular arrhythmias.

One might therefore anticipate that this patient population would benefit from antiarrhythmic drug therapy. However, this has not proved to be the case and studies of antiarrhythmic drugs have proved either negative or to have an adverse effect. The exception is beta-blockade, which has been shown to dramatically reduce sudden deaths (see above).

There is growing evidence to suggest a role for implantable defibrillators in this patient population. A number of studies have demonstrated a role for the implantable defibrillator in patients with impaired ventricular function and non-sustained ventricular tachycardia. More recently, implantable defibrillators have been shown to significantly reduce mortality in patients with an ejection fraction less than 30%.

As implantable defibrillators can be combined with ventricular resynchronization, there is likely to be a growing role for device therapy in the management of patients with severe heart failure.

ACUTE LEFT VENTRICULAR FAILURE

Acute pulmonary oedema is a life-threatening emergency. Characteristically, the patient is extremely breathless and frightened. The patient is unable to lie flat and prefers to sit bolt upright. In severe cases they may cough up blood-tinged, pink sputum.

Clinical features

- The patient is tachypnoeic and distressed, peripherally shutdown and perspiring profusely.
- Systolic pressure is frequently elevated.
- A marked tachycardia is evident with a gallop rhythm on auscultation.
- Crackles and wheeze are heard throughout the chest.

Investigations

- *Chest radiograph* shows diffuse haziness due to alveolar fluid. Changes are generally bilateral but occasionally may be unilateral.
- *Blood gases.* Arterial pO_2 falls. Initially pCO_2 also falls due to over-breathing, but in the later stages pCO_2 may rise due to impaired gas exchange.

Management

Management of acute LVF:

PRACTICE GUIDELINES

- *General.* A venous line should be inserted and the patient should be monitored. If there is an underlying cardiac rhythm disturbance, this should be corrected.
- *Oxygen.* This should be administered in high concentrations (60%) unless the patient has concomitant airways disease and a susceptibility to hypercapnia is suspected, in which case it it may be necessary to use a lower inspired oxygen concentration.
- *Diamorphine.* The standard dose of diamorphine is 5 mg given intravenously. It may be necessary to reduce this dose in elderly or frail patients. The diamorphine should be accompanied by an antiemetic, such as cyclizine.
- *Diuretics.* The patient should be given intravenous furosemide (frusemide). The usual dose would be 40 mg, but this may be increased in patients already on diuretic therapy. The immediate benefits of furosemide (frusemide) are related to a direct effect to reduce pulmonary pressures – the benefits from diuresis take longer to occur.
- *Nitrates.* Administration of a sublingual tablet of glyceryl trinitrate has an immediate effect of lowering pulmonary pressures and reducing pulmonary oedema. This may be followed, if necessary, by an infusion of the drug.
- *Inotropic therapy.* In cases of refractory pulmonary oedema, inotropic therapy should be considered. Aminophylline 250 mg i.v. over 10 min is frequently effective. Alternatively, patients may be started on a dobutamine infusion, beginning at 5 μg/kg/min.

CARDIOGENIC SHOCK

The terms *acute circulatory failure, low output state,* and *shock* are used to describe a syndrome comprising arterial hypotension, cold, moist and cyanosed extremities, a rapid weak pulse, a low urine output and a diminished level of consciousness. This pattern can arise as a result of impaired cardiac function, in which case, it is termed *cardiogenic shock.*

This clinical pattern is common to a number of other disorders and cardiogenic shock must be differentiated from other causes of shock, including:

- hypovolaemic shock, which is exemplified by haemorrhage and loss of fluid from burns, vomiting and diarrhoea
- septicaemic shock
- anaphylactic shock
- acute pancreatitis.

Shock is described as cardiogenic when it is clearly cardiac in origin. This may be due to many different causes, including myocardial infarction, massive pulmonary embolism, dissecting aneurysm, pericardial tamponade, rupture of a valve cusp, and arrhythmias. In cardiogenic shock, the central venous pressure is usually raised, in contrast to hypovolaemic shock, in which it is characteristically low.

Although the fall in cardiac output and blood pressure is an essential feature of shock, these abnormalities are insufficient to account for the syndrome. Falls of the same magnitude may be seen in some patients in whom the clinical features of shock are not seen and in whom the prognosis is good.

Clinical features

- In the first stage of shock, there is a fall in cardiac output and blood pressure, due to either a diminution in venous return or to an inability of the myocardium to expel an adequate stroke volume.
- As a consequence of the hypotension, there is a fall in renal blood flow, with oliguria.
- Reflex tachycardia occurs.
- Compensatory reflex arteriolar vasoconstriction further reduces blood flow to the kidneys, abdominal viscera, muscle and skin. Vasodilatation of the cerebral and coronary vessels permits the maintenance of a relatively good blood flow in these territories. If the vasoconstriction is sufficiently great, the blood pressure may be kept at or close to normal levels but at the expense of producing tissue hypoxia with consequent acidosis.

Management of cardiogenic shock

General management

If the patient is in severe pain or distress, opiates should be given intravenously (provided there is no contraindication) and high-flow oxygen administered, preferably by a tight-fitting face mask making use of the Venturi principle, or by mechanical ventilation. Unless there is pulmonary oedema, the patient should be laid flat, with the legs slightly raised. A catheter should be introduced to measure urinary output. Arterial blood gases and pH should be monitored. Although central venous monitoring may be adequate for the less severe cases of traumatic shock, a Swan–Ganz balloon-tip catheter should be used to obtain pulmonary artery and 'pulmonary capillary wedge' pressures if a cardiac or pulmonary cause is known or suspected. As measurement of blood pressure by a sphygmomanometer is unreliable in severe shock, direct arterial pressure monitoring should be undertaken, when possible.

Correction of hypovolaemia

Although left ventricular filling pressures are most commonly elevated in patients with cardiogenic shock, this is not always the case. Patients may have undergone a period of prior diuretic therapy resulting in fluid depletion. Alternatively, in cases of right ventricular infarction, the left ventricle may be under filled. A Swan–Ganz catheter (p. 72) enables pulmonary artery wedge pressure to be estimated to achieve an optimal pressure of between 18 and 20 mmHg. If the pressure is below this level, saline should be administered to increase the wedge pressure and optimize cardiac output

Inotropic agents

These drugs enhance myocardial contractility, but at the expense of increased oxygen consumption. Dopamine and dobutamine are most frequently used.

The effects of dopamine, a natural precursor of noradrenaline (norepinephrine), depend upon the dose. Administered intravenously in a dosage of 2–5 µg/kg/min, it causes dilatation of renal and mesenteric vessels; at doses of 5–10 µg/kg/min, it increases myocardial contractility and cardiac output. At higher doses, it causes vasoconstriction (it should not be infused directly into a peripheral vein as leakage may cause local necrosis). Dopamine may induce nausea and vomiting, and can lead to an excessive tachycardia and arrhythmias.

Dobutamine is a synthetic sympathomimetic agent whose predominant action is one of stimulating β_1 activity. It is less likely to cause vasoconstriction or tachycardia than dopamine. It is given by intravenous infusion at a rate of 2.5–10 µg/kg/min.

Mechanical support

The intra-aortic balloon pump is of value in acute myocardial infarction if shock has been caused by a surgically correctable lesion, such as a ventricular septal defect or papillary muscle rupture (see also p. 371).

Other extracorporeal and intracorporeal circulatory systems have been developed to provide longer term support in patients with cardiogenic shock. They do not as yet provide a long-term option for cardiac support and their role is to provide temporary support in a patient who may be suitable for other interventional options, particularly potential transplant recipients while awaiting a donor heart.

CARDIAC TRANSPLANTATION

Cardiac transplantation is now well established in the management of refractory heart failure, not amenable to other forms of treatment. The prognosis of transplant recipients has dramatically improved, since the introduction of ciclosporin for immunosuppression. One-year survival is now approaching 90%, with a 5-year survival in excess of 60%.

In the majority of transplant recipients, the cause of heart failure is either cardiomyopathy or end-stage ischaemic heart disease. In both cases, the indication for treatment is severe symptoms, refractory to medical therapy and not amenable to other forms of surgery. Such patients have a very limited life expectancy, which is dramatically improved by transplantation.

Selection criteria for transplantation include:

- patients not amenable to conventional surgery
- patients remaining severely symptomatic despite maximal medical treatment
- poor prognosis without transplantation
- freedom from other major diseases, particularly diabetes, peripheral vessel disease, renal impairment, malignancy and pulmonary hypertension
- likelihood of good prognosis and quality of life posttransplant.

The timing of transplantation is difficult. On the one hand, the patient must have severe enough impairment of left ventricular function to warrant a transplant. On the other, if the operation is undertaken at a stage when the patient has end-stage heart failure, causing failure of other organ systems, the success of transplantation decreases dramatically.

The success of cardiac transplantation has meant that the number of patients who could potentially benefit from transplantation exceeds the number of donor hearts available.

As a result, transplant waiting lists are relatively long and many patients die while awaiting a donor heart. In patients considered at high risk of arrhythmic death while awaiting a donor heart, the short-term use of an implantable defibrillator can be considered as a 'bridge to transplant'.

Immunosuppression

Immunosuppression is achieved by a combination of:

- ciclosporin
- corticosteroids
- azathioprine.

Using combined therapy, successful immunosuppression can be achieved with lower doses of each agent. This minimizes the side-effects of each. The degree of immunosuppression needs to be greatest in the earlier stages after transplantation, but can subsequently be reduced to a low maintenance level. Patients remain susceptible to episodes of rejection, but these can be managed by increasing immunosuppressive therapy when they occur.

Rejection

The recognition of episodes of rejection is important in transplant patients. The patient is generally non-specifically unwell. Clinical features may include the development of a third heart sound and atrial arrhythmias. The ECG may show reduction in QRS voltages, but this is a relatively late finding.

Diagnosis is based upon cardiac biopsy and this should be undertaken on suspicion of rejection. This is a simple procedure performed under local anaesthetic using either rigid biopsy forceps introduced into the jugular vein in the neck or using a biopsy catheter introduced into the femoral vein.

Complications

In addition to rejection, heart transplant recipients are subject to a number of other problems:

- *Infection.* This remains a major cause of death in transplant recipients. Viral infections, such as cytomegalovirus and herpes zoster, which produce relatively trivial infections in normal individuals, can be life-threatening in immunosuppressed patients. It is important that even minor symptoms should be investigated to detect and treat any infective illness early.
- *Accelerated atherosclerosis.* Heart transplant patients develop accelerated atherosclerosis. This occurs both in patients whose preoperative diagnosis was cardiomyopathy and in those with preoperative ischaemic heart disease. It is important that any contributory factor to atherosclerosis, such as hypercholesterolaemia, should be adequately controlled. Patients should also undergo regular assessment with coronary angiography or nuclear cardiography.
- *Ciclosporin nephrotoxicity.* Patients should be regularly reviewed with a check of their renal function and ciclosporin levels, to minimize the risk of nephrotoxicity.
- *Cushingoid features.* The features of Cushing disease are, in general, less troublesome with the advent of ciclosporin and reduction in steroid dosage.
- *Malignancy.* It is well recognized that there is an increased incidence of malignant disease, particularly lymphoproliferative disorders, in immunosuppressed patients.

Despite these difficulties, cardiac transplantation is a highly successful procedure, in patients fortunate enough to receive a transplant. The main limitation in the growth of transplantation continues to be availability of donor hearts.

Heart–lung transplantation

Heart–lung transplantation is still much less common than simple heart transplantation. Conditions requiring heart–lung transplantation include primary pulmonary hypertension and congenital cardiac abnormalities which have resulted in Eisenmenger's syndrome. These indications have now grown to include patients with end-stage pulmonary disease, particularly patients with cystic fibrosis.

The success rate for heart–lung transplantation is not yet as good as that for heart transplantation, with 1-year survival rates reported of approximately 70%.

FURTHER READING

Abraham, W. (2002) Cardiac resynchronisation therapy for heart failure; biventricular pacing and beyond. *Current Opinion in Cardiology* **17**:346.

CIBIS II investigators (1999) The cardiac insufficiency bisoprolol study II: a randomized trial. *Lancet* **353**:9.

Colucci, W. S. & Braunwald, E. (2001) Pathophysiology of heart failure. In: Braunwald, E., Zipes, D. & Libby, P. *Heart Disease: A Textbook of Cardiovascular Medicine*. Philadelphia: Saunders.

Digitalis Investigation Group (1997) The effect of digoxin on mortality and morbidity in patients with heart failure. *New England Journal of Medicine* **336**:525.

McMurray, J.J.V, Ostergren, J. & Swedberg, K. et al (2003) Effects of candesartan in patients with chronic heart failure and reduced left ventricular systolic function taking angiotensin-converting-enzyme inhibitors: the CHARM-added trial. *Lancet* **362**:767–771.

MERIT HF study group (1999) Beneficial effects of metoprolol in CCF. *Lancet* **353**:2001.

Miniati, D., Robbins, R. & Reitz, B. (2001) Heart and lung transplantation. In: Braunwald, E., Zipes, D., & Libby, P. *Heart Disease. A Textbook of Cardiovascular Medicine*. Philadelphia: Saunders.

National Institute for Clinical Excellence (2003) *Chronic Heart Failure. Management of Chronic Heart Failure in Adults in Primary and Secondary Care*. London: National Institute of Clinical Excellence. www.nice.org.uk

Packer, M., Coats, A., Fowler, M. et al (2001) Effect of carvedilol on survival in severe heart failure. *New England Journal of Medicine* **344**:1651.

Packer, M. (1993) The development of positive inotropic agents for chronic heart failure: How have we gone astray? *Journal of the American College of Cardiology* **22**:119.

Pitt, B., Zannad, F., Remme, W. et al (for the Randomised Aldactone Evaluation Study investigators) (1999) The effects of spironolactone on morbidity and mortality in patients with severe heart failure. *New England Journal of Medicine* **341**:709.

SOLVD Investigators (1991) Effect of enalapril on survival in patients with reduced left ventricular ejection fractions and congestive heart failure. *New England Journal of Medicine* **325**:293.

Disorders of rate, rhythm and conduction

DISTURBANCES OF RATE AND RHYTHM

Sinus node abnormalities

Sinus tachycardia

Sinus tachycardia is sinus rhythm at a rate faster than is normal (Fig. 9.1). In adults, this is commonly defined as being greater than 100/min. In children the heart rate, even at rest, frequently exceeds 100/min, and in infants may exceed 150/min. Amongst factors associated with disease which cause sinus tachycardia are:

- *anaemia*
- *hyperthyroidism*
- *fever*
- *blood loss and hypovolaemia*
- *heart failure*
- *drugs* such as adrenaline (epinephrine), isoprenaline, ephedrine, propantheline, atropine and thyroxine.

Sinus tachycardia is seldom harmful and may be a compensatory mechanism.

The patient with sinus tachycardia may complain of palpitation which is of gradual and explicable onset, unlike the abrupt and unexpected appearance of the symptom in paroxysmal tachycardia. The diagnosis is usually obvious when there is a regular pulse at a rate of more than 100/min. Frequently, the tachycardia subsides during the examination as anxiety diminishes. Carotid sinus pressure causes little slowing in contrast to its usually dramatic effect in atrial tachycardia or atrial flutter. The electrocardiogram (ECG) shows

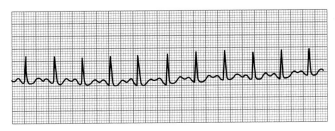

Fig. 9.1 Sinus tachycardia.

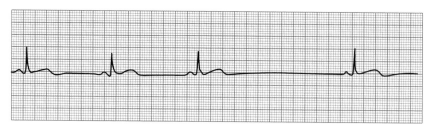

Fig. 9.2 Sinus bradycardia. A marked sinus bradycardia of 40 beats/min is followed by a 2.7 s pause before the next sinus beat.

P waves having a normal relationship to QRS complexes. The J point may be depressed; the ST then slopes upward.

Sinus tachycardia does not of itself require treatment although the underlying cause of tachycardia should be sought and, where necessary, treated.

Sinus bradycardia

Sinus bradycardia describes a slow heart in sinus rhythm (Fig. 9.2). This term is commonly applied to heart rates of less than 60/min, although such rates are frequently seen in healthy elderly people; in the highly trained athlete the heart rate may be less than 40/min. Amongst factors causing sinus bradycardia are:

- increased vagal tone (e.g. during carotid sinus massage)
- myxoedema
- hypothermia
- raised intracranial pressure
- drugs including digitalis and the beta-adrenergic blocking agents such as propranolol.

Sinus bradycardia seldom gives rise to symptoms or undesirable haemo-dynamic effects but, occasionally, in the elderly and in acute myocardial infarction, cardiac failure or hypotension may develop if the stroke output cannot be increased to compensate adequately for the slow rate. The heart can be accelerated by atropine 0.6 mg subcutaneously or intravenously. Oral sympathomimetics, such as long-acting isoprenaline, can also be used to treat sinus bradycardia, but in general pacing is preferable.

Sick sinus syndrome

Sinus bradycardia is a component of the sick sinus syndrome, a relatively common condition amongst the elderly. The bradycardia may be complicated by paroxysms of atrial tachyarrhythmias (tachycardia, flutter or fibrillation), the so-called bradycardia–tachycardia syndrome (Fig. 9.3). Syncope may result either from too slow or too fast a heart rate.

Sick sinus syndrome is seldom life-threatening, but frequently causes distressing symptoms of palpitations, dizziness or syncope. These can be treated by implantation of a pacemaker. Tachyarrhythmias may require antiarrhythmic drug therapy combined with a pacemaker to guard against bradycardia.

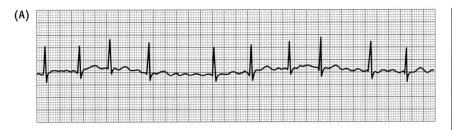

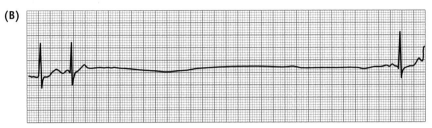

Fig. 9.3 Sick sinus syndrome with bradycardia and tachycardia. (A) Tachycardia due to atrial fibrillation. (B) Termination of atrial fibrillation is followed by a prolonged asystolic pause, eventually terminated by a sinus beat.

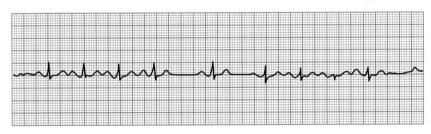

Fig. 9.4 Sinus arrhythmia. Acceleration of the sinus rate is evident during inspiration and slowing during expiration.

Sinus arrhythmia *(Fig. 9.4)*

Normally, the sinus node does not discharge with absolute regularity owing to variations in vagal tone. These variations are related to respiration, and it is characteristic in the young to find acceleration of the heart during inspiration with slowing during expiration. This phasic change in the rhythm of the heart is known as sinus arrhythmia. It is seldom clinically obvious in adults, but is occasionally seen in the healthy old person. It is of no clinical importance, but it must be differentiated from the other types of arrhythmia. Its relationship to respiration usually makes this easy.

Supraventricular arrhythmias

A variety of rhythm disturbances can arise in the atria and AV junctional area (that is, the AV node and adjacent specialized tissues). These may result from either increased automaticity or re-entry.

Atrial ectopic beats *(atrial extrasystoles, atrial premature beats)*

Atrial ectopic beats are common in normal individuals, but seldom give rise to symptoms, apart from an awareness of heart irregularity from time to time.

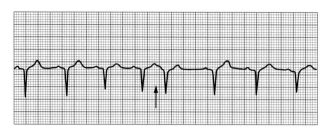

Fig. 9.5 Atrial ectopic beat. A premature P wave (arrowed) is followed by a QRS complex of normal appearance.

They cause an occasional irregularity in an otherwise normal pulse, and are usually abolished by exercise. The diagnosis is readily confirmed from the ECG (Fig. 9.5) which shows a premature beat occurring earlier than the next anticipated sinus beat. The P wave differs in configuration from that of a sinus beat, because depolarization of the atria takes place in an abnormal direction. The accompanying QRST complex is usually similar to that of previous beats of sinus origin because the pathway of ventricular depolarization is normal. Occasionally, the QRST complex is abnormally broad ('aberrant') because the impulse passes down only one of the bundle branches, the other still being refractory from the preceding beat. It then simulates the appearance of a ventricular ectopic beat (see p. 174) but is usually preceded by a P wave.

Atrial ectopic beats may presage the appearance of other atrial arrhythmias but they require no treatment.

Junctional (nodal) ectopic beats

Ectopic beats deriving from the junctional tissue are quite common and, like atrial ectopic beats, usually benign. They are responsible for an occasional irregularity in an otherwise regular pulse and cannot be diagnosed without an ECG, which shows the same features as with atrial ectopic beats except that the P wave is inverted in lead II and is either buried in the QRS complex, or precedes or follows it by a very short interval. No treatment is necessary.

Junctional (nodal) rhythm (Fig. 9.6)

In this condition the junctional tissue is acting as the pacemaker of the heart and the ECG appearance is that of a succession of junctional ectopic beats. It is usually a transient condition resulting from a depression of sinus node activity. It occurs in some normal individuals and may be provoked by digitalis or ischaemic heart disease. The heart rate is usually in the region of

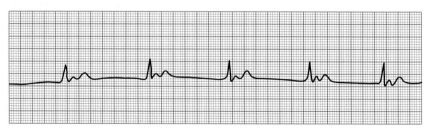

Fig. 9.6 Junctional rhythm. In this example, retrograde conduction into the atria is relatively slow and a P wave can be distinguished after the QRS complex, interrupting the ST segment.

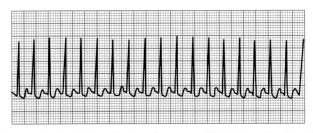

Fig. 9.7 Supraventricular tachycardia. Regular narrow QRS tachycardia at a rate of 220 beats/min.

50–60/min and no treatment is required. If the heart rate is undesirably slow, it can be accelerated by the use of atropine.

In patients with acute myocardial infarction treated with thrombolytic therapy, the occurrence of junctional rhythm is an indicator of successful reperfusion.

Paroxysmal supraventricular tachycardias (Fig. 9.7)

In its broadest sense, the term paroxysmal supraventricular tachycardia refers to any recurrent supraventricular arrhythmia. However, arrhythmias originating within the atrium (atrial tachycardia, atrial flutter and atrial fibrillation) are generally excluded. The term encompasses a number of different arrhythmias, which share certain characteristics – starting abruptly, usually being regular at a rate of 140–220/min, and being associated with narrow QRS complexes, closely resembling those seen in sinus rhythm. Aberrant conduction with broadening of the QRS may, however, occur, as may rates above and below those quoted.

Paroxysmal supraventricular tachycardias commonly arise from one of two mechanisms:

- In the commonest form, re-entry involves dual pathways within the AV node, which have different rates of conduction and refractoriness. This is called *AV node re-entry tachycardia*.
- The second common cause is the presence of an additional electrical connection (*accessory pathway*), linking atrium and ventricle – the best recognized form is *Wolff–Parkinson–White syndrome*, which is characterized in sinus rhythm by a short PR interval and delta wave (p. 166). During the common form of tachycardia, excitation passes from atrium to ventricle over the AV node and from ventricle to atrium via the accessory pathway. As the ventricles are excited over the normal route QRS complexes are narrow. The absence of a delta wave during sinus rhythm does not exclude the possibility of an accessory pathway, as some pathways only conduct retrogradely from ventricle to atrium. These pathways are hence '*concealed*' during sinus rhythm, but can still conduct retrogradely giving rise to a re-entrant tachycardia.

Attacks of paroxysmal SVT may last only seconds, but they often persist for minutes or hours or, much less commonly, for days. They may recur at short intervals or be separated from one another by weeks, months or even years. It is sometimes possible to identify provoking factors such as tobacco, coffee and alcohol. Paroxysms are most often encountered in otherwise normal people in whom they give rise to palpitation, but no serious haemodynamic effects. These tachycardias can, however, produce cardiac failure and hypotension in the presence of heart disease because of the increased workload of the heart and the inadequate filling time during diastole.

The patient usually complains of attacks of rapid regular palpitation of abrupt onset, sometimes accompanied by dizziness or even syncope. When the attack is prolonged or when it occurs in those with heart disease, there may be dyspnoea and ischaemic chest pain. There may also be polyuria.

The episodes are often so brief and infrequent that no doctor ever sees them; if the patient is observed at the time, the pulse is found to be regular at a rate between 140 and 220. Carotid sinus massage frequently terminates the attack, but if it fails to do so, it has no effect upon the pulse rate.

Investigations

The ECG in tachycardia reveals QRST complexes of normal or near normal configuration occurring rapidly and regularly. The presence and timing of a P wave is of diagnostic value (Fig. 9.8):

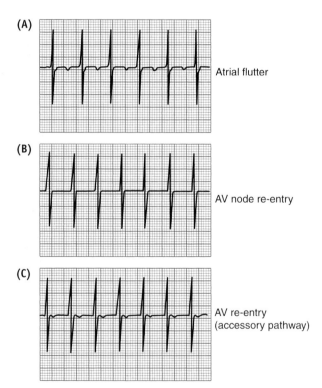

(A) Atrial flutter

(B) AV node re-entry

(C) AV re-entry (accessory pathway)

Fig. 9.8 Differential diagnosis of regular narrow QRS tachycardia. Schematic ECGs. (A) Atrial flutter with 2:1 AV block. Close examination of the trace reveals two flutter waves for every QRS complex. The second flutter wave is partly hidden in the terminal portion of the QRS complex. (See also Fig. 9.10.) (B) Atrioventricular nodal re-entry tachycardia. Atrial depolarization is generally synchronous with ventricular depolarization. The P wave is either lost within the QRS complex or is in the terminal portion of the QRS complex. (C) Atrioventricular re-entry tachycardia due to the presence of an accessory pathway. A P wave is evident after the QRS complex, reflecting retrograde atrial activation over the accessory pathway. (See also Fig. 9.9.)

- A P wave which is 'absent' (hidden in the QRS or in the terminal portion of the QRS) suggests *AV node re-entry* as the underlying mechanism of tachycardia.
- A P wave following the QRS suggests the presence of an *accessory pathway*.
- *Atrial flutter* with a 2:1 AV block should also be considered in the differential diagnosis of any regular narrow complex tachycardia (Fig. 9.8). Characteristically, the rate is in the range 140 to 160 beats/min.

It is difficult to obtain conventional ECG recordings of the attacks because of their unpredictability and brevity; the documentation of episodes is aided by dynamic electrocardiography (Holter monitoring), and by patient-activated ECG recorders.

Termination of the acute attack

In the treatment of the individual attack, the patient may be taught to carry out the *Valsalva manoeuvre* and the doctor can use carotid sinus massage. If these procedures prove unsuccessful, drug treatment should be considered. As the majority of tachycardias arise by re-entry either within or involving the AV node, drugs slowing AV nodal conduction are indicated. Generally, adenosine or verapamil are the drugs of choice (see p. 201).

In patients in whom the safety and efficacy of intravenous verapamil has been demonstrated, it is reasonable to provide the patient with a supply of oral verapamil to take a stat 120 mg dose in the event of an acute attack, hence avoiding the need for hospital attendance.

Prevention

Because of the repetitive paroxysmal nature of the tachycardia, prevention is often of greater importance than the treatment of the individual attack. When possible, a provoking factor such as strong coffee or tobacco should be identified and avoided. If episodes are infrequent and symptoms are not severe, drug treatment is not required and simple reassurance is all that is necessary. In other patients stat doses of verapamil as outlined above can obviate the need for continuous drug treatment. When drug therapy is required, a number of drugs can be considered, including beta-blockers, verapamil and class I antiarrhythmic drugs such as flecainide.

Another approach is radiofrequency ablation (p. 194). Ablation offers a definitive cure in the majority of patients and should be considered as the treatment of choice in patients with significant continuing symptoms despite drug therapy and in those intolerant of drug therapy or in whom drug therapy is contraindicated.

Pre-excitation (Wolff–Parkinson–White syndrome)

In this condition, an anomalous conduction pathway bypasses the AV node. This permits the abnormally early activation of part of one ventricle, the remaining ventricular muscle receiving its impulse normally. This leads to a short PR interval (less than 0.12 s) and a slurred upstroke and widening of the QRS (Fig. 9.9A).

The normal and abnormal conduction pathways are able to form part of a re-entry circuit. This facilitates the occurrence of paroxysmal tachycardia. In the common form of re-entry tachycardia the ventricles are excited

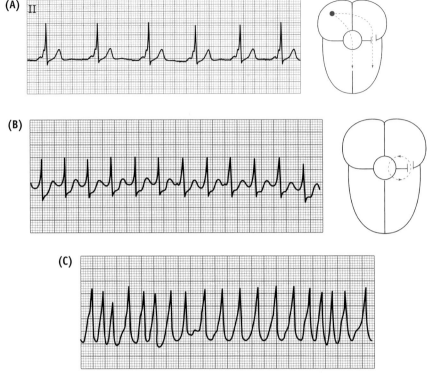

Fig. 9.9 ECG patterns in Wolff–Parkinson–White syndrome. (A) Sinus rhythm. A short PR interval and delta wave are evident. (B) Re-entrant tachycardia. This is the common form of re-entrant tachycardia conducting from atrium to ventricle over the AV node and retrogradely from ventricle to atrium over the accessory pathway. It results in a narrow QRS tachycardia with a loss of delta wave. (C) Atrial fibrillation. The characteristic features of atrial fibrillation in Wolff–Parkinson–White syndrome are apparent. 1. Irregular QRS complexes. 2. Varying QRS morphology, reflecting different degrees of activation over the AV node and accessory pathway. 3. Some very short RR intervals (less than 200 ms), reflecting rapid conduction over the accessory pathway.

normally through the AV node and His–Purkinje system. Consequently there is no pre-excitation during tachycardia and the delta wave disappears (Fig. 9.9B). On presentation, this narrow QRS tachycardia may be indistinguishable from other causes of paroxysmal supraventricular tachycardia.

Sudden death occasionally occurs in patients with Wolff–Parkinson–White syndrome. The danger lies not in re-entry tachycardia, but in atrial fibrillation (Fig. 9.9C). Normally in patients with atrial fibrillation, the ventricles are protected from the rapid rate of atrial depolarization by the gating effect of the AV node. In patients with an accessory pathway this protection is lost. If the refractory period of the pathway is short, impulses from the atrium can be conducted at very high rates to the ventricle and can result in ventricular fibrillation.

Atrial fibrillation, complicating Wolff–Parkinson–White syndrome, is an emergency and should be treated with a drug acting selectively on the accessory pathway to abolish pre-excitation (see p. 201).

In many patients, the identification of Wolff–Parkinson–White syndrome is an incidental finding at routine ECG. If the patient is asymptomatic, the risks of the condition are generally considered to be very low, and further investigation is generally unnecessary unless indicated on grounds of occupation or sporting activities. Information on speed of pathway conduction can sometimes be derived from exercise testing – if pre-excitation disappears during exercise this indicates a relatively slow conducting pathway, and the patient would not be able to sustain very high ventricular rates if atrial fibrillation should develop.

In patients with symptomatic arrhythmias, the advent of radiofrequency ablation has revolutionized the treatment of the condition and in general, radiofrequency ablation is the preferred option to drug therapy (p. 194).

Atrial tachycardia

The term atrial tachycardia refers to a tachycardia arising within the atria. Atrial tachycardias can arise in normal hearts and represent a relatively uncommon tachycardia mechanism in the category of paroxysmal supraventricular tachycardias discussed above. More commonly they occur in association with atrial enlargement or atrial structural abnormalities and hence may be indicative of other disease states.

Accelerated automaticity is often the underlying mechanism of tachycardia, although re-entrant mechanisms can occur. Tachycardias tend to be more variable in rate than other forms of paroxysmal supraventricular tachycardia. Some tachycardias are adenosine responsive, but others are not.

It is now recognized that many atrial tachycardias originate in the pulmonary veins. Atrial tachycardias from this location may have a particular role in the pathogenesis of forms of atrial fibrillation (see p. 170).

Atrial tachycardias are often difficult to treat. In the first instance a beta-blocker would often be appropriate. Radiofrequency ablation may be appropriate when drug therapy fails, but is frequently less successful and manifests higher recurrence rates than ablation for other types of supraventricular tachycardia.

Atrial flutter (Fig. 9.10)

In this arrhythmia, the atria beat regularly at a rate of 250–350/min – usually close to 300/min. In most cases the arrhythmia arises due to a re-entry circuit within the right atrium, due to an area of slow conduction in an isthmus of myocardium between the inferior vena cava, tricuspid valve and coronary sinus.

Some degree of AV block is almost invariable. In most instances the ventricles beat regularly because of a 2:1, 3:1 or 4:1 response to the regular atrial activity, but it is irregular if the degree of block varies from cycle to cycle. The commonest variety is that of 2:1 block which characteristically has a ventricular rate of 140–160. In cases with 2:1 block, flutter waves are not always obvious. Any regular, narrow QRS complex arrhythmia in this rate band should be closely scrutinized for the presence of flutter waves (Figs 9.8 and 9.10).

Atrial flutter is commonly a complication of underlying organic heart disease, although it occasionally occurs as a primary condition in patients with no definable cardiac abnormality. Common associations include:

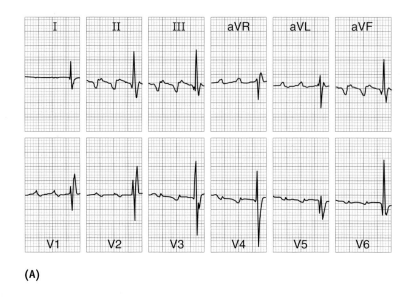

(A)

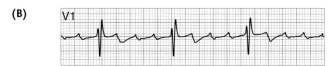

(B)

Fig. 9.10 Atrial flutter. (A) 12 lead ECG. Flutter waves are most readily apparent in the right-sided chest leads V1 and V2. They are also seen in inferior leads, III and aVF. A high degree of AV block is apparent with five to six flutter waves for every one QRS complex. (B) Rhythm strip lead is V1.

- rheumatic heart disease
- ischaemic heart disease
- myocarditis
- hyperthyroidism.

It may be persistent or occur in paroxysms which are usually self-limited to hours or days, but it may progress to atrial fibrillation. The symptoms resemble those of atrial tachycardia, with palpitation, dizziness or syncope. The arrhythmia often provokes cardiac failure.

The pulse is usually regular at a rate of 140–160/min. It may be possible to see venous 'flutter' waves in the neck. Carotid sinus massage leads to a transient increase in the atrioventricular block, with a slowing of the ventricular rate only as long as the pressure is maintained.

Investigations

The electrocardiogram is diagnostic with 'flutter' waves of a sawtooth appearance, best seen in leads VI and III occurring at approximately 300/min. The sawtooth nature of the complexes may be obscured by the QRS complexes when there is 2:1 block, but it is readily revealed when carotid sinus massage is applied.

Treatment

Drug treatment is seldom effective in restoring sinus rhythm. Digitalis increases the AV block, brings the heart rate under control, and sometimes abolishes the arrhythmia. Intravenous amiodarone slows the ventricular response rate and occasionally restores sinus rhythm. Class I antiarrhythmic agents are best avoided because of the risk of slowing the flutter rate, enabling 1:1 conduction of the flutter waves into the ventricle, with consequent haemodynamic deterioration. DC cardioversion is preferable to drug therapy if immediate correction is necessary, and is almost invariably effective.

Prevention

In the patient liable to paroxysms of atrial flutter, beta-blockers, particularly sotalol, may be of some value. If this is ineffective, oral amiodarone is an alternative, but carries a risk of serious long-term side-effects. Radiofrequency ablation provides an alternative treatment strategy (see p. 194).

Anti-coagulation

Just as for atrial fibrillation (see below), patients with atrial flutter are at increased risk of stroke and other thromboembolic complications. The risk is probably lower than for atrial fibrillation but is not negligible and anticoagulant therapy should be considered (see below). Just as for atrial fibrillation, patients undergoing cardioversion are at risk of thromboembolic complications and prior anticoagulation should be considered unless the arrhythmia is known to be of new onset and present for less than 24 h.

Atrial fibrillation (Fig. 9.11)

In this arrhythmia, irregular atrial impulses occur at rates over 300/min. It may be due to multiple foci of ectopic activity or to wavelets of excitation following variable courses through the atrial myocardium depending upon the location of patches of excitable and refractory muscle. It is recognized that in some patients, atrial fibrillation arises due to a rapidly firing focus or foci, most often in the origin of the pulmonary veins. Some degree of AV block is invariable; the ventricular rhythm is slower than the atrial but it is also irregular.

The presence of atrial fibrillation suggests that there has been either a pathological process involving the atria, as in rheumatic heart disease, or that there has been a rise in pressure with atrial dilatation secondary to

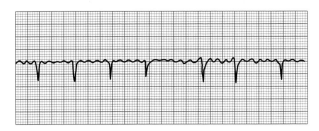

Fig. 9.11 Atrial fibrillation. The rhythm strip shows narrow QRS complexes which are irregularly irregular.

mitral valve or left ventricular disease. Common causes of atrial fibrillation include:

- rheumatic mitral valve disease
- ischaemic heart disease, particularly acute myocardial infarction
- alcohol
- thyrotoxicosis
- hypertension
- acute infections, particularly when these affect the lungs
- cardiopulmonary surgery.

It is a rare complication of many other types of heart disease. In a substantial proportion of patients, no evidence of organic heart disease can be found – 'lone' atrial fibrillation. The incidence of lone atrial fibrillation is greater amongst younger patients. A focal source in the pulmonary veins may be of particular importance amongst patients with lone atrial fibrillation.

Atrial fibrillation may be paroxysmal, with attacks lasting for a few minutes or hours. This is particularly likely in acute myocardial infarction, in chest infections, and in the early stages of thyrotoxicosis and mitral valve disease. In rheumatic cases, the arrhythmia usually becomes established eventually and persists for the rest of the patient's life.

Adverse effects of atrial fibrillation

Atrial fibrillation leads to untoward effects for three major reasons:

- *Rapid ventricular response* – the ventricular response may be so fast that there is inadequate time for diastolic filling and the cardiac output falls.
- *Loss of A-V synchrony* – the atrial contribution to ventricular filling is lost.
- *Stasis of blood* in the ineffectively contracting atrium encourages thrombosis. As a consequence, embolism is common, particularly in patients with mitral valve disease. Emboli from the right atrium produce pulmonary artery obstruction; those from the left atrium may lodge in cerebral, renal or other peripheral vessels.

Investigations

In the ECG, the P wave disappears but atrial activity produces an irregular undulation of the base line (Fig. 9.11). The QRS complexes are totally irregular in timing, except in the rare situation of atrial fibrillation complicated by complete heart block. In most cases of untreated atrial fibrillation, the ventricular rate lies between 100 and 160/min, but rates above or below this are not uncommon.

Assessment of underlying cause

It is important to consider possible underlying disease states which may have played a contributory role to the development of atrial fibrillation. All patients should undergo an echocardiogram to assess ventricular function, possible ventricular hypertrophy and valvular status. Occasionally atrial fibrillation can be a manifestation of underlying ischaemic heart disease, and in some patients, it may be appropriate to undertake further investigation to exclude coronary disease. Thyroid function should also be checked in all patients presenting with atrial fibrillation, as the arrhythmia may be a manifestation of thyrotoxicosis.

Treatment

There are four aspects to the treatment of atrial fibrillation:

- the control of ventricular rate
- the restoration of sinus rhythm
- the maintenance of sinus rhythm
- prevention of embolism.

Control of the ventricular rate. Control of the ventricular rate is a priority because it is the fast ventricular rate that is most deleterious, rather than the atrial fibrillation *per se*, and also because the arrhythmia may terminate spontaneously. Depending upon the severity of the clinical situation, digoxin may be given intravenously or orally. In most cases, oral administration is satisfactory, and brings the heart rate under control within 2–3 h. When full digitalization has been achieved, the ventricular rate at rest should be held at about 70–80/min. If the heart rate cannot be reduced to this level, a beta-adrenoceptor blocking drug or verapamil may be added.

Restoration of sinus rhythm. When atrial fibrillation has been present for many years, and there is associated and untreatable severe heart disease, there is little to be gained by trying to restore normal rhythm because this is not likely to be maintained. Even if it is, the atrial muscle has usually atrophied and is functionally ineffective. When the arrhythmia is of relatively recent onset, and particularly when the heart disease has been alleviated or some complicating condition such as thyrotoxicosis or pulmonary infection corrected, the patient is likely to benefit from its termination.

In some patients, sinus rhythm can be restored by pharmacological means. Amiodarone is frequently used for this purpose. Class I antiarrhythmic drugs, such as flecainide, have also been used successfully, but should be restricted to patients with no evidence of underlying heart disease.

DC cardioversion (p. 193) is the most reliable means of restoring sinus rhythm and is effective in most instances, at least initially. However, there is a considerable relapse rate within the succeeding months. DC cardioversion should not be undertaken without a prior period of anticoagulation, unless the atrial fibrillation is known to be of new onset and to have been present for less than 24 h.

The maintenance of sinus rhythm presents a difficult problem, particularly in patients with paroxysmal atrial fibrillation:

- Amiodarone is the most effective agent. However, its long-term use may give rise to serious side-effects and the risks of therapy have to be weighed against the benefits.
- Class I agents such as flecainide are also effective, but there are serious concerns regarding the potential proarrhythmic effects and their use should be restricted to patients with no underlying heart disease.
- Beta-blockers are generally less effective, but are nonetheless a reasonable choice for first line drug therapy because they have less troublesome side-effects.

Drug selection must therefore be tailored to the severity of the problem posed by recurrent episodes of atrial fibrillation. Digoxin is of no value in preventing recurrences of atrial fibrillation.

Non-pharmacological treatments may also play a role in maintaining sinus rhythm.

Permanent pacing is effective in some individuals in maintaining sinus rhythm (see also p. 193). Unfortunately, it is difficult to identify in advance those individuals who will benefit from pacing. Patients whose episodes of atrial fibrillation appear to be bradycardia-related, particularly those who experience a majority of their episodes in bed overnight, seem to benefit most from pacing.

There is currently great interest in *radiofrequency ablation* as a treatment for individuals with a focal origin to their atrial fibrillation. This approach requires identification of the focal sources, which are most commonly within the pulmonary veins, followed by current application in these areas. Success rates are lower than for other types of radiofrequency ablation. There are also concerns that ablation in the pulmonary veins may lead to pulmonary vein narrowing at the ablation sites. For these reasons, it is probably best at present to reserve this type of approach for the most severely affected patients.

Anticoagulation. Patients with atrial fibrillation complicating rheumatic heart disease should be anticoagulated. Recent evidence has shown that patients with non-rheumatic atrial fibrillation, but with demonstrable underlying heart disease, also benefit from anticoagulation. In patients with lone atrial fibrillation the risks of thromboembolism are low and the benefits of anticoagulation remain uncertain. In this group, aspirin may be considered as an alternative. Curent guidelines identifying those patients at increased risk of thromboembolism who should be considered for long-term anticoagulant therapy are reproduced in Table 9.1.

Table 9.1 Recommendations for antithrombotic therapy in patients with atrial fibrillation based on thromboembolic risk stratification (adaptation of ACC/AHA/ESC Guidelines JACC 2001;38:1231)

Patient features	Anti-thrombotic therapy recommendation
Age < 60, no heart disease (lone atrial fibrillation)	Aspirin or no therapy
Age < 60, heart disease but no risk factors[a]	Aspirin
Age > 60, no risk factors[a]	Aspirin
Age > 60, diabetes or coronary disease	Warfarin, addition of aspirin optional
Age > 75, especially women	Warfarin
Heart failure	Warfarin
Ejection fraction < 35%	Warfarin
Thyrotoxicosis	Warfarin
Hypertension	Warfarin
Rheumatic heart disease (mitral stenosis)	Warfarin
Prosthetic heart valves	Warfarin
Prior thromboembolism	Warfarin
Persistent atrial thrombus on transoesophageal Echo	Warfarin

[a] Risk factors for thromboembolism: heart failure, LV ejection fraction < 35%, history of hypertension.

In patients undergoing cardioversion, anticoagulation for a period of 1 month before and 1 month after cardioversion is indicated. This may be omitted if the arrhythmia is of very recent onset (less than 24 h). In patients in whom a delay of 1 month for anticoagulation prior to cardioversion is thought undesirable, transoesophageal echocardiography (see p. 53) can be used to exclude the presence of atrial thrombus, prior to cardioversion. However, anticoagulation is still required postcardioversion, as it may take some weeks for normal atrial contractile activity to be resumed.

The carotid sinus and arrhythmias

The carotid sinus is situated at the bifurcation of the common carotid artery and is sensitive to changes in arterial pressure. Impulses arising from the stretch receptors in the carotid sinus pass to the medulla and reflexly slow the heart by stimulating the motor nucleus of the vagus nerve and by inhibiting cardiac sympathetic action. Usually, external pressure on the carotid sinus leads to a slight slowing of the heart rate by reducing the activity of the sinus node. In some individuals in whom the carotid sinus is hypersensitive, external pressure leads to extreme bradycardia and hypotension with resulting syncope.

Carotid sinus pressure plays an important part in the recognition and management of cardiac arrhythmias. It is best to locate the carotid artery on one side first and then to stroke it gently, but firmly. If this is ineffective, the manoeuvre should be repeated on the other side. The effects of carotid sinus massage are as follows:

- *Sinus tachycardia.* Carotid sinus massage causes only slight slowing of the ventricular rate in patients with sinus tachycardia.
- *Atrial fibrillation.* Carotid sinus massage causes slight slowing of the ventricular response.
- *Paroxysmal supraventricular tachycardia.* Carotid sinus massage causes an abrupt termination of the arrhythmia, if it has any effect at all.
- *Atrial flutter.* Carotid sinus massage produces an increase in atrioventricular block, temporarily decreasing the ventricular rate which rises again when the massage is discontinued (Fig. 9.12).
- *Ventricular tachycardia.* Carotid sinus massage has no effect.
- *Carotid sinus hypersensitivity.* Carotid sinus massage causes a profound bradycardia or asystole, frequently dizziness or syncope.

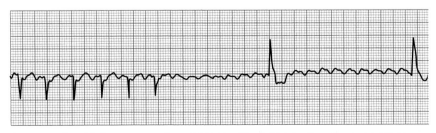

Fig. 9.12 Carotid sinus massage in atrial flutter. The initial tracing shows atrial flutter with 2:1 atrioventricular block. Carotid sinus massage causes a high degree of atrioventricular block, enabling the individual flutter waves to be clearly distinguished. The subsequent QRS complexes are ventricular escape beats.

It is best to carry out carotid sinus massage with ECG control, as excessive bradycardia and even ventricular arrhythmias may result from this procedure. Other dangers include reflex hypotension and cerebrovascular insufficiency. In patients with peripheral arterial disease there is a small risk of precipitating a transient ischaemic attack or stroke.

Ventricular arrhythmias

Ventricular ectopic beats (extrasystoles, premature beats)

An ectopic focus in the ventricles may arise because of ventricular escape, enhanced automatic activity, or re-entry. Ventricular ectopic beats are not uncommon in normal individuals but are encountered frequently in organic heart disease, especially in myocardial infarction. If they occur every second beat (bigeminy or 'coupling') they are frequently due to digitalis therapy.

Patients are seldom aware of ventricular ectopic beats, but may complain of the heart seeming to stop briefly, or of an occasional heavy beat. The diagnosis may be suspected from an irregularity of the pulse interrupting an otherwise regular rhythm, but cannot be made without an ECG, in which there are bizarre and broadened QRS complexes followed by T waves pointing in the direction opposite to that of the main QRS component (Fig. 9.13). The QRS complexes are not preceded by a P wave and are usually succeeded by a long period (the compensatory pause) before the next sinus-activated beat appears.

The importance of ventricular ectopic beats depends upon their context. In normal individuals they are virtually of no consequence. Such individuals should undergo clinical examination, echocardiography and exercise testing, as appropriate, to rule out structural heart disease or coronary disease. Ventricular ectopic beats are associated with an impaired prognosis in ischaemic heart disease. But there is no evidence that suppression of ventricular ectopics with antiarrhythmic drugs improves prognosis. On the contrary, the class I antiarrhythmic drugs flecainide and encainide have been shown to increase mortality in patients with ventricular ectopic beats following myocardial infarction, despite reducing the frequency of ectopic beats.

Sustained ventricular tachycardia (Fig. 9.14)

In this condition a tachycardia arises in the ventricles at a rate of 120–220/min; the atria usually remain under the control of the sinus node. It

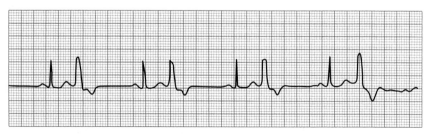

Fig. 9.13 Ventricular ectopic beats. Each sinus beat is followed by a broad complex ventricular ectopic beat. The constant coupling in this example is termed ventricular bigeminy.

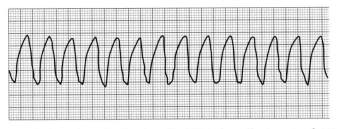

Fig. 9.14 Ventricular tachycardia. Regular wide QRS tachycardia at a rate of 170/min.

may be a consequence of either re-entry or enhanced automaticity of ventricular pacemaker cells. It is nearly always a complication of serious heart disease, although occasionally seen in an otherwise normal individual. The attacks are liable to occur in paroxysms lasting for seconds or minutes, but may continue for several hours. Ventricular tachycardia is a frequent complication in patients with severe heart failure (see p. 152).

As with supraventricular tachycardia, the first symptom may be that of rapid and regular palpitations, but because of the more serious effects on the circulation, acute breathlessness and ischaemic chest pain tend to be more severe. On examination there is a rapid, regular but small pulse. The independent atrial activity may be responsible for dissociated 'a' waves in the venous pulse and a variation in the intensity of the first heart sound, but these physical signs are difficult to elicit.

Electrocardiogram
The ECG shows rapidly occurring broad QRS complexes resembling those of bundle branch block (see Fig. 9.14). *Dissociated P waves* may be identified at a rate different from that of the ventricles (Fig. 9.15). The RR intervals are usually equal, but may vary by up to 0.03 s from one another. The lack of response to carotid pressure assists in the differentiation from atrial tachycardia with bundle branch block (see also pp. 173 and 176).

Treatment of acute episodes
Most instances of ventricular tachycardia call for immediate action, particularly in the context of acute myocardial infarction. Haemodynamically compromised patients should be cardioverted. Drug treatment may be considered in patients without immediate haemodynamic compromise (see p. 199)

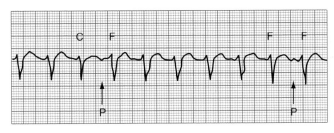

Fig. 9.15 Features of ventricular tachycardia. The ECG shows a slow ventricular tachycardia at a rate of 120/min. Several diagnostic features of ventricular tachycardia are evident: dissociated P waves (P), narrow complex 'capture' beats, and intermediate morphology 'fusion' (F) beats.

Long-term treatment

Ventricular tachycardia is a very serious arrhythmia and in many cases is indicative of severe underlying heart disease. Although antiarrhythmic drug therapy may be of value in some individual cases in preventing recurrence, it has not been shown in clinical trials to improve prognosis. As many of these patients are at risk of sudden death, all individuals who have presented with sustained ventricular tachycardia should be considered for an *implantable defibrillator* (see p. 194) to terminate the arrhythmia should it recur.

The UK guidelines laid down by the National Institute of Clinical Excellence (NICE) relating to patients with sustained ventricular tachycardia advise implanting a defibrillator in two groups of patients:

- Patients presenting with *haemodynamically compromising VT* causing collapse, hypotension, left ventricular failure or angina.
- Patients presenting with sustained VT without the above features but with an *ejection fraction < 35%*.

In practice the substantial majority of patients with sustained ventricular tachycardia arising as a consequence of previous myocardial infarction fall into one or other of these two categories.

In patients with frequent, symptomatic episodes of ventricular tachycardia, *radiofrequency ablation* (p. 194) may offer a way of reducing the frequency of attacks. However, ablation has not been shown to be of prognostic benefit and should be considered as an adjunct rather than an alternative to defibrillator therapy.

The differentiation of supraventricular from ventricular tachycardia

The rapid rate associated with some supraventricular tachycardias may result in bundle branch block, causing a broad QRS complex tachycardia which is difficult to distinguish from ventricular tachycardia. It is occasionally possible to distinguish between the two on clinical grounds:

- In ventricular tachycardia, atrial activity is usually dissociated from that of the ventricles. There may be irregular cannon waves in the jugular veins (see p. 29) and variation in the intensity of the first heart sound. In junctional tachycardia, cannon waves may occur with every beat.
- The response to carotid sinus massage is sometimes diagnostic (see p. 173), as this manoeuvre frequently abolishes supraventricular tachycardia but leaves ventricular tachycardia unaffected. However, one should delay applying this test if possible until a 12-lead ECG is available, as one may otherwise miss the opportunity of verifying the nature of the arrhythmia by obtaining an ECG.

Commonly, a clinical diagnosis is not possible. A 12-lead ECG may provide additional formation. ECG evidence of atrial dissociation confirms a diagnosis of ventricular tachycardia (Fig. 9.15). The following findings are diagnostic:

- *Dissociated P waves.*
- *Capture beats* – the dissociated atrial activity 'captures' the ventricle over the normal conduction pathway, giving a single beat with narrow QRS morphology.

- *Fusion beats* – the dissociated atrial activity is conducted into the ventricles fusing with the tachycardia beats and giving a QRS morphology intermediate between a supraventricular morphology and the tachycardia morphology.

However, these classical diagnostic features are frequently absent and their absence should not be used to infer a supraventricular origin. There are a number of other ECG features which may be helpful in reaching a diagnosis (Fig. 9.16):

- *QRS width.* A tachycardia with a QRS width greater than 140 ms (3.5 small squares) is very likely to be ventricular.
- *QRS axis.* A tachycardia demonstrating left axis deviation is similarly likely to be ventricular.

If doubt remains, it is important to remember that ventricular tachycardia is much more common than supraventricular tachycardia with bundle branch block. When in doubt, a tachycardia is best treated as ventricular.

Intravenous adenosine may also prove of value in distinguishing supraventricular tachycardia with aberration from ventricular tachycardia, as it terminates the majority of supraventricular tachycardias, but is without effect on ventricular tachycardia.

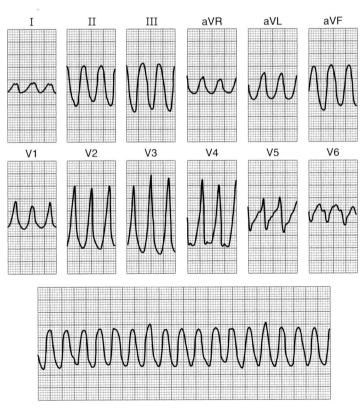

Fig. 9.16 Ventricular tachycardia. The QRS width (200 ms) suggests that the tachycardia is ventricular in origin. For further discussion see text.

Non-sustained ventricular tachycardia

Non-sustained ventricular tachycardia is defined as three or more ventricular complexes occurring in succession at a rate greater than 100 beats/min. It is frequently a manifestation of underlying ventricular damage. In such patients it is a serious adverse prognostic risk factor for sudden death. Episodes may be asymptomatic or cause only minor palpitations, but should nonetheless be taken seriously.

Antiarrhythmic drug treatment has not been found to be effective in preventing sudden death. Two trials have shown that patients with non-sustained VT and impaired ventricular function (ejection fraction <35%) as a consequence of previous infarction may benefit from an implantable defibrillator. NICE recommends that such patients should undergo electrophysiological testing and that patients in whom sustained ventricular tachycardia can be induced should receive an implantable defibrillator (p. 194)

Benign ventricular tachycardias

Although ventricular tachycardia is most commonly indicative of serious underlying heart disease, there are some uncommon types of ventricular tachycardia which arise in patients with no discernible underlying cardiac pathology.

The commonest form is *right ventricular outflow tachycardia*. This shows a characteristic ECG morphology with left bundle branch block, and an axis directed inferiorly (leads II, III and AVF positive) (Fig. 9.17). Characteristically, episodes of tachycardia are provoked by adrenergic stress and exercise. Accordingly, the best means of treatment is beta-blockade. In patients with refractory symptoms, the arrhythmia is readily amenable to radiofrequency ablation.

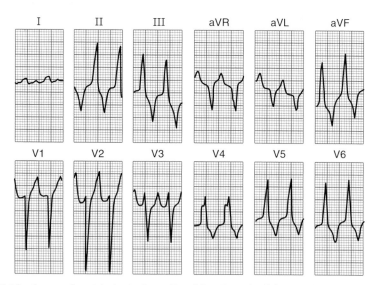

Fig. 9.17 A case of ventricular tachycardia arising from the right ventricular outflow tract. The characteristic features of left bundle branch block and an inferior axis in the frontal plane are evident.

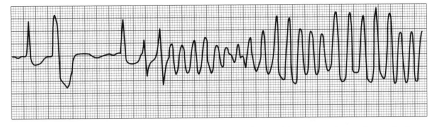

Fig. 9.18 Torsades de pointes. This is a form of polymorphic ventricular tachycardia in which the QRS axis undergoes progressive change. As a result the amplitude of the QRS complexes waxes and wanes.

Less commonly, a further form of benign ventricular tachycardia arises within the left ventricle, characteristically within the posterior fascicle of the left bundle and is termed *fascicular tachycardia*. The resultant arrhythmia consequently shows a right bundle branch block morphology accompanying left axis deviation. The arrhythmia is once again amenable to radiofrequency ablation.

Torsades de pointes (Fig. 9.18)

This distinctive type of ventricular tachycardia is associated with a long QT interval, which most frequently arises due to the action of such drugs as tricyclic antidepressants and type Ia antiarrhythmics, often in the presence of hypokalaemia. Its characteristic ECG feature is 'twisting of the points' of the QRS complexes. It usually occurs in repetitive bursts lasting a few seconds; it may progress to ventricular fibrillation.

It is particularly important to recognize this arrhythmia pattern for two reasons:

- Recognition should lead to a search for any underlying cause with withdrawal of any contributory drug or correction of hypokalaemia.
- Anti-arrhythmic drug therapy should be avoided. The problem is best treated by rapid atrial or ventricular pacing at 90–100/min.

The arrhythmia also occurs in a congenital form in the *hereditary long QT syndrome*. This is a group of single gene disorders of ion channels, resulting in prolongation of repolarization and a susceptibility of affected individuals to torsades de pointes and sudden death. It should be considered as a potential cause of sudden death in patients with ostensibly normal hearts. The disorder is most commonly dominantly inherited and relatives of affected individuals should be screened.

Ventricular fibrillation (Fig. 9.19)

In this condition, there is a chaotic electrical disturbance of the ventricles, with impulses occurring irregularly at a rate of 300–500/min. Ventricular contraction is uncoordinated and ventricular filling and emptying cease. The cardiac output falls precipitously to zero.

Ventricular fibrillation is the commonest cause of sudden death. It may occur as a primary arrhythmia or as a complication of acute myocardial infarction.

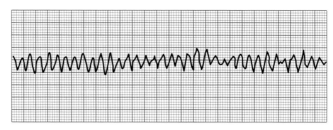

Fig. 9.19 Ventricular fibrillation.

It may also result from drowning, electrocution and overdosage of drugs including digitalis, adrenaline (epinephrine) and isoprenaline. Self-terminating episodes are rare but may complicate complete heart block.

Because of its catastrophic effects, ventricular fibrillation gives rise to the clinical features of cardiac arrest, with sudden disappearance of arterial pulses, cessation of respiration, loss of consciousness and dilatation of the pupils. Although it cannot be diagnosed clinically, it is to be suspected in any patient dying with apparent suddenness, particularly in the context of acute myocardial infarction. On the ECG, there is a chaotic rhythm with ventricular complexes of varying amplitude and rate (Fig. 9.19). Eventually asystole ensues.

Ventricular fibrillation is almost invariably fatal, and immediate treatment is necessary if death is to be prevented. As with other forms of cardiac arrest, an effective circulation and ventilation must be obtained with 4 min if irreversible brain damage is not to occur. Sinus rhythm can usually only be restored by electric shock, which should be administered as soon as possible. If an electrical defibrillator is not immediately available, the standard treatment of cardiac arrest should be started with closed chest cardiac compression and artificial ventilation (see p. 202).

In any patient who has had a cardiac arrest due to ventricular fibrillation, the cause of the arrhythmia and likelihood of recurrence must be considered. In some cases, for example ventricular fibrillation complicating the acute phase of myocardial infarction, recurrence may be unlikely. In others, a drug or metabolic cause may be established and corrected. However, in many individuals, ventricular fibrillation may be a manifestation of serious under-lying heart disease which is not correctable. Just as for ventricular tachy-cardia, antiarrhythmic drug therapy is largely discredited in this situation, and an implantable defibrillator should be considered.

DISORDERS OF CONDUCTION

Sinoatrial block and sinus arrest

In sinoatrial block, an impulse from the sinus node fails to activate the atria. This results in a dropped beat; on the ECG, a complete PQRST complex is absent, but the next sinus beat comes in at the predicted time (Fig. 9.20). It is of little clinical importance except that it may be a manifestation of intoxication by digoxin or other antiarrhythmic drugs. It may be a

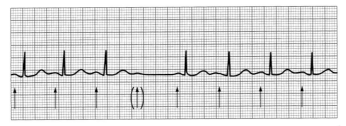

Fig. 9.20 Sinu-atrial exit block. The P waves are regular (arrowed). One P wave is absent (bracketed arrow), but the P wave rhythm is maintained without change in cycle length. The sinus discharge rate has therefore been maintained, although the impulse has failed to exit the sinus node.

component of the sick sinus syndrome (see p. 160). If it is prolonged, syncope occurs. In sinus arrest, the sinus node fails to initiate an impulse; after a pause, junctional or ventricular escape occurs. Its significance is similar to that of sinoatrial block.

Atrioventricular (heart) block

The term atrioventricular (AV) block implies that there is some defect in conduction of the impulse from the atria to the ventricles:

- In *first-degree AV block*, all the impulses reach the ventricles but they are delayed in their passage and the PR interval exceeds 0.20 s.
- In *second-degree block*, some impulses reach the ventricles while others fail to do so.
- In *complete heart block*, no impulses reach the ventricles from the atria, and the ventricles are under the control of a lower pacemaker situated in the junctional tissue, bundle of His, the bundle of branches or Purkinje tissue.

First-degree AV block (Fig. 9.21)

First-degree AV block occurs occasionally in normal individuals; it is a characteristic feature of the carditis of acute rheumatic fever and of digitalis overdosage. It cannot be diagnosed clinically and its recognition depends on observing a PR interval of greater than 0.20 s in the ECG. Its only importance is as an index of digitalis intoxication and as a precursor of the more advanced degrees of AV block.

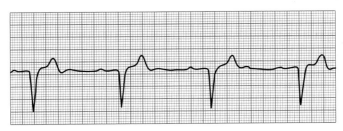

Fig. 9.21 First-degree AV block. The PR interval is prolonged at 320 ms. In this example, bradycardia (rate 40) and QRS widening (130 ms) are also evident.

Second-degree AV block

There are two types of second degree heart block:

- In the first type (sometimes referred to as *Mobitz type 1* or *Wenckebach block*) the PR interval becomes progressively more prolonged from beat to beat until one P wave is not succeeded by a QRS complex (Fig. 9.22). The next atrial complex is followed at a normal or near normal interval by a QRS complex and the cycle of events recurs. The pulse is correspondingly irregular. Second degree heart block may occur in many types of cardiac disease. It is particularly seen in inferior myocardial infarction and may also be indicative of digitalis toxicity.
- In the second type (*Mobitz type 2*), block occurs without progressive prolongation of the PR interval (Fig. 9.23). This is much rarer than Wenckebach block. Whereas Wenckebach block is indicative of diseased conduction in the AV node, sudden dropped beats, without progressive PR prolongation, suggest disease lower in the His–Purkinje system.
- In 2:1 block there is no opportunity to observe progressive PR prolongation and consequently it is difficult to categorize the site of conduction disturbance.

The main significance of second degree heart block lies in the liability of the patient to develop complete heart block and the Adams–Stokes syndrome. The more distal the site of block in the conduction system, the less reliable becomes the escape pacemaker if complete heart block develops. For this reason, the two types of second degree AV block are of differing significance:

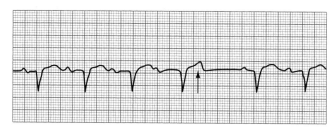

Fig. 9.22 Second-degree AV block: Wenckebach. Progressive PR prolongation is evident, culminating in a P wave (arrowed) which fails to conduct to the ventricle.

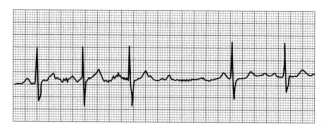

Fig. 9.23 Second-degree AV block: Mobitz 2. A P wave fails to conduct to the ventricles, without any progressive PR prolongation beforehand. The tracing is taken from a Holter recording and high frequency artefact is apparent.

- *Sudden dropped beats (Mobitz 2)* indicate disease low in the conduction system and a risk of a poor escape rhythm, should complete heart block develop. They are therefore an indication for pacing.
- *Progressive PR prolongation (Mobitz 1)*, on the other hand, indicate AV node disease, is more likely to be succeeded by a satisfactory ventricular escape rhythm, should complete block occur. Pacing, therefore, generally is unnecessary.

Occasionally, the slow heart rate accompanying second-degree AV block is responsible for clinical deterioration and the heart must be accelerated. This may be achieved by administering atropine or by artificial pacing.

Complete AV (heart) block (Fig. 9.24)

The ventricular rate is slow (25–50/min). There are cannon waves in the venous pulse (see p. 29) and a varying first heart sound (see p. 34).

Acute complete heart block is most commonly a complication of myocardial infarction, but may also result from cardiac surgery and myocarditis. In myocardial infarction, it usually follows occlusion of the right coronary artery which is responsible for the blood supply of the junctional tissue and bundle of His (see also p. 123). The severely damaged heart may not be able to compensate adequately for the bradycardia by increasing its stroke volume; heart failure and hypotension may ensue.

In most cases of chronic complete heart block, there is fibrosis of both bundle branches of unknown cause. This variety is most commonly seen in the elderly. A congenital form occurs either as an isolated finding or in association with other congenital heart defects. Heart block can also complicate rheumatic or ischaemic heart disease, or follow trauma to the conducting tissue at surgery.

A proportion of patients with chronic complete heart block survive for years with no symptoms, but once heart failure or syncopal attacks of the Adams–Stokes variety develop, the expectation of life, if left untreated, is usually only a few months. For this reason, an artificial pacemaker is indicated when symptoms arise.

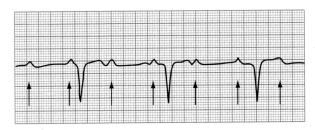

Fig. 9.24 Complete heart block, P waves (arrowed) are completely dissociated from the QRS complexes.

Bundle branch block

In this condition, either the right or the left branch of the bundle of His is not conducting impulses.

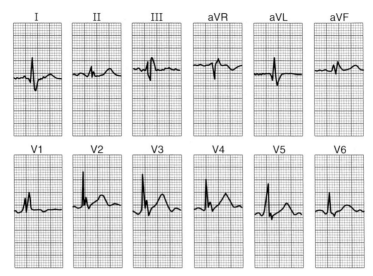

Fig. 9.25 Right bundle branch block and RsR' pattern is evident in lead V1. There is a late S wave in lead V6.

Right bundle branch block

Block of the right bundle branch gives rise to a characteristic electrocardiographic appearance (Fig. 9.25). This is often an isolated congenital lesion of no importance but may be associated with other congenital heart defects, particularly atrial septal defect (p. 278); in middle or advanced age, it is usually due to ischaemic heart disease or idiopathic fibrosis. Right bundle branch block may be partial, with QRS width of less than 0.12 s, or complete, in which case the QRS is of 0.12 s duration or more. It may be suspected clinically because the block leads to a delayed activation, and therefore contraction, of the right ventricle. This results in late closure of the pulmonary valve which can be recognized by a wide splitting of the second heart sound (p. 34).

Right bundle branch block is generally of minor clinical significance, except as an indicator of possible heart disease, and as a precursor of complete heart block (especially if associated with left or right axis deviation indicating block in one of the fascicles of the left bundle (see p. 124). There is, however, one newly recognized and very rare condition in which right bundle branch block is accompanied by ST elevation in leads V2 and V3 (Fig. 9.26) This condition, named *Brugada syndrome* after the brothers who originally described it, is associated with serious ventricular arrhythmias and sudden death. Patients with this ECG appearance are likely to require specialist referral for further investigation.

Left bundle branch block

Left bundle branch block is rare in the otherwise normal individual and is most commonly seen in ischaemic heart disease. It is difficult to recognize clinically, although there may be reversed splitting of the second heart sound (p. 34); it is readily identified on the ECG (Fig. 9.27). Because it is associated with severe ventricular disease (usually ischaemic) it carries a more serious prognosis than right bundle branch block.

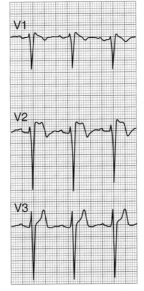

Fig. 9.26 Brugada syndrome. The pattern of right bundle branch block is accompanied by ST elevation in leads V1 and V2

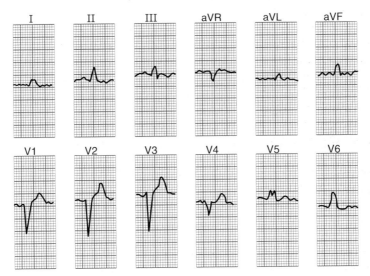

Fig. 9.27 Left bundle branch block.

INVESTIGATION OF RHYTHM ABNORMALITIES

Many disturbances of heart rhythm are transient and are not evident on a standard 12 lead ECG recording. One approach to detect intermittent disturbances of rhythm is 24 hour ECG recording. A continuous recording of two or more leads of the ECG is made for a period of 24 h. The technique is of value in the investigation of patients with unexplained palpitations, dizzy episodes or blackouts. The patient can carry out normal activities during the recording period and indeed should be encouraged to do whatever has provoked their symptoms in the past. An example of the usefulness of this investigation is shown in Figure 9.28.

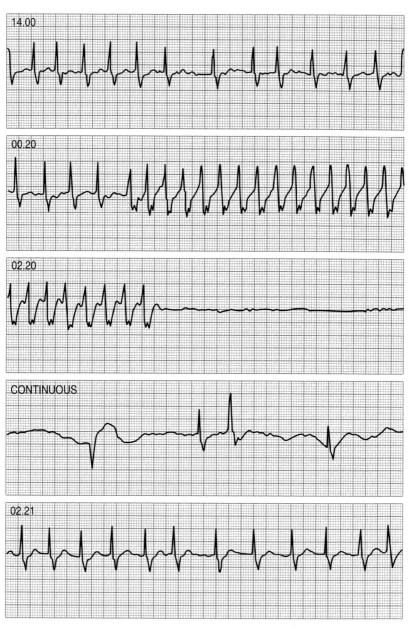

Fig. 9.28 The patient had a history of palpitations and syncope. On commencement of the tape (14.00) he was in atrial fibrillation. At 00.20 he developed sustained ventricular tachycardia. This lasted for 2 hours. On termination of the tachycardia (02.20) there was a prolonged asystolic pause followed by a ventricular escape beat. The patient subsequently continued in atrial fibrillation.

Syncope due to cardiac rhythm disturbance is characterized by sudden collapse with rapid recovery of consciousness within a few seconds. These episodes may also be referred to as *Adams–Stokes attacks*. Such episodes are most commonly due to bradycardia, frequently to the development of complete heart block. It is particularly common during the progression from second-degree to complete heart block because the ventricular pacemaker necessary for survival may not have become firmly established. In some cases, the Adams–Stokes attack is due not to ventricular asystole but to a short burst of ventricular tachycardia or fibrillation.

The presenting symptom is syncope with or without a preceding period of dizziness. The attack usually lasts some 10–30 s and convulsions may occur. During the attack the patient is pulseless, pale or cyanosed. Consciousness returns rapidly with reappearance of the heart beat, the patient then flushing as blood courses through capillaries dilated by the hypoxia of the attack. Attacks of the Adams–Stokes variety may be separated from one another by a number of months, but occasionally, a series occurs over a period of minutes or hours.

The diagnosis should be considered in any patient presenting with syncope, but can be very difficult to make because of the difficulty in recording an ECG at the time of the episode. Conduction disturbance with PR prolongation or bundle branch block in the ECG recorded between episodes may provide some clue as to the cause of the attacks. Twenty-four hour ECG monitoring may also prove helpful, but frequently the cause of the syncopal episodes remains unexplained.

In these circumstances, an implantable ECG loop recorder is of particular value. These devices, which are implanted prepectorally under local anaesthetic continuously record the ECG, which is looped through the memory of the device. Should the patient experience a syncopal attack, it is possible to 'freeze' the memory of the device on recovery. Subsequent interrogation should then be able to reveal whether there was any cardiac rhythm disturbance at the time of the syncopal episode.

MANAGEMENT OF BRADYARRHYTHMIAS – CARDIAC PACING

Control over the electrical activity of the heart may be obtained by the use of an artificial pacemaker (Fig. 9.29). A pacemaking system consists of a pulse generator (containing batteries and electronic circuitry) and one or more

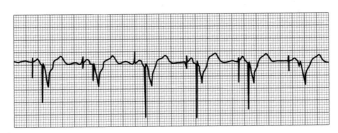

Fig. 9.29 Paced ECG. A dual chamber pacemaker is present, pacing both atrium and ventricle. The first pacing spike is followed by a P wave and the second by a QRS complex.

electrodes. If pacing is to be maintained for only a short period of time, an external power source is used; if long-term pacing is necessary, the pulse generator is implanted.

Electrical pacemaking is potentially hazardous. If the electrical impulse is of sufficient magnitude and falls during the period of ventricular repolarization, i.e. on the T wave of the ECG, ventricular fibrillation may be induced. This problem is overcome by the use of a 'demand' pacemaker which senses the patient's spontaneous beats and operates only when there is no ventricular complex generated by the patient's own heart. In the absence of a complex, the pacemaker discharges after a selected interval.

External pacing

In an emergency, pacing can be established through large patch electrodes applied to the skin. An electric current is passed through the chest from these external skin electrodes and the voltage gradually increased until it is of sufficient magnitude to cause myocardial depolarization and pace the heart. Unfortunately, this is inevitably accompanied by extensive skeletal muscle contractions, which are extremely uncomfortable for the patient. Consequently, external pacing should only be used as a short-term measure in emergency situations until an endocardial temporary pacing wire can be passed.

Temporary pacing

Temporary pacing is employed in situations requiring urgent pacing. It can also be used when the requirement for a temporary pacemaker is not thought to be long term, for example in the treatment of heart block in acute inferior myocardial infarction. The temporary pacing wire is generally introduced via the subclavian or jugular vein under radiological screening and its tip positioned in the apex of the right ventricle.

PRACTICE GUIDELINES

A description of the procedure for temporary pacing via the subclavian route follows. Where available, ultrasound guidance may be used to help locate the subclavian vein. The skin is anaesthetized about 1 cm below the mid-point of the clavicle, a local anaesthetic infiltrated upwards underneath the clavicle and then medially towards the sternal notch. A longer needle attached to a saline-filled syringe is then substituted and passed in the same direction, whilst aspirating. When the subclavian vein is entered, a guidewire is passed through the needle and along the vein, under fluoroscopic guidance to the right atrium. The needle is then withdrawn and an introducer passed over the guidewire. The guidewire itself is then withdrawn and a bipolar temporary pacing wire passed through the sheath. The pacing wire is passed to the right atrium. In general, it is difficult to advance the pacing wire directly across the tricuspid valve and this can only be achieved by forming a loop in the right atrium. The wire should be positioned along the floor of the ventricle with its tip in the apex. The pacing threshold is then determined by attaching the wire to an external pacemaker box. In general, the threshold should be less than 1 V, at a pulse duration of 0.5 ms. Occasionally, particularly in patients with a right ventricular infarction, it may be necessary to accept higher thresholds.

Complications of temporary pacing

- *Pneumothorax.* After any subclavian venous puncture, a chest radiograph should be requested to check for a pneumothorax. Angling the exploring needle as close as possible to the undersurface of the clavicle minimizes the risk of pneumothorax. In patients with severe respiratory disease, in whom a pneumothorax might provoke respiratory failure, alternative pacing routes should be considered (see below).
- *Subclavian artery puncture.* Even in the most experienced hands it is possible to puncture the subclavian artery rather than the subclavian vein. If arterial puncture should occur, serious consequences are rare. The exception, however, is in thrombolysed patients, where severe bleeding may result. As the subclavian artery is inaccessible to apply pressure, bleeding may be difficult to control. For this reason, where possible, subclavian access should be avoided, when temporary pacing becomes necessary following thrombolysis in acute myocardial infarction. Venous access for pacing can also be achieved by the antecubital vein, the femoral vein or the jugular vein.
- *Lead displacement.* This results in a loss of capture or variable capture and necessitates reposition of the pacing wire.
- *Lead perforation.* This may occur acutely during lead positioning or due to gradual erosion over a number of days. It causes a rise in the threshold and may result in loss of pacing. The threshold should be checked every day in a patient with a temporary wire to detect any change in the threshold which might indicate perforation. When perforation occurs it may result in pericardial pain and may, occasionally, cause cardiac tamponade. Diaphragmatic twitching in time with pacing impulses should raise suspicion of perforation.

Temporary pacing is only a short-term measure. Where subsequent permanent pacing is required, this should be undertaken as soon as possible.

Permanent pacing

Permanent pacing is one of the most effective treatments in the whole of medicine. This relatively modest procedure has the ability to be life-transforming, and in some instances, life-saving.

Pacemaker implantation is generally undertaken under local anaesthetic. After a prepectoral incision, the pacing electrode(s) are introduced into either the cephalic vein or the subclavian vein and then positioned under radiological guidance in the heart. Electrodes are positioned in the ventricle and in the atrium as appropriate for the particular patient (see p. 190). The pacemaker generator sits in a prepectoral pocket on the front of the chest.

After implant, most pacemakers are relatively trouble-free. Battery life is generally of the order of 6 to 8 years. Patients require follow-up on a regular basis to check on remaining battery life and on the satisfactory function of the device.

All pacemakers currently implanted are programmable, that is the cardiologist can choose the particular type of pacing programme that is most suitable for an individual patient. Programmable functions include:

- *Stimulus voltage and duration.* These factors are programmable to provide an adequate safety margin, exceeding the patient's threshold voltage. Excessive voltages should be avoided as these are an unnecessary drain on the generator and may lead to skeletal muscle twitching.
- *Sensing threshold.* In patients with an underlying spontaneous rhythm, the threshold voltage for detection of sensed electrograms can be determined. The sensitivity of the pacemaker is then programmed to provide an adequate margin of safety for detection of these electrograms. Problems may, however, arise if the pacemaker unit is made excessively sensitive – musculoskeletal potentials may be detected and misinterpreted as cardiac activity, inhibiting pacing. Most pacemakers have noise detection circuits which switch to fixed rate pacing when electrical noise is detected to guard against this possibility. Some pacemakers are *unipolar*, that is they record the heart's electrical activity between a single electrode in the heart and the can of the pacemaker device. Because of the wide separation of the two, these devices are more prone to skeletal muscle interference. More commonly nowadays, the pacing electrode incorporates a *bipolar* pacing electrode within the heart and such devices are much less susceptible to skeletal muscle interference than unipolar devices.
- *Pacing rate.* This sets the rate at which the generator unit will discharge impulses. Many units feature, in addition, *hysteresis*, that is the heart rate must fall to a lower value than the generator's discharge rate, before pacing will be initiated. For example, a rate of 70/min with hysteresis of 20/min would mean that a pacemaker will only start pacing when the spontaneous heart rate falls below 50/min, at which time pacing will commence at 70/min.

Hazards of pacemaking include infection and failure of the components of the pacemaking unit, such as batteries, circuitry and electrodes.

Dual-chamber pacing

Ventricular pacing successfully prevents bradycardias, but it fails to substitute for the heart's normal pacemaker function in two ways. First, the rate of the pacemaker is fixed and cannot adapt to the differing needs of the body, as for example during exercise. Second, the normal sequence of atrial and ventricular contraction is lost, which leads to a fall in cardiac output.

In patients who continue to have a normal atrial rhythm, these problems can be prevented by insertion of a dual-chamber pacemaker. Dual chamber pacing involves the use of two intracardiac leads, one in the atrium and one in the ventricle. This system ensures the maintenance of normal AV synchrony. The AV interval is a programmable function. The pacemaker may operate in a number of modes. In one, it paces both atrium and ventricle. In another, the patient's underlying spontaneous atrial activity is sensed and this is followed, after the AV delay, by a ventricular impulse. This system has the advantage that the rate of discharge of ventricular impulses is determined by the patient's own intrinsic atrial rate. Heart rate, therefore, increases appropriately to meet the varying demands of the body.

Dual-chamber pacing improves the exercise tolerance of patients with complete heart block in comparison with single chamber pacing. It also prevents the occurrence of pacemaker syndrome. *Pacemaker syndrome* is a problem which arises in occasional individuals with single chamber ventricular pacemakers. Patients experience transient hypotension and dizziness with the onset of pacing. It occurs particularly in patients with intact retrograde conduction from the ventricle to the atrium over the AV node. The retrograde V-A conduction consequent on pacing causes a 'negative atrial kick' and results in a more profound haemodynamic disadvantage than simple loss of AV synchrony.

Rate-responsive pacing

In some patients, particularly those with atrial fibrillation, dual-chamber pacing is not possible. A variety of rate-responsive pacing systems have been developed, to enable heart rate to rise with exercise in a single chamber ventricular pacing system. These pacemakers detect the onset of exercise and increase the ventricular pacing rate. Sensed parameters include the mechanical detection of vibrations, changes in QT interval of the ECG, changes in temperature of the blood returning to the right atrium and changes in respiratory rate. Rate-responsive systems have the advantage of increasing the patient's exercise capacity, in comparison with fixed-rate pacemakers.

Rate response may also be of value in patients with dual chamber pacing systems if the response of the patient's own sinus node to exercise is inadequate (*chronotropic incompetence*). Dual chamber rate-responsive pacemakers enable the normal sequence of AV synchrony to be maintained, with an accompanying increase in heart rate with exercise.

Pacing modes

The international pacemaker code

A three-letter alphabetical code is used to describe the mode of a pacemaker's operation. Each of the three letters of this code presents specific information:

- The first letter refers to the site of cardiac pacing – **A**trium, **V**entricle or **D**ual (both).
- The second letter refers to the site of sensing – **A**trium, **V**entricle, **D**ual or no sensing (designated O).
- The third letter refers to the response to sensing – **I**nhibited, **T**riggered, **D**ual (both inhibited and triggered) and no response (designated O).
- Additional letters can be added to this basic three-letter code to indicate a rate-adaptive pulse generator (**R**) or to provide information on the type of pacing lead.

Although numerous pacing modes are theoretically possible, in practice, relatively few modes are actually used. Examples are as follows:

- *VVI mode.* This represents single-chamber ventricular-demand pacing. A sensed impulse in the ventricle inhibits the output of the pacemaker. VVI pacing and VVIR (rate-responsive) pacing are the commonest choice of pacemaker worldwide.

- *AAI mode.* This is exactly the same as the VVI mode except that the pacemaker senses and paces the atrium instead of the ventricle. This mode is reserved for patients with sick sinus syndrome with normal AV conduction and hence no need to pace the ventricle.
- *DDD mode.* This represents a dual-chamber pacemaker and is the most sophisticated mode of dual-chamber pacing. The pacemaker can be considered as an AAI pacemaker which paces or senses the atrium with an added AV counter, which emits a ventricular stimulus if no ventricular impulse has been sensed by the end of the AV period. AV synchrony is therefore maintained during atrial pacing while the pacemaker will also 'track' the rate of atrial activity enabling the ventricular rate to respond to physiological changes in sinus rate. This, however, also represents a shortcoming of DDD pacing: the pacemaker will sense atrial arrhythmias and could result in an excessive ventricular tracking rate. To guard against this, a maximum tracking rate is programmed to limit ventricular response at high atrial rates. This can be achieved either by imposing a Wenckebach-type block in ventricular response or by programming the pacemaker to switch to VVI mode. This is termed *mode switching.* In patients with intact VA conduction, a pacemaker-mediated tachycardia can be generated by conduction of a paced ventricular impulse back into the atrium. This is sensed as an atrial event by the pacemaker, leading to ventricular stimulation and completing a tachycardia loop. This complication can generally be avoided by careful programming.
- *VDD mode.* The device senses in the atrium but does not pace. This mode is useful in the management of patients with AV block and normal sinus node function. This mode has the further advantage that it can be used in combination with a single-lead system in which an atrial cavity electrode is present on a ventricular lead. The cavity electrode senses atrial activity, but is not able to pace the atrium.

Choice of pacemaker and pacing mode

- *Sinus node disease.* In general, dual-chamber pacing is indicated. Single-chamber ventricular pacing is unsatisfactory as intermittent ventricular pacing may cause hypotension and dizziness, termed pacemaker syndrome. In patients in whom AV nodal conduction is not in question, single-chamber atrial pacing is satisfactory.
- *AV block.* Dual-chamber pacing is optimal. In patients with a satisfactory sinus node activity, VDD pacing can be substituted. Single-chamber ventricular pacing is in general suboptimal because of loss of AV synchrony, but may be acceptable in more elderly or sedentary patients.
- *Carotid sinus sensitivity.* As for sick sinus syndrome, dual-chamber pacing is indicated.

New indications for pacing

Pacemaker devices are increasingly being considered for a number of indications in addition to merely preventing bradyarrhythmias. Examples are:

- *Cardiac resynchronization therapy.* This is a new pacing indication, used in the management of patients with advanced heart failure. In addition to a conventional right ventricular pacing electrode, a second electrode is used to pace the left ventricle. As a result there is a more synchronous spread of excitation over the left ventricle, resulting in a more efficient pump performance. This technique is described in more detail in Chapter 8.
- *Pacing to prevent atrial fibrillation.* Some patients with paroxysmal atrial fibrillation can be benefited by pacing. Patient selection is difficult as it is only those patients with bradycardia-induced atrial fibrillation who consistently benefit. In addition, new pacemakers are becoming available with sophisticated anti-atrial fibrillation algorithms. These pacemakers are able to detect the onset of atrial ectopics, which in some individuals precede the development of atrial fibrillation, and then pace the atrium to suppress the ectopics.

GENERAL MANAGEMENT OF TACHYARRHYTHMIAS

A range of treatment options are available in the management of tachyarrhythmias. These include shock therapy, ablation and antiarrhythmic drugs.

Direct current (DC) shock therapy

The DC shock must be timed to avoid the vulnerable period. It is customary to arrange for the defibrillator to discharge 0.02 s after the peak of the R wave. A synchronized discharge of this kind is not possible when there is ventricular fibrillation.

PRACTICE GUIDELINES

Because the procedure is a painful one, an anaesthetic is usually given, except when there is ventricular fibrillation (because the patient is unconscious). One electrode, smeared with electrode jelly, is placed in the right parasternal region and the other either in the left axilla or posteriorly below the left scapula. The machine is charged to the chosen level and discharged by pressing a button on the electrode.

Many new defibrillators have the capability of delivering a *biphasic shock*. This decreases the current energy required to terminate arrhythmias and is associated with higher success rates in restoring sinus rhythm. The strength of shock needed varies with the arrhythmia being treated. It also varies between defibrillators because of differences in the nature of the biphasic shock profile in machines from different manufacturers.

Apart from slight skin burns, the procedure is usually free from undesirable effects. However, there is a danger of producing serious arrhythmias in the patient with digitalis intoxication, and it is wise to discontinue this drug for 1–2 days prior to electric shock administration if possible.

The indications for electric shock therapy are discussed under the individual arrhythmias, but electric shock therapy is generally effective for all types of tachycardia including atrial flutter, atrial fibrillation, ventricular tachycardia and ventricular fibrillation. Some cases of chronic atrial fibrillation are resistant to external shock therapy. A proportion of these patients can be reverted to sinus rhythm with a shock delivered internally via a catheter in the heart.

The implantable defibrillator

Implantable defibrillators have been developed which can deliver a DC shock to the heart to terminate episodes of ventricular tachycardia or ventricular fibrillation. The shock is delivered between the can of the device sitting in front of the left shoulder and either one or two endocardial electrodes within the heart (Fig. 9.30)

Device implantation is very similar to implantation of a simple pacemaker, but requires induction of ventricular fibrillation to ensure that the arrhythmia can be both detected and terminated by the device. This is carried out under sedation or general anaesthesia to minimize patient discomfort from the shock. Much lower energies are required than for external defibrillation. Shocks of 10–20 J are generally sufficient to defibrillate the heart and restore sinus rhythm. In patients with ventricular tachycardia, this can frequently be terminated by antitachycardia pacing, without the need to resort to a shock (Fig. 9.30)

Implantable defibrillators also have a pacing capability and are hence protective against bradyarrhythmias as well as tachyarrhythmias. Just as for simple pacemakers, single and dual chamber devices are available.

Implantable defibrillators are particularly expensive. Their use should be restricted to patients at high risk of sudden death. These patients fall into two categories: secondary prevention and primary prevention.

Secondary prevention indications include:

- patients resuscitated from cardiac arrest due to ventricular tachycardia or ventricular fibrillation
- patients with haemodynamicly compromising ventricular tachycardia
- patients with ventricular tachycardia with a background of severe ventricular impairment (ejection fraction <35%).

Primary preventon indications include:

- *patients with severe ventricular impairment* (ejection fraction < 35%), non-sustained ventricular tachycardia and inducible ventricular arrhythmias on electrophysiological testing. Recent evidence has suggested that the primary prevention category should be simplified and based solely on ventricular impairment (ejection fraction < 30%)
- *patients at high risk of sudden death* due to conditions such as hypertrophic cardiomyopathy (p. 226), right ventricular dysplasia (p. 232), long QT syndrome (p. 179) and Brugada syndrome (p. 184).

Catheter ablation (Fig. 9.31)

Catheter ablation has revolutionized the management of a number of arrhythmias. Radiofrequency current is passed down an electrode catheter positioned in contact with the endocardium, producing a small area of thermal tissue destruction. The technique can be used in the management of a number of arrhythmias:

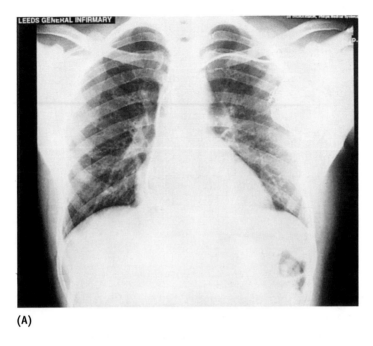

(A)

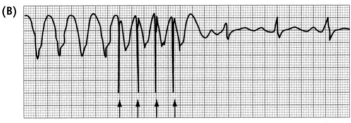

(B)

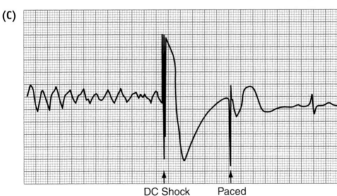

(C)

DC Shock   Paced

Fig. 9.30 Implanted defibrillator. (A) Chest X-ray in a patient with a prepectoral defibrillator. The shock is delivered between the coil in the right ventricle and the 'active' can of the device. (B) Ventricular tachycardia terminated by a train of four extrastimuli. (C) Ventricular fibrillation terminated by a DC shock delivered by the device (arrowed). The first beat after delivery of the shock is paced.

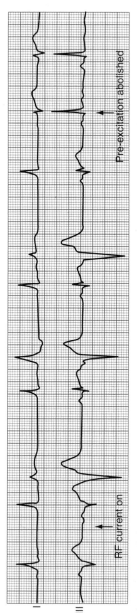

Fig. 9.31 Radiofrequency ablation of an accessory pathway in a patient with Wolff–Parkinson–White syndrome. Six seconds after commencing current application accessory pathway conduction is abolished, with loss of the delta wave and prolongation of the PR interval.

- *Accessory pathways*, whether *overt* (in patients with Wolff–Parkinson–White syndrome) or *concealed* (only conducting from ventricle to atrium and hence not causing pre-excitation) can be successfully destroyed thereby preventing arrhythmia recurrence.
- *AV node re-entrant tachycardia*, the re-entry circuit can be interrupted by destroying one of the pathways through the AV node. With this technique, there is a small risk of complete destruction of the AV node, resulting in complete heart block and the need for permanent pacing.
- The common form of *atrial flutter* is amenable to ablation by inducing a line of conduction block across the isthmus between the inferior vena cava and the tricuspid valve ring.
- *Benign ventricular tachycardias*, such as right ventricular outflow tachycardias (p. 178) are readily amenable to ablation. Success has also been reported for the other more common forms of ventricular tachycardia arising as a result of scar formation following myocardial infarction, but these generally involve widespread abnormalities in the ventricles and consequently recurrence rates are high.
- *Total AV node ablation* is an option in patients with refractory atrial fibrillation in whom drugs fail to provide satisfactory rate control. By ablating the bundle of His, complete heart block is produced. The atria continue to fibrillate but the ventricles are protected from the fast rate. Permanent pacing is necessary and dictates the rate of ventricular contraction.
- There is currently great interest in ablation to attempt to cure *atrial fibrillation*. Most commonly, this involves ablation at the ostia of the pulmonary veins at the sites of origin of atrial ectopic activity. In addition, in some patients, linear ablation is required within the body of the atria.

Antiarrhythmic drugs

The role of antiarrhythmic drug therapy has decreased in recent years, This reflects both the growth in alternative successful treatments for many arrhythmias and a growing understanding of the problems which may be encountered with antiarrhythmic drug therapy.

Before commencing a patient on therapy with an antiarrhythmic drug, it is essential to consider the advantages and disadvantages of drug treatment. As a group, antiarrhythmic drugs have the potential to do harm as well as to do good. It is well established that under some circumstances antiarrhythmic drugs may exacerbate existing arrhythmias or even create new ones. Particular caution is required in patients with structural heart disease in whom antiarrhythmic drugs can have unforeseen adverse consequences.

Antiarrhythmic therapy is used to:

- suppress or prevent arrhythmias
- slow the ventricular response rate in the case of supraventricular arrhythmias.

Antiarrhythmic drug classification (Box 9.1)

There are four main classes of antiarrhythmic drug action:

- *Class I 'membrane-stabilizing'* drugs, which also have a local anaesthetic action, block the inflow of sodium into the cell and, therefore, the rate of

Box 9.1

Classification of antiarrhythmic drugs

Class I Membrane-stabilizing drugs
Subgroup   (A)   Quinidine
                 Procainamide
                 Disopyramide
            (B)   Lidocaine (Lignocaine)
                 Mexiletine
            (C)   Flecainide
                 Propafenone
Class II Anti-sympathetic drugs
Beta-blockers
Class III Drugs that prolong action potential duration
Amiodarone
Bretylium
Sotalol
Dofetilide
Azimilide
Class IV Calcium antagonists
Verapamil

depolarization. This has the effect of reducing the automaticity of ectopic pacemaker foci and of slowing conduction, which may abolish a re-entry circuit.

- *Class II 'antisympathetic' drugs* – notably those that block beta-adrenoceptors.
- *Class III drugs that prolong action potential duration.* Amiodarone is the main drug in this category, although sotalol and bretylium also have class III actions; dofetilide and azimilide are two new drugs in this category but are not yet generally available.
- *Class IV drugs that block the inflow of calcium into the cell.* This affects the activity of certain cells, particularly those of the atrioventricular node, which are dependent more on the calcium inflow than on sodium. Verapamil belongs to this group.

PRACTICAL ARRHYTHMIA MANAGEMENT

Acute tachycardia management

For all tachyarrhythmias, if the patient is severely compromised haemo-dynamically, cardioversion is the most appropriate treatment. In less severely compromised patients, drug management may be considered. Drug selection is determined by the nature of the arrhythmia. A simple diagnostic algorithm to aid in the diagnosis of a number of common arrhythmias is presented in Fig. 9.32.

Ventricular tachycardia

Rapid ventricular tachycardias cause cardiac arrest and management is similar to ventricular fibrillation, with urgent DC shock in the case of haemodynamically compromised patients. In less severely compromised patients, intravenous drug treatment should be considered:

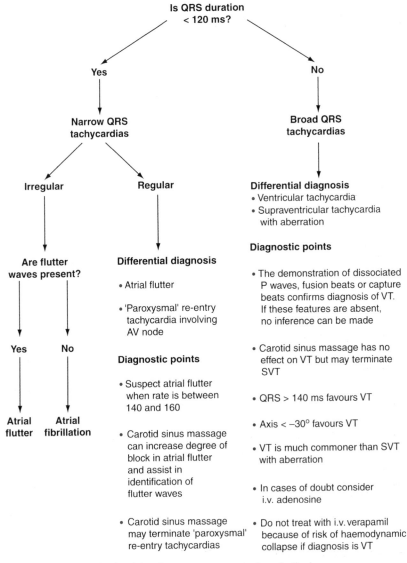

Fig. 9.32 Diagnostic algorithm for some common tachyarrhythmias.

- Intravenous amiodarone is one option as in the cardiac arrest protocol (see p. 205).
- Intravenous lidocaine (lignocaine) is a second option. Lidocaine (lignocaine) is relatively non-toxic and is unlikely to cause haemodynamic deterioration or to exacerbate the arrhythmia.

Undiagnosed broad complex tachycardias

The majority of broad complex tachycardias are ventricular in origin. A minority are supraventricular, with accompanying bundle branch block. The diagnostic features of ventricular tachycardia are described on p. 176. If the diagnosis remains in doubt, the patient should be

Table 9.2 Response to adenosine

Arrhythmia	Response
'Paroxysmal' supraventricular tachycardia	Termination
Atrial fibrillation, atrial flutter	Transient increase in AV block
Ventricular tachycardia	No effect
Atrial fibrillation in Wolff–Parkinson–White syndrome	No effect on ventricular rate, but increased pre-excitation

given intravenous adenosine. This terminates the majority of supraventricular tachycardias and is without effect on ventricular tachycardias (Table 9.2).

Adenosine should be administered as a series of increasing intravenous boluses, successive doses being determined by response of the arrhythmia. The recommended initial bolus dose for adults is 3 mg over 2 s. If the tachycardia does not terminate within 1–2 min, a second bolus dose of 6 mg should be given. If after a further 1–2 min, this too is unsuccessful, a third bolus dose of 12 mg should be given.

Transient side-effects, particularly chest discomfort and dyspnoea, are common. Occasionally there may be excessive bradycardia and heart block, but this generally lasts only a few seconds. Adenosine is best avoided in patients on therapy with dipyridamole and may be ineffective in patients receiving theophylline. Adenosine can provoke bronchospasm in predisposed individuals and is contraindicated in asthmatics.

Torsades de pointes tachycardia
This arrhythmia is generally a manifestation of drug toxicity or metabolic disturbance. It is frequently multifactorial in origin. Episodes causing collapse and loss of consciousness may require DC shock, although the arrhythmia generally takes the form of recurrent, self-terminating episodes of tachycardia. The precipitating cause should be identified and corrected. Correction of hypokalaemia is particularly important. In many cases, bradycardia contributes to the genesis of the arrhythmia. This should be treated by pacing, at a rate of 90–100 beats/min. Atrial pacing is satisfactory but is more prone to lead displacement than ventricular pacing, which is more commonly chosen. If pacing cannot be easily instituted, then an isoprenaline infusion should be considered as an alternative.

Atrial fibrillation
If the patient is severely compromised haemodynamically, cardioversion may be appropriate. However, in many cases atrial fibrillation occurs because the patient is ill in other ways and, in these circumstances, the arrhythmia is likely to recur after cardioversion.

In most cases, drug treatment of the arrhythmia is appropriate. A number of options are possible. These options are alternatives – different antiarrhythmic drugs should not be combined:

- digoxin 1 mg i.v. in 100 ml saline over 2 h (or 0.5 mg orally, repeated after 2 h). Digoxin limits the ventricular response rate but has no direct action to restore sinus rhythm
- flecainide up to 2 mg/kg i.v. over 10 min. Flecainide is effective in restoring sinus rhythm in many patients with acute onset atrial fibrillation. However, the drug should not be used in patients with underlying structural heart disease or coronary disease because of its negative inotropic effects and potential proarrhythmic action
- amiodarone 300 mg i.v. over 30 min followed by up to 1200 mg in 24 h. Amiodarone is effective in restoring and maintaining sinus rhythm. The drug has the disadvantage of causing thrombophlebitis when given via a peripheral line and should hence be administered via a central line.

It should be appreciated that many cases of atrial fibrillation terminate spontaneously without the need for any treatment. This is particularly true following myocardial infarction. Episodes of atrial fibrillation related to alcohol abuse are also, in general, self-limiting and specific antiarrhythmic treatment is unnecessary.

When intervening either pharmacologically or with cardioversion to restore sinus rhythm, the possibility of systemic embolism should be considered. There is a risk of thrombus formation in the fibrillating atria, particularly during prolonged episodes of fibrillation, with subsequent embolism on restoring sinus rhythm. If atrial fibrillation is not causing haemodynamic compromise, a safer approach may be to control the ventricular response rate and anticoagulate the patient with warfarin, prior to elective cardioversion in 1 month.

Atrial flutter
The same agents used for ventricular rate control in atrial fibrillation can also be used for rate control in atrial flutter. However, pharmacological treatment is less often successful in restoring sinus rhythm and hence cardioversion may be more appropriate. In some patients it is possible to terminate the arrhythmia by atrial pacing.

Paroxysmal supraventricular tachycardia
This term encompasses a number of different arrhythmias, due to re-entry tachycardia involving conduction through the AV node (p. 163). Carotid sinus massage will terminate a proportion of these arrhythmias and should be attempted before drug therapy. If the patient is severely compromised cardioversion is appropriate. In most instances, the patient is sufficiently well to consider drug treatment. Intravenous adenosine is an appropriate treatment (Fig. 9.33). Verapamil 5 mg i.v. over 30 s (repeated after 1 min if necessary) is an alternative.

Atrial fibrillation in Wolff–Parkinson–White syndrome
Patients are frequently severely compromised haemodynamically. Cardioversion may well be necessary. In patients well enough to consider drug treatment, flecainide (up to 2 mg/kg i.v. over 10 min, maximum total dose 150 mg) is the most appropriate therapy.

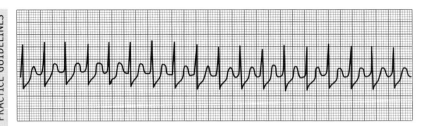

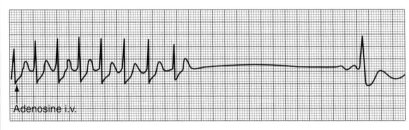

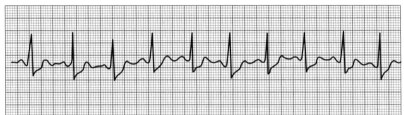

Fig. 9.33 A narrow complex supraventricular tachycardia is terminated by a bolus of intravenous adenosine. There is a 3-second pause on restoration of sinus rhythm. With resumption of sinus rhythm a delta wave is apparent, revealing the underlying diagnosis of Wolff–Parkinson–White syndrome. Continuous rhythm strips.

CARDIAC ARREST

Basic life-support

The term basic life-support refers to the simple resuscitative measures which any individual can undertake, without the use of specialist equipment, to restore an adequate ventilation and circulation following a cardiac arrest. It comprises:

- initial assessment
- airway maintenance
- mouth to mouth ventilation
- chest compression.

The purpose of basic life-support is to maintain the circulation until more definitive treatment of the arrest, generally in the form of a defibrillator, is available. The majority of cardiac arrests occur outside hospital and in this setting the provision of basic life-support pending the arrival of a defibrillator is of the utmost importance to improve the chances of a successful outcome.

The following sequence of basic life-support measures have been proposed by the United Kingdom Resuscitation Council.

Check responsiveness

The subject should be gently shaken while asking 'What's the problem?' or 'Are you all right?' If there is no response the rescuer should shout for help and continue with the resuscitative measures below.

Check the airway

It is necessary to open the airway by tilting the head backwards and lifting the chin. Any obvious obstructions such as dentures or vomitus should be removed.

Check for breathing and initiate respiration

The rescuer should look for chest movements, listen at the victim's mouth for breath sounds and feel at the mouth for any air movements. If the victim is not breathing help should be summoned, even if this means leaving the victim to call for help. Mouth to mouth resuscitation should be commenced with two *effective* rescue breaths. The chest should be seen to rise and fall with each breath. While pinching the subject's nose and maintaining chin lift, the rescuer should blow into the victim's mouth for 1½–2 s. If resuscitation aids are available, these should be used. Some rescuers may be reluctant to undertake mouth to mouth resuscitation on an unknown cardiac arrest victim. In these circumstances, there is still benefit to be gained from chest compression alone.

Assess for signs of circulation

After two effective breaths the rescuer should check for signs of a circulation, by checking the carotid pulse. If a pulse is detected the rescuer should continue rescue breathing until the victim breathes unaided. When this is happening, the victim should be turned on to the side into the recovery position to help to safeguard the airway.

If no pulse is detected within 10 s, chest compression should be commenced. For external cardiac massage the patient must be lying on a firm surface, either on the floor or on a board placed behind the chest. The heel of one hand should be placed on the lower part of the sternum and the heel of the other hand placed immediately on top of it. The sternum should then be rhythmically depressed, by about 3–5 cm, 100 times per minute. The action should be forceful and must be applied only to the sternum. Pressure by the fingers or the hand on the ribs may lead to fractures which may cause serious respiratory embarrassment or damage the liver and spleen. If the cardiac compression is effective, pulses can be felt in the carotid or femoral arteries and the pupils become smaller.

Rescue breathing should be combined with chest compression. After every 15 compressions, two effective breaths should be administered.

After every minute of cardiopulmonary resuscitation, chest compressions and breathing should be briefly interrupted to check for the return of a pulse and spontaneous respiration.

Advanced life-support

Basic life-support is a holding measure until definitive treatment of the patient's underlying rhythm disturbance can restore cardiac output.

Out-of-hospital ambulance paramedics equipped with defibrillators can provide definitive treatment. In hospital, this is the role of the cardiac arrest team.

Guidelines for the sequence of resuscitative procedures in advanced life support have been suggested by the United Kingdom Resuscitation Council. Patients can be divided into three categories according to their presenting arrhythmia in cardiac arrest:

• ventricular fibrillation
• apparent asystole
• electromechanical dissociation.

Although the specific treatment given to the patient will differ according to the mode of arrest, there is a considerable overlap of the general procedures which should be applied during advanced life-support. The most recent guidelines emphasise these common features and advocate a single algorithm (Fig. 9.34). Patients with ventricular tachycardia and ventricular fibrillation follow the right-hand side of the algorithm. Patients with asystole and electromechanical dissociation are treated together as 'non-VT/VF' on the right-hand side of the algorithm.

The route of access to this algorithm will vary from patient to patient. In some, basic life-support may have been ongoing for some time. In others, for example those monitored on a coronary care unit, clinical and electrocardiographic detection of arrest are likely to be simultaneous.

In patients who have had a witnessed collapse, a precordial thump is advocated prior to the attachment of monitor/defibrillator leads or if there is any delay in the administration of the first defibrillating shock. With many defibrillators, application of the paddles to the chest wall enables an ECG strip to be recorded, categorizing the underlying rhythm disturbance. In other instances, the rhythm should be established by attaching the patient to a cardiac monitor.

If ventricular tachycardia or ventricular fibrillation is confirmed, a defibrillator shock should be given as rapidly as possible. The patient should receive up to three shocks in rapid succession. For defibrillators with a monophasic waveform, these should be successively 200 J, 200 J and 360 J. For defibrillators with a biphasic waveform, the optimal shock energy is as yet undetermined and probably varies with the different waveforms employed in different units – the manufacturer's instructions should be followed.

If these initial shocks do not restore sinus rhythm, cardiopulmonary resuscitation should be commenced and continued for 1 min before the rhythm is again assessed and a further sequence of three shocks applied, assuming the patient continues in ventricular fibrillation.

While the sequential loops of the left-hand side of the algorithm are continuing, other resuscitative measures should be put in place. These should include:

• attempts to secure the airway with an endotracheal tube
• chest compressions at a rate of 100/min uninterrupted except for defibrillation and pulse checks
• ventilation at approximately 12 breaths/min

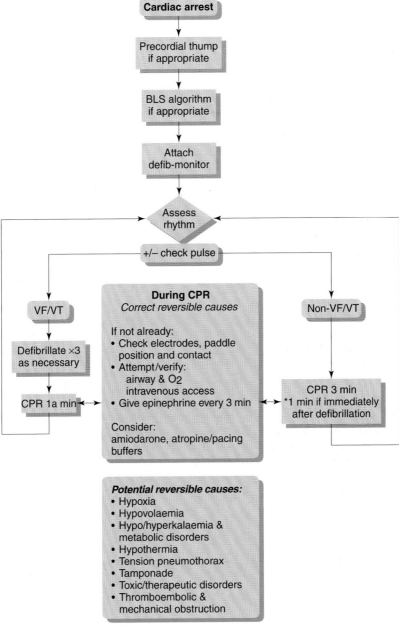

Fig. 9.34 Algorithm for advanced life support management. BLS = Basic life support. (Reproduced from Advanced Life Support Course manual, published by the Resuscitation Council [UK]).

- the establishment of intravenous access
- the intravenous administration 1 mg of adrenaline (epinephrine), repeated every 3 min throughout the resuscitation
- in the case of shock-refractory cardiac arrest due to VF or VT, amiodarone should be considered. 300 mg may be administered in this

emergency situation into a peripheral vein. Lidocaine (lignocaine) should not be used if the patient has received amiodarone, but can be considered as an alternative if amiodarone is not available

- intravenous magnesium (8 mmol = 4 ml 50% magnesium sulphate), which should be administered if there is any reason to suspect hypomagnesaemia, as for example in patients on diuretic therapy
- the use of bicarbonate (50 mmol), which can be considered if the arterial pH is less than 7.1 or if the cardiac arrest is associated with tricyclic overdose or hyperkalaemia
- changing the defibrillator paddle positions or substituting an alternative defibrillator may also be apropriate.

If the patient remains in VF after 1 min of cardiopulmonary rescuscitation, then three further shocks at 360 J or the biphasic equivalent are administered. The loop on the left-hand side of the algorithm is then followed, with each sequence of three shocks being followed by cardiopulmonary rescuscitation for 1 min.

Asystole
True asytole is uncommon early in cardiac arrest. When asystole does occur, it is generally the result of prolonged arrest and indicates a very poor prognosis. On occasions it is possible to be misled and to interpret ventricular fibrillation as asystole, if the gain control has been turned back on the monitor or if the leads are attached incorrectly. For this reason, unless the physician is certain that the underlying rhythm is true asystole, the patient should be defibrillated.

In cases of true asystole, patients should be given 3 mg of atropine i.v., in addition to the standard advanced life-support algorithm. Emergency pacing should be considered if facilities are available for this.

Electro-mechanical dissociation
Electromechanical dissociation is frequently a late event in cardiac arrest and indicates a poor prognosis. When electromechanical dissociation is the presenting feature it suggests the possibility of an underlying left ventricular rupture and it is unlikely that the patient will be resuscitated. However, there are also other causes of electromechanical dissociation which should not be overlooked, as these disorders are potentially remediable. Treatable causes of electromechanical dissociation include:

- hypoxia
- hypovolaemia
- hypothermia
- hyperkalaemia
- tension pneumothorax
- tamponade
- thromboembolism
- therapeutic or toxic substances.

Appropriate treatment depends on recognition of the specific underlying cause.

Management post-arrest

After resuscitation from a cardiac arrest, the patient should be carefully monitored, preferably on a coronary care unit. If the patient remains unconscious, it will certainly be necessary to protect the airway and it may be necessary to provide ventilatory support. Blood gases should be checked frequently. Electrolytes should also be checked and hypokalaemia corrected. Following an arrest due to ventricular fibrillation, potassium should be maintained in the high normal range.

FURTHER READING

Rescuscitation Council (UK) (2002) *Advanced Life Support Course*, 4th edn. London: Resuscitation Council (UK). Website: www.resus.org.uk

Bennett, D. (2002) *Cardiac Arrhythmias*. Oxford: Butterworth-Heinemann.

Almendral, J., Ormaetxe, J. & Delcan, J.L. (1992) Idiopathic ventricular tachycardia and fibrillation: Incidence, prognosis and therapy. *PACE* **15**:627.

Bernstein, A.D., Camm, A.J., Fletcher, R.D. et al (1987) The NASPE/BPEG generic pacemaker code for antibradyarrhythmia and adaptive-rate pacing and antitachyarrhythmia devices. *PACE* **10**:794.

Clark, M., Surtton, R., Ward, D. et al (1991) Recommendations for pacemaker prescription for symptomatic bradycardia. *British Heart Journal* **66**:185.

Fuster, V., Ryden, L.E. et al (2001) ACC/AHA/ESC guidelines for the management of patients with atrial fibrillation. *Journal of the American Collage of Cardiology* **38**:1231.

Griffith, M.J., Garratt, C.J., Mounsey, P. et al (1994) Ventricular tachycardia as default diagnosis in broad complex tachycardia. *Lancet* **343(8894)**:386.

Ellenbogen, K., Hayes, D. & Wood, M.A. (2001) *Cardiac Pacing and ICDs*. Oxford: Blackwell.

Huang, S.K. & Wilber, D.J. (2000) *Radiofrequency Catheter Ablation of Cardiac Arrhythmias*. New York: Futura.

Moss, A.J., Zareba, W., Hall, W.J. et al (2002) Prophylactic implantation of a defibrillator in patients with myocardial infarction and reduced ejection fraction. *New England Journal of Medicine* **346**:877–883.

National Institute for Clinical Excellence (2000) Guidance on the use of implantable cardioverter defibrillators for arrhythmias. *NICE Technology Appraisal Guidance – No. 11*. Website: www.nice.org.uk

Singer, I., Barold, S.S. & Camm, A.J. (1998) *Nonpharmacological Therapy of Arrhythmias for the 21st Century*. New York: Futura.

Taylor, F., Cohen, H. & Ebrahim, S. (2001) Systematic review of long term anticoagulation or anti-platelet treatment in patients with non-rheumatic atrial fibrillation. *British Medical Journal* **322**:321.

CHAPTER 10

Diseases of the pericardium

The pericardium has several functions: it helps to fix the heart and prevent excessive movement, it acts as a barrier against the spread of infection and malignancy from adjacent organs, and it reduces friction between the heart and its neighbouring tissues. It also limits acute cardiac dilatation and plays a part in the distribution and equalization of hydrostatic forces on the heart, being responsible for 'diastolic coupling', such that the diastolic pressures in the two ventricles are closely correlated when the pericardium is intact, but not when it is absent.

PATHOLOGY

Pericardial disease, which may be acute or chronic, is usually associated either with a generalized disorder or with pulmonary disease. Pericarditis may be fibrinous, purulent or constrictive and have the following pathological characteristics:

- In acute fibrinous pericarditis, the serous pericardium is inflamed and covered with an adherent layer of fibrin. There may be an accompanying effusion.
- In purulent pericarditis, there is usually a thick fibrinous exudate containing polymorphonuclear cells and organisms.
- In pericardial constriction, the pericardium is a dense mass of fibrous tissue which is often heavily calcified. Sometimes a mixed picture of effusion and constriction is seen ('effusive–constrictive pericarditis').

ACUTE PERICARDITIS

The causes of acute pericarditis are diverse (Box 10.1). Frequently no cause is identified. It seems probable that most idiopathic cases are due either to an unrecognized viral infection or or to autoimmune mechanisms. The viruses most frequently identified have been of the Coxsackie B group, but influenza, measles, mumps, chickenpox and human immunodeficiency virus (HIV) may also be responsible. Purulent pericarditis usually results from the spread of infection from adjacent lung. Tuberculous pericarditis is preceded by infection in contiguous mediastinal lymph nodes.

Box 10.1

Causes of pericarditis

Infective
Viral – Coxsackie B, influenza, measles, mumps, chickenpox, human immunodeficiency virus
Pyogenic
Fungal
Tuberculous

Connective tissue disorder
Rheumatic fever (p. 341)
Rheumatoid arthritis
Systemic lupus erythematosus (p.353)
Polyarteritis
Scleroderma
Sarcoid (p. 353)

Acute myocardial infarction

Autoimmune
Post-myocardial infarction (Dressler) syndrome
Post-pericardiotomy syndrome

Neoplastic invasion

Metabolic and endocrine
Uraemia
Gout

Trauma

Clinical features

Chest pain is the commonest symptom of acute pericarditis and is characterized as follows:

- Its distribution simulates that of acute myocardial infarction, being central and sometimes radiating to the shoulder and upper arm. The pain may be most severe in the xiphisternal or epigastric regions.
- It is often sharp and severe, but may be aching or oppressive.
- Unlike ischaemic cardiac pain, pericardial pain is commonly accentuated by inspiration, by movement and by lying flat.

The most definitive sign of pericarditis is a *pericardial rub*, although this is not always present. A to-and-fro scratchy or grating noise may be heard in systole, mid-diastole and presystole, or in only one of these phases. It is often localized to a small area but varies in position from time to time. It is usually accentuated if the patient leans forward, with the breath held in expiration, but is sometimes heard better towards the end of inspiration. Although the rub may disappear with the development of the pericardial effusion, it does not necessarily do so. Other signs may include those of pericardial effusion and, occasionally, of pericardial tamponade.

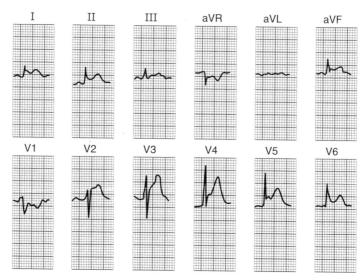

Fig. 10.1 Acute pericarditis. There is widespread ST elevation, with characteristic upward concavity of the ST segments.

Investigations

- *Electrocardiogram (ECG)* In the early stages, the ECG usually shows widespread ST elevation with the ST segment concave upwards (Fig. 10.1). After a few days the ST segment returns to the iso-electric line and the T wave becomes inverted. The ECG may simulate that of myocardial infarction, but Q waves are not seen and the ST segment elevation is of a different configuration (see Fig. 1.9).
- *Echocardiography* is frequently of value in the detection of a pericardial effusion, but the absence of a pericardial effusion does not exclude the diagnosis of acute pericarditis.
- *Blood tests* may be of value depending on the aetiology of the pericarditis. Viral and other infective causes of pericarditis are generally associated with a raised C-reactive protein (CRP). Even in the case of viral pericarditis, viral titres are generally normal in the acute phase and only become raised when the patient is convalescent. Autoimmune markers may be abnormal in cases of pericarditis associated with connective tissue diseases.
- Cardiac enzymes may be elevated if there is an associated myocarditis.

Differential diagnosis

Acute pericarditis is most likely to be confused with:

- *Acute myocardial infarction.* In differentiating it from acute myocardial infarction, the following points are of importance. The character of the pain, the absence of pre-existing angina, and commonly, the history of an upper respiratory infection or of pyrexia preceding the onset of chest pain are all distinguishing features. Q *waves* are absent and the concave pattern of ST elevation differs from the characteristic convex pattern of infarction.

Cardiac enzymes may show some degree of elevation if there is an associated myocarditis. However, this is generally modest and with a different time course from the enzyme elevation in acute myocardial infarction.

- *Pneumothorax*. In pneumothorax, the diagnosis can sometimes be made clinically by the detection of hyper-resonance and absent breath sounds over the affected lung or more reliably by the radiological demonstration of air in the pleural space. There is sometimes a coexistent pneumomediastinum which can cause a crunching or crackling sound with each heart beat.
- *Pleurisy*. The pain of pleurisy bears some similar characteristics to the pain of pericarditis. In some cases, a pleural rub may be evident on clinical eamination. More commonly, radiological evidence of a pleural effusion may provide the diagnosis. Pleurisy and pericarditis commonly coexist.

Aetiological diagnosis

Viral pericarditis should be suspected if there is a history of an upper respiratory infection and fever preceding the chest pain, and can be confirmed by the demonstration of changing titres of viral antibodies in the blood, or the culture of viruses from the stools.

Tuberculous pericarditis may be difficult to diagnose, because there is often no evidence of either pulmonary or miliary infection. Usually, however, there is a history of malaise and weight loss for some weeks prior to the pericarditis. Tuberculosis is unlikely if tuberculin skin tests are negative. If necessary the diagnosis may be confirmed by pericardial aspiration or biopsy.

In pericarditis due to staphylococci, streptococci or pneumococci, there is usually infection in the lungs or elsewhere in the body. In rheumatic fever, there is accompanying evidence of the rheumatic process as well as of myocarditis and endocarditis. In pericarditis due to hypersensitivity or autoimmunity, there is no preceding respiratory infection but there is often a history of similar episodes in the past.

Acute pericarditis may also occur in patients with acquired immune deficiency syndrome (AIDS). Some cases are idiopathic, while others are related to specific viral pathogens, particularly cytomegalovirus. Tuberculous pericarditis may also occur in patients with AIDS.

Treatment

This consists of the symptomatic relief of pain with antiinflammatory analgesics such as indometacin or ibuprofen and the treatment of the underlying cause when this is possible.

No specific therapy is usually necessary for *viral* or *allergic pericarditis*. Corticosteroids may be used to terminate the acute course, but their value remains uncertain. It is rare for acute pericarditis to be associated with a constrictive effusion, but in such cases, drainage may be necessary to relieve tamponade.

Tuberculous pericarditis requires prolonged treatment with antituberculous drugs; corticosteroids are indicated in patients with evidence of constriction. Pericardial constriction is common and pericardial resection may be necessary even during the acute phase if constriction develops.

Bacterial pericarditis should be treated with the appropriate antibiotics; surgical removal of pericardial pus may be necessary.

PERICARDIAL EFFUSION

Pericardial effusion may result from:

- *transudation* (in cardiac failure)
- *exudation* of serous fluid or pus (in pericarditis)
- *blood* (from trauma or malignant disease).

It is also a feature of myxoedema. The hydropericardium of cardiac failure causes few, if any, symptoms, although it may cause compression of the lungs and reduce the vital capacity. Pericardial effusion due to other causes may produce pain and pericardial tamponade.

Clinical features

Heart sounds are generally soft on auscultation. Pericardial friction rubs are uncommon in chronic effusions. If the effusion is constricting, there may be the associated signs of cardiac tamponade (see below).

Investigations

- The *chest radiograph* is valuable in diagnosis, particularly if several films are taken over a period of days – a sudden increase in the cardiothoracic ratio being very suggestive of pericardial effusion. When there is a considerable effusion, the cardiac silhouette is enlarged and rounded, with loss of the normal demarcation between the cardiac chambers (Fig. 10.2). Similar abnormalities may be seen in some cases of cardiac failure, but the

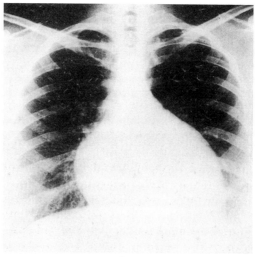

Fig. 10.2 Chest X-ray of pericardial effusion. The cardiac contour is markedly enlarged with a rounded appearance.

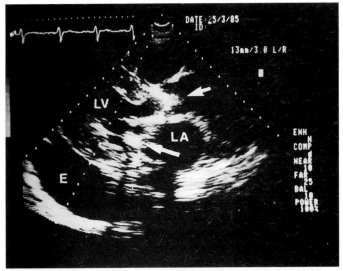

Fig. 10.3 Cross-sectional echocardiogram in the long axis parasternal view of a patient with a large pericardial effusion. An echo-free space is seen behind the posterior left ventricular wall. (LV: left ventricle; LA: left atrium; E: pericardial effusion). The arrows point to a thickened aortic valve and a calcified mitral valve.

presence of a very large heart shadow in the absence of pulmonary vascular congestion makes the diagnosis of pericardial effusion likely.

- *Pericardial effusion* produces low-voltage ECG complexes which may vary considerably in amplitude from cycle to cycle ('electrical alternans'), reflecting changes in the position of the heart within the pericardial effusion.
- *Echocardiography* is the most useful diagnostic method. When fluid separates the contracting and relaxing posterior wall of the heart from the stationary posterior pericardium, an echo-free space is produced (Fig. 10.3). Similarly, the anterior wall of the heart is separated from the chest wall.

Treatment

Paracentesis may occasionally be required for diagnostic purposes, e.g. to identify a causative organism. No specific treatment is required for a pericardial effusion unless there is tamponade. Otherwise treatment is of the underlying condition.

PERICARDIAL TAMPONADE

The pericardium does not normally impede ventricular distension during diastole. An accumulation of pericardial fluid, or pericardial fibrosis or calcification may prevent adequate filling. This may develop acutely, as when the pericardium fills with fluid, or slowly, as in chronic pericardial constriction. Probably the commonest causes are neoplasm and idiopathic or viral pericarditis, but it may develop in such conditions as uraemia, myocardial infarction, and after a traumatic cardiac catheterization, perforation by a pacing wire, cardiac surgery and chest injury.

The inability of the ventricles to fill during diastole leads to raised diastolic pressures in right and left ventricles, an increase in systemic and pulmonary venous pressures, and a fall in cardiac output.

Clinical features

Clinical features include:

- *sinus tachycardia*
- *elevation of jugular venous pulse*. A further rise may occur during inspiration – *Kussmaul's sign*
- *hypotension* and shock in severe cases
- *pulsus paradoxus* – variation in systemic blood pressure in relation to the respiratory cycle.

Pulsus paradoxus is an exaggeration of the normal respiratory variation in pulse amplitude. It can be detected on clinical examination. A major artery (carotid or femoral) should be palpated. In pulsus paradoxus, there is a respiratory variation in pulse amplitude, with a decrease on inspiration. A more reliable approach is to assess variation in systolic blood pressure using a sphygmomanometer. The cuff of the sphygmomanometer is inflated to 20 mmHg above systolic pressure and very gradually deflated. The Korotkoff sounds will be first heard in expiration. With further deflation of the cuff, the sounds will be heard equally in expiration and in inspiration. The difference between the two pressures is the magnitude of pulsus paradoxus.

Investigations

Echocardiography is the most important investigation in pericardial tamponade. Echocardiographic findings include:

- right and left atrial diastolic collapse
- right ventricular diastolic collapse
- inspiratory increae in tricuspid flow
- inspiratory increase in right ventricular dimensions and decrease in left ventricular dimensions.

Management of cardiac tamponade

General management

The management of cardiac tamponade depends upon clinical circumstances. In many cases, haemodynamic compromise may be relatively mild and no action may be required other than simple observation. Patients with cardiac tamponade require high right-sided filling pressures. Diuretics and vasodilators should be avoided. Further elevation of right-sided pressures with intravenous fluids may be of value and gain a temporary improvement in cardiac output while awaiting more definitive therapy.

In other cases of more severe haemodynamic compromise, intervention may be necessary. If the patient is not critical and if there is an underlying cause of tamponade which is likely to recur, formal surgical drainage with the formation of a pericardial window to the pleural cavity is most appropriate.

In cases of severe haemodynamic compromise, where urgent action is required, pericardial aspiration is indicated. In all but the most severe emergencies, the pericardial effusion should be defined with an echocardiogram. This facilitates assessment of the best approach for drainage, which in most cases will be subcostal. In a few cases, however, there may be a greater separation of pericardium from myocardium over the apex, and in these circumstances, an apical approach should be considered.

Pericardial aspiration – subcostal approach:
- The procedure should be undertaken under sterile conditions, preferably in a cardiac catheter laboratory.
- The patient should be sitting at an angle of 45° with the back supported. Local anaesthetic is infiltrated just to the left of the xiphisternum. An 18- or 16-gauge aspiration needle is then inserted, directed towards the left shoulder. Prior echocardiography can demonstrate the correct angulation of the needle.
- In cases with a small effusion where there is a significant risk of the needle perforating the myocardium, the procedure should be carried out under ECG guidance – a sterile, insulated wire with a crocodile clip at each end is attached to the needle and to a V lead of an appropriate ECG machine.
- The needle is advanced slowly, applying gentle suction until either pericardial fluid is aspirated or ST elevation becomes apparent on the ECG recorded from the needle – ST elevation indicates that the needle has contacted the myocardium (Fig. 10.4). A sudden 'give' will usually be felt when the pericardial space is entered.
- If blood is withdrawn, it should be observed for clotting to determine whether the fluid might have been aspirated from a pericardial chamber – fluid from a haemopericardium will not clot.
- Once the needle is in the pericardial space, a guidewire is passed and the needle replaced by a blunt cannula or a catheter such as a pigtail catheter.
- The catheter may be left in place for up to 24 h to facilitate drainage.
- Samples of aspirate should be sent to microbiology, cytology and for haemoglobin estimation.

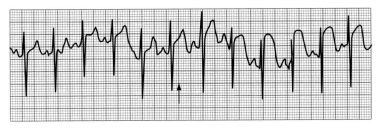

Fig. 10.4 Pericardial aspiration. An ECG has been recorded by attaching the V lead of an ECG machine to the aspiration needle. The development of marked ST elevation indicates that the tip of the needle is in contact with the myocardium.

PERICARDIAL CONSTRICTION ('CONSTRICTIVE PERICARDITIS')

Constriction of the heart by a fibrosed or calcified pericardium is relatively uncommon. In most patients, no identifiable cause can be found, although in some communities a tuberculous infection is responsible for the majority of cases. Constriction can also be a late complication of other types of infection, neoplastic invasion and intrapericardial haemorrhage, including previous cardiac surgery.

Adequate filling of the ventricles during diastole is prevented by thick, fibrous and, often, calcified pericardium. Although extension of the disease process may affect the superficial areas of the myocardium, the rest of the heart is usually normal.

Clinical features and diagnosis

The inability of the ventricles to distend during diastole leads to an increase in diastolic pressure and to a consequent rise in pressure in the left and right atria and in both pulmonary and systemic veins. The stroke volume is low and there is a compensatory tachycardia.

The onset may be subacute or chronic. Symptoms resemble those of right-sided cardiac failure. The presenting complaint is often that of abdominal swelling due to ascites, but dyspnoea and ankle swelling are also common. The clinical features are as follows:

- *The pulse* is of small volume and may exhibit paradox. Sinus tachycardia is usually present, but atrial fibrillation develops in the advanced case.
- *The neck veins* are grossly engorded and show two characteristic features; a rapid 'y' descent (Fig. 3.4, p. 30) and an increase in pressure on inspiration.
- *The first and second heart sounds* are soft, and there is nearly always an early diastolic sound heard best at the lower end of the sternum. This is an unusually early third heart sound associated with rapid but abbreviated ventricular filling.
- *The liver* is enlarged and often tender, although it may be difficult to feel because of gross ascites. In contrast with the severity of the ascites, peripheral oedema is comparatively slight.

Investigations

One of the most characteristic features of pericardial constriction is a shell-like rim of calcified pericardium, which is particularly well seen in lateral radiographs of the heart (Fig. 10.5). However, calcification is not invariable, nor does its presence necessarily imply constriction. The heart is usually small or of normal size, but is occasionally large. Computed tomography (CT) and magnetic resonance imaging (MRI) are of value, demonstrating thickening of the pericardium in almost all cases.

The ECG is not diagnostic, but usually shows low-voltage QRS complexes associated with flattened or slightly inverted T waves. If atrial fibrillation is not present, the P waves are often broad and bifid.

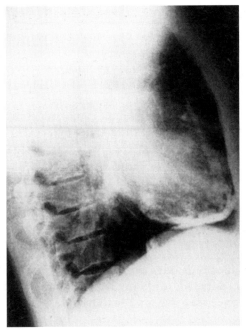

Fig. 10.5 Lateral chest X-ray showing a rim of calcification over the inferior aspect of the ventricles.

Cardiac catheterization reveals:

- raised left ventricular diastolic, left atrial, pulmonary arterial, right ventricular diastolic and right atrial pressures. Characteristically, the diastolic pressures are identical in all four cardiac chambers
- the right ventricular pressure pulse shows an early diastolic dip followed by a plateau (Fig. 10.6). This appearance is not specific to pericardial constriction and may be seen in restrictive cardiomyopathy.

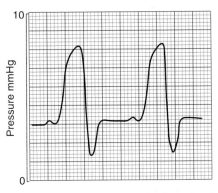

Fig. 10.6 Characteristic right ventricular pressure pulse in pericardial constriction. Note early diastolic dip, followed by a plateau.

Differential diagnosis

Pericardial constriction is suggested by a small and paradoxical pulse, a high venous pressure, a quiet heart with an early third heart sound and pericardial calcification, although not all these features are necessarily present. An important clue to the diagnosis is the combination of advanced right-sided failure with a normal-sized heart.

Pericardial constriction may be difficult to diagose. A number of other disorders should be considered in the differential diagnosis:

* restrictive cardiomyopathy
* other causes of heart failure
* pulmonary disease and cor pulmonale
* tricuspid stenosis and regurgitation
* superior vena cava obstruction
* hepatic disease.

The greatest difficulty is often encountered in distinguishing pericardial constriction from restrictive cardiomyopathy. Features which may help in distinguishing between the two are listed in Table 10.1.

Treatment

The medical treatment of the failure associated with pericardial constriction is seldom successful, although some improvement may follow the use of diuretics. Digoxin is of value only if atrial fibrillation supervenes.

The only effective treatment is surgical removal of the thickened pericardium. However, pericardial constriction sometimes occurs during the acute or subacute phase of tuberculous pericarditis, and preliminary treatment should then be undertaken with antituberculous drugs and corticosteroids. In some patients the pericardium may be densely calcified and adherent to the underlying heart muscle. In such cases, ultrasonic debridement can provide a useful surgical adjunct.

Progress following pericardiectomy is usually satisfactory but may not be so if there has been extensive myocardial involvement or severe liver damage. In such patients, a low output syndrome may ensue, resulting in a high

Table 10.1 Distinguishing features of constrictive pericarditis and restrictive cardiomyopathy

	Constrictive pericarditis	Restrictive cardiomyopathy
S3 gallop	Absent	May be present
Palpable apical impulse	Absent	May be pesent
Pericardial calcification	Frequently present	Absent
CT / MRI findings	Thickened pericardium	Normal pericardium
RV and LV pressures	Usually equal	LV > RV
Rate of LV filling	Rapid early diastolic filling	Reduced early diastolic filling

operative mortality rate. Pericardiectomy should probably not be attempted routinely in such patients.

FURTHER READING

Spodick, D. (2001) Pericardial diseases. In: Braunwald, E., Zipes, D., & Libby, P. *Heart Disease. A Textbook of Cardiovascular Medicine*. Philadelphia: Saunders.

Hancock, E. (2001) Differential diagnosis of restrictive cardiomyopathy and constrictive pericarditis. *Heart* **86**:343.

CHAPTER 11

Cardiomyopathy and myocarditis

The myocardium is involved in most types of heart disease. The terms *myocarditis* and *cardiomyopathy* are reserved for those relatively uncommon types of myocardial disease which cannot be attributed to coronary atherosclerosis, congenital or valvar heart disease or hypertension.

Myocarditis is used to describe inflammatory disorders of the myocardium due to infection and toxins. *Cardiomyopathy* is used for chronic disorders of heart muscle; the term may be restricted to those disorders whose cause is unknown, and the term 'specific heart muscle disease' for those of identified aetiology.

MYOCARDITIS

Myocarditis usually forms part of a generalized infection (particularly viral) but can also be due to physical and chemical agents (see Box 11.1). It is often associated with pericarditis. Occasionally, septicaemia may lead to focal suppurative lesions. Myocarditis is an important component of acute rheumatic fever (see Chapter 17).

Mild forms of myocarditis occur in a large number of infectious diseases but often cause only sinus tachycardia and non-specific electrocardiogram (ECG) changes. They may, however, give rise to arrhythmias such as atrial fibrillation or supraventricular tachycardia without producing other overt cardiac effects.

Pathology

There are three basic ways by which an infectious agent can lead to myocardial damage:

- direct invasion of the myocardium
- toxin production, e.g. diphtheria
- immunologically mediated damage.

In the case of viral myocarditis, immune mechanisms are predominantly responsible for myocardial damage, rather than direct damage caused by the virus itself.

Box 11.1

Causes of myocarditis

Infective
Viruses – Coxsackie B, cytomegalovirus, infectious mononucleosis, human immunodeficiency virus

Mycoplasma
Bacteria
Spirochaetes

Rickettsiae
Fungi
Parasites and protozoa

Radiation

Drugs – Sulphonamides, doxorubicin, lithium, emetine, cyclophosphamide

Heavy metals

Hypersensitivity states

Insect stings

Clinical features

The clinical expression of myocarditis varies widely from a subclinical, asymptomatic state to a fulminant and rapidly fatal congestive heart failure. Clinical features are as follows:

- *Chest pain* is common, but usually attributable to associated pericarditis.
- *Heart rate.* Tachycardia is common and may be out of proportion to any accompanying pyrexia or heart failure. In diphtheria, there may be a bradycardia due to heart block.
- *Heart failure.* The symptoms and signs of left and right cardiac failure may develop, with dyspnoea, gallop rhythm, cardiac enlargement and murmurs due to dilatation of the ventricles.

Investigations

- *Echocardiography and radionuclide imaging.* These may be useful in demonstrating ventricular dysfunction.
- *ECG.* Minor ECG abnormalities are common, but such changes may occur in infections even in the absence of myocarditis. Occasionally, there is ST elevation (due to pericarditis) or depression, or inversion of T waves, or disturbances of conduction and rhythm.
- *Laboratory investigations.* There may be enzyme evidence of myocardial necrosis. In cases of suspected viral myocarditis, evidence of an associated viral infection should be sought, although it is relatively uncommon to identify a responsible organism.

- *Myocardial biopsy.* Myocardial biopsy may be of value in confirming the diagnosis Characteristically, a biopsy shows an inflammatory cell infiltrate, accompanied by evidence of myocardial damage.

There is a risk of acute circulatory failure (shock) and of serious ventricular arrhythmias and sudden death.

Viral myocarditis

In Europe and the USA, most cases of myocarditis are thought to be viral in origin. In South America, Chagas' disease (caused by *Trypanosoma cruzi*, p. 347) is the commonest cause of myocarditis. A large number of viruses may cause viral myocarditis. Coxsackie B is a particularly common cause, but other possibilities include cytomegalovirus, infectious mononucleosis, influenza and human immunodeficiency virus (HIV). Myocarditis characteristically develops several weeks after the original viral infection, suggesting that damage is immunologically mediated.

The diagnosis of viral myocarditis may be supported by the isolation of a virus from tissue or fluid specimens, or by increases in the titre of virus-neutralizing, complement-fixing or haemagglutination-inhibiting antibodies. Endomyocardial biopsy is of some limited value in confirming the diagnosis.

There is a spectrum of clinical expression of myocarditis, ranging from mild local inflammation which may only be inferred from ST segment changes in the ECG, to fulminant congestive cardiac failure. The outcome after viral myocarditis is similarly variable. In most cases, the myocarditis is self-limiting and recovery is complete. However, in a small minority of patients, myocarditis may culminate in dilated cardiomyopathy as a consequence of virally mediated immunological damage.

Management

There is no specific treatment. Therapy is primarily supportive, treating the complications of heart failure and arrhythmias if they occur. Bed rest is advisable, followed by a period of restricted activity for approximately 6 months.

The role of corticosteroids remains controversial. Corticosteroids are frequently administered to patients with progressive disease who have evidence of an inflammatory cell infiltrate on endomyocardial biopsy, although the benefits of such treatment are not proven. Nonsteroidal antiinflammatory agents are contraindicated during the acute phase because they increase myocardial damage.

HIV

Clinically apparent cardiac involvement occurs in about 10% of patients with acquired immune deficiency syndrome (AIDS). Manifestations include myocarditis, pericarditis, endocarditis, dilated cardiomyopathy and metastatic involvement from Kaposi's sarcoma. Most cases of myocarditis are thought to be related to the HIV itself, although myocarditis secondary to opportunistic pathogens may also occur.

The term *cardiomyopathy* refers to a disease process involving heart muscle. A number of different definitions of the term are in common usage. The most widely recognized has been proposed by the World Health Organization (WHO) and restricts the application of the term cardiomyopathy solely to diseases of heart muscle in which the cause is unknown. This definition specifically excludes heart muscle disease arising as a consequence of other known pathologies or as part of a more generalized systemic disorder.

A more useful definition may be to divide cardiomyopathies into primary and secondary:

- *Primary cardiomyopathy*. Disease confined to heart muscle and not arising from any other identifiable disease processes.
- *Secondary cardiomyopathy*. Heart muscle diseases arising as part of a more generalized disorder, which closely resemble the clinical characteristics of a primary cardiomyopathy.

Systemic diseases associated with heart muscle involvement and resulting in secondary cardiomyopathy are listed in Box 11.2.

The commonest cause of heart muscle disease is damage as a result of myocardial infarction. This is sometimes loosely referred to as *ischaemic cardiomyopathy*, but differs from the true cardiomyopathies in the focal nature of the myocardial abnormality. Ischaemic cardiac damage following myocardial infarction is considered separately in Chapter 7.

Functional categories

Three types of functional impairment are observed in patients with cardiomyopathy (Fig 11.1):

- *Dilated*. The ventricles are dilated with impaired function.
- *Hypertrophic*. The left ventricle is inappropriately thickened, but contractile function is preserved.
- *Restrictive*. Diastolic filling is impaired.

Dilated cardiomyopathy

Dilated cardiomyopathy is not a single specific disease entity, but a final common pathway which is the end result of myocardial damage produced

---

Box 11.2 **Systemic disorders causing secondary cardiomyopathy**

Connective tissue disorders (systemic lupus erythematosus, scleroderma and polyarteritis)
Amyloidosis
Sarcoidosis
Neuromuscular diseases (Friedreich's ataxia, progressive muscular dystrophy and myotonic dystrophy)
Haemochromatosis
Glycogen storage diseases

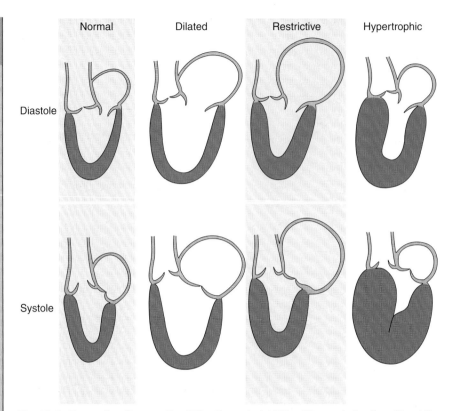

Fig. 11.1 Types of cardiomyopathy. (After Boon et al 1999, with permission from Churchill Livingstone.)

Box 11.3

Some causes of dilated cardiomyopathy

Infection
  Viral myocarditis
  Human immunodeficiency virus

Toxins and drugs
  Ethanol
  Anthracyclines (e.g. doxorubicin, daunorubicin)
  5-Fluorouracil

Nutritional and related deficiencies
  Thiamine deficiency
  Hypocalcaemia
  Hypophosphataemia

Pregnancy

---

by a variety of different mechanisms. In many patients no aetiological agent can be identified, but it is likely that a substantial proportion follow a viral myocarditis. Alcohol abuse is an important factor in many cases. Other causes of dilated cardiomyopathy are listed in Box 11.3.

Dilated cardiomyopathy can be familial. Although this is much rarer than the sporadic form of the disease, a detailed family history should be taken in all patients and, where appropriate, screening of other family members.

Clinical features
The major physiological defect is the decreased contractile force of the left ventricle, with slow and inadequate systolic emptying. The ventricle dilates and the pressure rises in the left atrium. Subsequently, pulmonary hypertension and right ventricular failure occur.

Patients usually present with dyspnoea and oedema whose onset may be abrupt or insidious. Clinical features are as follows:

- Tachycardia is common as are ventricular ectopic beats and atrial fibrillation.
- The venous pressure is raised and there may be systolic venous pulsation from tricuspid regurgitation.
- Cardiac enlargement is common and may affect both left and right ventricles.
- Third and fourth heart sounds are common.
- There may be the pansystolic murmurs of mitral or tricuspid regurgitation.

Investigation
- *ECG.* The ECG frequently demonstrates arrhythmias, as well as abnormalities of the ST segment and T waves. The absence of Q waves (suggesting previous myocardial infarction) is an important negative finding in ruling out ventricular damage due to previous myocardial infarction. Bundle branch block is common.
- *Radiograph.* The chest radiograph confirms cardiac enlargement affecting all chambers.
- *Echocardiography.* This reveals dilated, poorly contracting ventricles. Contractile impairment is global, in contrast to the regional impairment which occurs following myocardial infarction. Mitral and tricuspid regurgitation are common as a result of functional regurgitation from ventricular enlargement.
- *Cardiac catheterization.* The role of cardiac catheterization lies chiefly in excluding underlying coronary disease. In patients with severe ventricular impairment, catheterization may be necessary to assess the possibility of cardiac transplant.
- *Endomyocardial biopsy.* This is occasionally of value in confirming an underlying aetiology, but most often simply shows an end-stage fibrotic process, without providing clues as to the pathogenesis.

Treatment
As dilated cardiomyopathy is an end-stage process and not a single disease, there is no single, specific treatment. Alcohol should be severely restricted or forbidden. In secondary cases, where an underlying cause can be identified, treatment should be directed at the underlying disease process. More commonly, there is no specific treatment and management is the general

management of heart failure (Ch. 8). Drug therapies that may be considered include:

- *diuretics* which control the symptoms of both right and left heart failure. Loop diuretics are commonly used
- *Spironolactone* which conserves potassium and improves prognosis
- *angiotensin-converting enzyme (ACE) inhibitors* which are of value to control symptoms and to improve prognosis
- *beta-blockers* which are surprisingly well tolerated. They improve symptoms and may also improve prognosis. They should be excluded only in patients with the most severe degrees of failure
- *anticoagulants* which should be considered in all patients with dilated cardiomyopathy and are particularly indicated in the presence of atrial fibrillation.

Cardiac transplantation is indicated if disability is severe and life expectancy short (p. 155). Patients with life-threatening ventricular arrhythmias should be considered for an implantable cardioverter defibrillator (p. 194). Patients with a wide QRS, particularly those with left bundle branch block, may benefit from ventricular resynchronization using a biventricular pacemaker (p. 150).

Prognosis

The prognosis of patients with dilated cardiomyopathy is extremely variable. Many patients have minimal or no symptoms and have a reasonable long-term prognosis. In those with more severe or progressive symptoms, deterioration can be rapid. Amongst newly diagnosed patients referred to major centres, the 1-year mortality rate is 25% and the 5-year mortality rate 50%. Greater ventricular enlargement and more severe impairment of function correlate with poor prognosis.

Alcoholic cardiomyopathy

Excessive alcohol consumption is one of the commonest causes of dilated cardiomyopathy in the Western world. Myocardial damage may arise by three basic mechanisms:

- direct toxic effects of alcohol
- nutritional deficiencies, particularly thiamine deficiency
- toxic effects of additives (e.g. cobalt) in alcoholic beverages.

Identification of the aetiological role of alcohol is of particular importance because, in contrast to other causes of dilated cardiomyopathy, ceasing alcohol consumption can halt the progression of the disease and may lead to an improvement in ventricular function. In patients with associated thiamine deficiency, thiamine administration may improve ventricular function.

Hypertrophic cardiomyopathy

In this condition, there is massive hypertrophy of the ventricles. The hypertrophy arises in the absence of any obvious cause, that is in the absence of underlying aortic stenosis or hypertension. The increased stiffness of the left ventricle results in impaired diastolic filling. This in turn leads to an increase in left ventricular end diastolic pressure with resulting pulmonary congestion and dyspnoea, the commonest symptom in hypertrophic cardiomyopathy.

The ventricular septum is often the site of the most conspicuous hypertrophy, which may obstruct the left ventricular outflow tract (hypertrophic obstructive cardiomyopathy). The obstruction increases as systole progresses, and the more vigorously the ventricle contracts the more severe is the obstruction. An outflow gradient is present in approximately one-quarter of patients with hypertrophic cardiomyopathy.

Pathogenesis

The characteristic macroscopic feature of hypertrophic cardiomyopathy is heterogeneity in the degree of hypertrophy in different regions of the left ventricle. Characteristically, hypertrophy is more marked in the interventricular septum and anterolateral wall of the left ventricle compared with the posterolateral free wall. The left ventricle is generally more involved than the right. The left atrium is often enlarged as a result of impaired left ventricular compliance. Other patterns of hypertrophy seen more rarely are symmetrical hypertrophy with uniform thickening of the septum and free wall, and hypertrophy confined to the apex. The latter, apical hypertrophic cardiomyopathy, is particularly common in Japan.

Histological features demonstrated on microscopy include disorganization of the muscle bundles (*myofibrillar disarray*). This finding is present in almost all patients with hypertrophic cardiomyopathy. This disarray is evident both in grossly hypertrophied muscle segments and also in macroscopically normal segments.

Genetics

Considerable progress has been made in understanding the genetic disorders underlying this myofibrillar disarray. In about 50% of cases autosomal dominant Mendelian inheritance is present. Many of the sporadic forms may be due to spontaneous mutations.

The disorder is not due to a single gene. At least five different genes on four different chromosomes are involved. The first gene identified was localized to the long arm of chromosome 14, and subsequently recognized as coding for the beta cardiac myosin heavy chain (*CMH1* gene). The myosin heavy chain is the most frequent site of genetic abnormalities, accounting for about 30% of familial cases. Mutations of the cardiac troponin T gene and the alpha-tropomyosin gene account for another 15% and 3% respectively. The remainder of cases relate to abnormalities of as yet unidentified genes.

Even when the abnormal gene can be identified, there is a wide range of variation of phenotypic expression in different individuals, with a range of degree of hypertrophy and clinical symptoms. Nonetheless gene typing may be of value in predicting prognosis. Troponin T mutations cause particular concern, because they are associated with modest hypertrophy and yet carry a poor prognosis with a high risk of sudden death.

Family screening is an important part of the assessment of any patient with hypertrophic cardiomyopathy. In families in whom a particular gene

Cardiomyopathy and myocarditis

abnormality has been identified, this is of considerable value, enabling, for example, affected individuals to be identified in childhood, even before the disease becomes clinically evident. However, the fact that a number of different gene mutations can result in the phenotypic expression of hypertrophic cardiomyopathy and that many of these genes are as yet unidentified, means that there is no single genetic marker that enables the diagnosis to be excluded.

Pathophysiological consequences

The commonest abnormality in hypertrophic cardiomyopathy is impaired diastolic function. In a minority of individuals, there may also be a pressure gradient within the left ventricle. Two factors contribute to this gradient: a muscular sphincter action in the outflow and the abutment of the anterior leaflet of the mitral valve against the hypertrophied septum in systole. Outflow gradients in hypertrophic cardiomyopathy are characteristically dynamic, increasing under conditions of adrenergic stimulation.

Clinical features

The clinical features in patients with hypertrophic cardiomyopathy vary widely. Many are asymptomatic or minimally symptomatic, and may only be identified during screening of a relative with the disease. In more severely affected individuals, symptoms are often similar to those that occur in aortic stenosis, including dyspnoea, angina and syncope. Arrhythmias are common and there is a high risk of sudden death.

Physical signs are very variable, ranging from normal examination findings in asymptomatic patients without gradients to prominent abnormalities in patients with gradients. Physical signs include:

- a steep pulse upstroke due to the rapid ejection of blood by the hypertrophied ventricle during early systole
- the venous pulse which may show a large 'a' wave, reflecting impaired right ventricular complicance secondary to hypertrophy of the interventricular septum
- a possible double impulse on apical palpation, reflecting forceful atrial systole, or even a triple impulse, with the third component due to late systolic bulging of the left ventricle
- in patients with left ventricular outflow obstruction, evidence of an ejection systolic murmur, which is best heard at the apex or the left sternal border. The murmur is characteristically labile and increases with a Valsalva manoeuvre
- a pansystolic murmur of mitral regurgitation, which is additionally heard in some patients
- third and fourth heart sounds which are common.

The 'a' wave, fourth heart sound and presystolic apical impulse are due to forceful atrial contraction against the non-compliant hypertrophied ventricle.

Investigations

- *ECG.* The ECG is commonly abnormal. It may show ST/T wave abnormalities or criteria of left ventricular hypertrophy. The P wave may reflect left atrial enlargement.

Echocardiographic features of hypertrophic cardiomyopathy

- Non-concentric hypertrophy with asymmetrical hypertrophy of the septum (ASH); cross-sectional echocardiography demonstrates the asymmetrical hypertrophy and the obliteration of the ventricular cavity during systole
- In cases with a left ventricular gradient, systolic anterior movement of the mitral valve (SAM) and mid-systolic closure of the aortic valve may be evident (Fig. 11.2)
- Doppler echo can be used to measure any intraventricular pressure gradient
- Abnormal diastolic relaxation
- The presence of mitral regurgitation

- *Echocardiogram.* This is of great value. Abmormal features which may be seeen are listed in Box 11.4. Some of these features are evident in Figure 11.2.
- *Cardiac catheterization.* A systolic pressure difference can frequently be demonstrated between the body and the outflow tract of the left ventricle if there is obstruction. This difference is increased by drugs such as isoprenaline, which increase myocardial contractility, and may be abolished by drugs such as propranolol, which decrease myocardial contractility. Left ventricular angiography demonstrates a small left ventricular cavity with narrowing of the outflow tract and, often, mitral regurgitation.

Differential diagnosis

The murmur of obstructive cardiomyopathy has usually to be differentiated from other types of left ventricular outflow obstruction, most particularly aortic stenosis:

- In *valvar aortic stenosis*, the pulse is usually small and flat and there is either an early systolic click or calcification of the aortic valve. There may be accompanying aortic regurgitation.

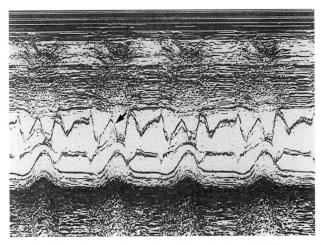

Fig. 11.2 M-mode echocardiogram in hypertrophic cardiomyopathy. The arrow indicates a systolic anterior movement of the mitral valve (SAM). The interventricular septum is grossly thickened.

- In *congenital subaortic stenosis*, the pulse is small and flat and there is frequently aortic regurgitation, which is not a feature of obstructive cardiomyopathy.
- The systolic murmur of *hypertrophic cardiomyopathy* characteristically increases during a Valsalva manoeuvre, in contradistinction to the murmur of aortic stenosis which decreases in intensity.

It is also important to distinguish hypertrophic cardiomyopathy from the 'physiological' hypertrophy of trained athletes (see also p. 357). Factors favouring hypertrophic cardiomyopathy over athlete's heart include:

- unusual and unequal distribution of hypertrophy (e.g. septal hypertrophy)
- decreased left ventricular cavity size
- left atrial enlargement
- abnormal ECG; although ECG abnormalities can also be seen in trained athletes
- family history of hypertrophic cardiomyopathy
- the persistence of hypertrophy on detraining.

Natural history and prognosis

The clinical course of hypertrophic cardiomyopathy is extremely variable. Clinical deterioration is usually slow. About 10% of patients develop left ventricular dilatation and progress to a dilated cardiomyopathy.

The greatest threat is sudden death. Identification of patients at particular risk of sudden death is extremely difficult; risk factors include:

- a family history of sudden death
- a history of recurrent syncope
- marked asymmetrical septal hypertrophy
- a fall in blood pressure on exercise testing
- non-sustained ventricular tachycardia on 24-h ECG monitor.

Management

A number of drugs may be useful in patient management:

- Beta-blockers are helpful in relieving symptoms of chest pain and shortness of breath.
- Calcium antagonists are an alternative to beta-blockade. Verapamil is most commonly used.
- In patients with frequent ventricular arrhythmias, on 24-h ECG recording, amiodarone is indicated, as there is some limited evidence that amiodarone treatment can prevent sudden death. Amiodarone is also indicated for the maintenance of sinus rhythm in patients developing atrial fibrillation.

There are in addition a number of non-pharmacological management options:

- In patients with refractory symptoms, surgical resection of part of the interventricular septum is occasionally indicated.
- An altenative approach is septal ablation. An injection of phenol is given directly into the septal branch of the left anterior descending coronary artery. This results in 'controlled infarction' of the septum thereby reducing outflow obstruction.

- Some patients appear to derive benefit from dual-chamber pacing. This can be thought of as changing the ventricular activation sequence, such that the body of the ventricle is activated earlier than the septal region responsible for outflow obstruction. A short AV delay is required to minimize activation over the His–Purkinje system, while maintaining normal AV synchrony. Although anecdotally, some patients seem to derive considerable benefit, this has not been borne out on a population basis in clinical trials.
- Patients thought to be at high risk of sudden cardiac death should be considered for an implantable cardioverter defibrillator (p. 194).

Patients should be advised to refrain from vigorous competitive sports to minimize the risk of sudden death. Patients should also be advised that the condition carries a risk of bacterial endocarditis and that antibiotics are indicated for dental procedures (p. 273).

Restrictive and infiltrative cardiomyopathies

Restrictive cardiomyopathy is the least common of the three major functional categories of cardiomyopathy (dilated, hypertrophic and restrictive). In restrictive cardiomyopathy, the ventricles are abnormally stiff and impede ventricular filling, with the result that there is abnormal diastolic function. Systolic function, by contrast, may remain normal.

While the cause of restrictive cardiomyopathy frequently remains obscure, it may arise secondarily to a number of pathological processes (Box 11.5). These may involve infiltration of the myocardium or endomyocardial scarring.

Differentiation from constrictive pericarditis

The haemodynamic presentation and clinical features closely resemble constrictive pericarditis (p. 216). Differentiation from cases of constrictive pericarditis may be extremely difficult, but is important because of the possibility of successful surgical treatment in cases of constriction. A number of features may help to distinguish restrictive cardiomyopathy from constrictive pericarditis:

Box 11.5

Causes of restrictive cardiomyopathy

Infiltrative
  Amyloid
  Sarcoid

Storage diseases
  Haemochromatosis
  Glycogen storage diseases

Endomyocardial
  Endomyocardial fibrosis
  Hypereosinophilic syndrome
  Carcinoid

- There is frequently cardiac enlargement in patients with restrictive cardiomyopathy, whereas it is unusual for the heart to be enlarged in constrictive pericarditis. An increase in left ventricular wall thickness may be evident on echocardiography in some cases of restriction.
- Computed tomography (CT) or magnetic resonance imaging (MRI) scan generally shows pericardial thickening in constrictive pericarditis and a normal pericardium in restrictive cardiomyopathy.
- Endomyocardial biopsy may show an underlying abnormality in cases of restriction.

Clinical features

Shortness of breath is the commonest presenting symptom. Other patients may present with signs of right heart failure. Features on clinical examination include:

- tachycardia. Because of compromised ventricular filling, heart rate increases to maintain cardiac output
- elevated jugular venous pulse, with a further increase on inspiration (Kussmaul's sign)
- enlarged liver, ascites and peripheral oedema
- S3, S4 or both.

Conduction disturbances and arrhythmias may occur if the disease process involves the conduction system. Sudden death is common.

Management

There is no specific therapy. Treatment is seldom effective and disease is commonly progressive. Use of low doses of diuretics and vasodilators may provide symptomatic benefit. Caution is necessary as decreased ventricular filling pressures may reduce cardiac output and cause excessive hypotension. In patients with eosinophilia, steroids and cytotoxic drugs may be helpful.

Arrhythmogenic right ventricular dysplasia

This is a rare form of cardiomyopathy involving predominantly the right ventricle. The aetiology is unknown, although some cases are familial. The disease differs from other forms of cardiomyopathy in that arrhythmias are the commonest presenting feature. Patients commonly present with features of palpitations, dizziness or syncope, although features of heart failure may also occur. In some cases, there may also be left ventricular involvement.

Diagnosis of arrhythmogenic right ventricular dysplasia is frequently very difficult. A number of investigations may prove helpful:

- *ECG.* The diagnosis should be considered in patients with ventricular tachycardia with a left bundle branch block morphology, suggesting a right ventricular origin. In advanced cases abnormalities may become apparent in the sinus rhythm ECG, typically T wave inversion in leads V2 and V3.
- *Echocardiography.* Echocardiography is frequently normal, but may show evidence of right ventricular enlargement.

- *Myocardial biopsy.* The diagnosis can be confirmed using myocardial biopsy to demonstrate characteristic fatty infiltration of the myocardium. However, the disease is patchy and is not excluded by a negative biopsy.
- *MRI.* is the most important single test in reaching a diagnosis, demonstrating abnormal infiltration, wall thinning and abnormal contraction patterns (see Fig. 4.27).

Management, in general, involves the control of any arrhythmias. Beta-blockers, particularly sotalol, are useful, although class I antiarrhythmics or other class III antiarrhythmics may be necessary. In occasional patients with localized disease, this may be amenable to radiofrequency ablation. The disease may result in sudden death, and in patients who are thought to be at increased risk, an implantable defibrillator should be considered.

FURTHER READING

Boon, N.A., Fox, K.A.A., Bloomfield, P. (1999) Diseases of the cardiovascular system. In: Hasslet, C., Chilvers, E.R., Hunter, J.A.A., Boon, N.A. *Davidson's Principles and Practice of Medicine* 18th edn. Edinburgh: Churchill Livingstone.

Cooper, L. & Gersh, B. (2002) Viral infection, inflammation, and the risk of idiopathic dilated cardiomyopathy; can the fire be extinguished? *American Journal of Cardiology* **90**: 751.

Gemayel, C., Pelliccia, A. & Thompson, P. (2001) Arrhythmogenic right ventricular cardiomyopathy. *Journal of the American College of Cardiology* **38**: 1773.

Louie, E.F. & Edwards, L.C. (1994) Hypertrophic cardiomyopathy. *Progress in Cardiovascular Diseases* **36**: 275.

Maron, B. (2002) Hypertrophic cardiomyopathy: a systematic review. *Journal of the American Medical Association* **287**: 1308.

Shaw, T., Elliott, P. & McKenna, W. (2002) Dilated cardiomyopathy; a genetically heterogeneous disease. *Lancet* **360**: 654.

Wynne, J. & Braunwald, E. (2001) The cardiomyopathies and myocarditides In: Braunwald, E., Zipes, D. & Libby, P. *Heart Disease. A Textbook of Cardiovascular Medicine.* Philadelphia: Saunders.

Disorders of the cardiac valves

Disorders of the cardiac valves may be secondary to a number of inflammatory, degenerative or infective processes. As a result of disease, a valve may become stenotic (when it fails to open normally) or regurgitant (when it fails to close normally). The causes and consequences of stenosis and regurgitation of each of the four heart valves are discussed below. This is followed by a description of infective endocarditis which may involve any of the heart valves.

MITRAL VALVE DISEASE

The normal mitral valve (Fig. 12.1) consists of the valve ring, two unequal cusps (leaflets), chordae tendineae and papillary muscles. The larger anteromedial (or aortic) cusp is interposed between the mitral and aortic orifices, and forms part of the outflow tract of the left ventricle (Fig. 12.2). The circumference of the valve is approximately 10 cm and the length of the commissure (where the two leaflets are in contact with each other) is approximately 4 cm. The papillary muscles arise from the ventricular wall opposite the commissures and are attached to the cusps on either side of the commissures by the chordae tendineae (Fig. 12.3). The chordae are collagenous strands, which, when tensed by the contracting papillary muscles, prevent the cusps from prolapsing into the left atrium during ventricular systole.

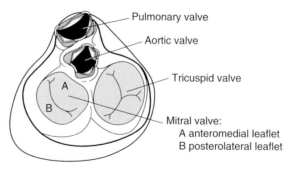

Fig. 12.1 Appearances of the heart valves during systole, with the atria and great vessels removed. The heart is viewed from above, with the left ventricle and mitral valve on the left.

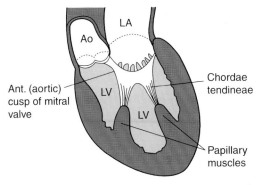

Fig. 12.2 Diagrammatic representation of relationships of left atrium (LA), left ventricle (LV) and aorta (Ao). Note the aortic cusp of the mitral valve separates the mitral valve orifice from the outflow tract of the left ventricle.

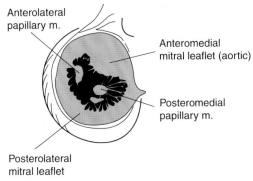

Fig. 12.3 Open mitral valve viewed from the left atrium. Note that the papillary muscles arise opposite the commissures and are attached to the cusps on either side of the commissures by the chordae tendineae.

Chronic mitral valve disease may take the form of mitral stenosis with or without some degree of regurgitation, in which case it is virtually always the consequence of rheumatic endocarditis. Pure mitral regurgitation in Western countries is seldom rheumatic in origin; mitral valve prolapse is the common abnormality. Regurgitation may also be due to ruptured or defective chordae tendineae, papillary muscles or valve cusps, or to dilatation of the valve ring following left ventricular enlargement from a variety of causes.

Mitral stenosis

Pathology
Mitral stenosis is usually the result of recurrent rheumatic inflammation followed by healing. The leaflets adhere at their commissures, leaving a central orifice. In some instances the valve cusps remain pliant and mobile; in others fibrosis and calcification make them rigid. In about 10% of cases severe shortening of the chordae tendineae produces a funnel-shaped orifice.

Pathophysiology
Serious haemodynamic consequences develop only when the mitral valve orifice is reduced from the normal size of approximately 5 cm^2 to about

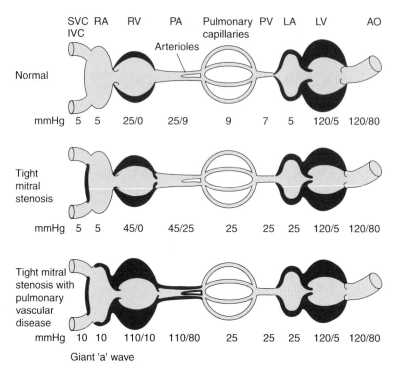

	SVC RA IVC	RV	PA	Pulmonary capillaries	PV	LA	LV	AO
Normal			Arterioles					
mmHg	5 5	25/0	25/9	9	7	5	120/5	120/80
Tight mitral stenosis								
mmHg	5 5	45/0	45/25	25	25	25	120/5	120/80
Tight mitral stenosis with pulmonary vascular disease								
mmHg	10 10	110/10	110/80	25	25	25	120/5	120/80

Giant 'a' wave

Fig. 12.4 The haemodynamic effects of mitral stenosis. In the normal heart, the pressure in the left atrium is similar to that of the left ventricle during ventricular diastole. With the development of mitral stenosis, the pressure in the left atrium rises, and this rise is transmitted to the pulmonary veins, capillaries and arteries. When pulmonary vascular disease develops, there is a narrowing of the pulmonary arterioles which leads to a disproportionate rise in the pulmonary arterial and right ventricular systolic pressures. With right ventricular failure, both the right ventricular end-diastolic pressure and the mean atrial pressure may rise to 10 mmHg.

1 cm^2. In severe mitral stenosis, the orifice is a slit less than 1 cm long and 0.5 cm across.

In the normal heart there is little pressure difference across the mitral valve between its opening in early ventricular diastole and its closure. In mitral stenosis, a pressure difference develops which depends upon the area of the mitral valve orifice and the volume of blood flowing through it (Fig. 12.4).

When the stenosis is relatively mild, the mean pressure in the left atrium may be normal at rest (i.e. less than 12 mmHg) but increases on exercise as the cardiac output rises. In more severe stenosis, the pressure is raised even at rest, and in the most severe grades is persistently elevated to 25 mmHg or more. The left ventricular pressure is normal, provided there is no disease affecting this chamber.

When the stenosis is slight, the cardiac output may be normal, but as the narrowing increases, the cardiac output diminishes to about half the normal value, and may not rise in response to exercise.

The pressure in the pulmonary veins and capillaries parallels that in the left atrium. If the pulmonary capillary pressure rises rapidly to 30 mmHg, pulmonary oedema develops as the hydrostatic pressure exceeds plasma osmotic pressure. If the process takes place slowly, fluid exudes into the alveolar wall and a physical barrier eventually develops between capillaries and alveoli consisting of a thickened capillary basement membrane, increased collagen and oedema. These changes increase the tissue tension of the alveolar wall and limit the exudation of fluid. As a consequence, patients with mitral stenosis can sometimes tolerate high pulmonary capillary pressures without developing severe pulmonary oedema. Because of the increased fluid in the interstitial tissues, the lymphatics become engorged.

As the pulmonary capillary pressure increases, there is a concomitant rise in pulmonary arterial pressure. However, in many cases of tight mitral stenosis, pulmonary arterial hypertension is much more severe than can be accounted for by this passive rise. The disproportionate elevation of pulmonary arterial pressure is largely due to an increase in tone in the small pulmonary arteries. Severe pulmonary arterial hypertension is disadvantageous in that it leads to right ventricular hypertrophy and failure. However, the increased resistance of the pulmonary arterial vessels prevents an abrupt rise in right ventricular output on exercise and therefore protects the lungs from a sudden increase in pulmonary capillary pressure.

The pulmonary vascular congestion typical of mitral stenosis leads to increased rigidity (decreased compliance) in the lungs. As a consequence, patients with severe mitral stenosis may have to double or treble the work of breathing.

Complications

- Atrial fibrillation develops sooner or later in most cases of mitral stenosis. At first this may be paroxysmal, but it is usual for it to become permanent. At its onset, the ventricular rate is often more than 140 beats/min and the patient may be rapidly precipitated into acute pulmonary oedema. It is an important complication, both because it contributes to the development of cardiac failure and because it is responsible for atrial stasis and the consequent risk of thrombosis and embolism.
- Pulmonary embolism and infarction frequently occur, especially when the disease is far advanced, as thrombosis is encouraged by atrial fibrillation, cardiac failure and bed rest.
- Systemic embolism is common and often follows the onset of atrial fibrillation. The embolism is cerebral in a high proportion of cases but may involve the mesenteric, renal or other arteries.
- The congested respiratory tract makes the patient liable to attacks of acute bronchitis and to the development of chronic bronchitis.
- Infective endocarditis is rare in pure mitral stenosis but is commoner as a complication of mixed mitral stenosis and regurgitation.

Symptoms

The patient with mitral stenosis, who is often symptom-free for many years, eventually develops features of left-sided cardiac failure and, later, those of right-sided failure. Various factors, such as pregnancy and the onset of atrial fibrillation, may suddenly precipitate the patient from one of these stages into the next.

The major symptom of mitral stenosis is shortness of breath. This occurs at first only on strenuous exercise, but as time passes less and less exertion is required to evoke it. Eventually, orthopnoea develops and the patient is liable to attacks of paroxysmal nocturnal dyspnoea and acute pulmonary oedema. Acute pulmonary oedema is less likely when severe pulmonary arterial hypertension has developed.

Haemoptysis occurs in some 10–20% of patients with mitral stenosis but is seldom severe. In some cases, the sputum is frothy and pink due to acute pulmonary oedema, but frankly bloody sputum may be expectorated by a patient who is almost free of breathlessness. This is probably due to the rupture of dilated pulmonary or bronchial veins. Another important cause of haemoptysis is pulmonary infarction.

Patients may also complain of palpitations, cough and angina pectoris. Severe breathlessness and orthopnoea have usually been present for years before right-sided heart failure develops. The earliest symptom of this is oedema of the legs, but abdominal discomfort due to engorgement of the liver or to ascites also occurs.

Physical signs

Patients with long-standing mitral stenosis often have a characteristic facies – a dusky malar discoloration. This may be attributed to peripheral cyanosis associated with a low cardiac output and vasoconstriction.

The arterial pulse is usually normal in volume but may be small, and is often irregular due to atrial fibrillation. In the earlier stages, the venous pressure is normal, but rises with the onset of right-sided heart failure. When there is severe pulmonary hypertension, there may be a large venous 'a' wave due to forceful right atrial contraction against the hypertrophied non-compliant right ventricle.

The apex beat is usually in the normal place but may be deviated to the left by right ventricular hypertrophy. It often has a tapping quality, which is associated with the characteristic loud first heart sound. In more advanced cases, right ventricular hypertrophy produces a heaving impulse to the left of the lower sternum. Mid-diastolic and presystolic thrills may be present at, or internal to, the apex beat.

There are four cardinal auscultatory features of mitral stenosis (Fig. 12.5):

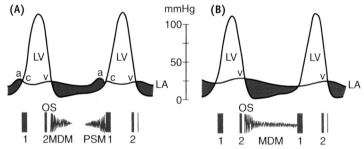

Fig. 12.5 (A) The pressure pulses in left ventricle and left atrium and the phonocardiographic appearances in mitral stenosis. A pressure difference is present throughout diastole (shaded area), and is accentuated by atrial contraction ('a' wave). Mid-diastolic and presystolic murmurs result. (B) Atrial fibrillation has developed with loss of the 'a' wave and of the presystolic accentuation of the murmur.

- a loud first sound
- an opening snap
- a mid-diastolic murmur
- a presystolic murmur.

The first sound is accentuated and the opening snap loud when the cusps are mobile; these signs may disappear with the development of rigidity and calcification of the valves. A mid-diastolic murmur is usually present, and its length, but not its intensity, gives an indication of the severity of the lesion. The presystolic murmur is often an early sign but may not be heard unless the patient is exercised and then turned into the left lateral position. A mitral systolic murmur signifies concomitant mitral regurgitation.

The second sound splits normally, but the pulmonary component is often accentuated because of pulmonary hypertension. An apical third heart sound is impossible in significant mitral stenosis because the rapid filling of the left ventricle necessary for its production cannot occur.

Investigations

- Electrocardiogram (ECG). If sinus rhythm is present, there is usually P mitrale (Fig. 12.6). Atrial fibrillation is common; other atrial and ventricular arrhythmias occur occasionally. Evidence of right ventricular hypertrophy develops in cases with severe pulmonary hypertension.
- *Radiological appearances.* The most characteristic radiological feature of mitral stenosis is the selective enlargement of the left atrium, which, in the posteroanterior view, produces a bulge below the pulmonary artery on the left border of the heart, and a rounded dense shadow within or outside the middle part of the right border of the heart (see Fig. 5.4). Left atrial enlargement can be confirmed by observing the displacement of the barium-filled oesophagus in the lateral view. Other radiological features may include calcification of the mitral valve, a normal or small left ventricle, and a normal or small aorta. The upper pulmonary veins are usually prominent. When the pulmonary capillary pressure is high, horizontal septal lines (Kerley's B lines) appear in the costophrenic angles, and the radiological features of pulmonary oedema may be seen. Haemosiderosis may produce mottling of the lungs. Pulmonary artery, right ventricular and, occasionally, right atrial enlargement may also be present when there is pulmonary arterial hypertension (Fig. 12.7).

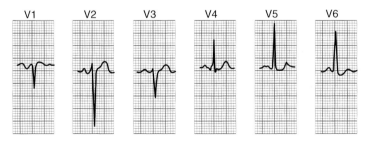

V1   V2   V3   V4   V5   V6

Fig. 12.6 P mitrale. There is a biphasic P wave in lead VI, with deep inversion of the terminal segment. In the left-sided leads the P wave is bifid, most clearly seen in leads V4 and V5 in this example.

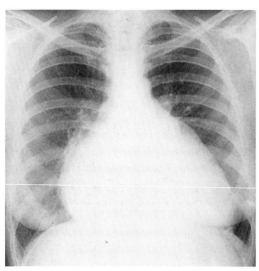

Fig. 12.7 Mixed mitral valve disease. Gross cardiac enlargement in a severe case of mixed mitral valve disease.

- *Echocardiography.* Echocardiography is the investigation most commonly used to confirm the diagnosis of mitral stenosis and to assess its severity. Two-dimensional echocardiography will demonstrate thickened mitral valve leaflets with restricted opening (Fig. 12.8). The left atrium is usually enlarged and there may be a 'swirling' appearance in the left atrium which has been termed 'spontaneous contrast'. This appearance is caused by red cell aggregation in the slow moving blood. If present, this appearance indicates severe mitral stenosis, although it is not specific for mitral valve disease and can occur in other conditions of low cardiac output. In some patients with severe mitral stenosis, left atrial thrombosis may be visible on two-dimensional echocardiography (Fig. 12.9). Analysis of the mitral leaflet motion with the M-mode cursor shows three characteristic abnormalities in mitral stenosis:

1. a reduction in the diastolic closure rate of the anterior mitral valve leaflet (Fig. 12.10)
2. increased echogenicity of both leaflets
3. the anterior and posterior leaflets, which are fused together at the commissures, appear to move in the same direction (anteriorly) during diastole.

Doppler examination allows assessment of the functional severity of the stenosis. In a normal heart, the opening of the mitral valve at the onset of diastole is followed by a period of rapid ventricular filling as blood flows through the open mitral valve into a compliant left ventricle. This results in rapid equalization of the pressures in the left atrium and left ventricle. In mitral stenosis, antegrade flow through the stenotic mitral valve is impeded; in mild mitral stenosis, the left atrial and left ventricular pressures will take longer to equilibrate, whereas in severe mitral stenosis the pressures will not equilibrate during diastole and a gradient will still be present at the end of diastole. Using pulsed-wave Doppler examination, blood velocity through the mitral valve can be measured and

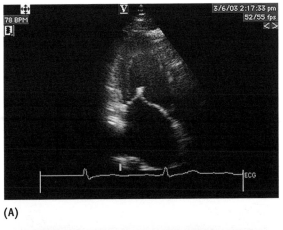

(A)

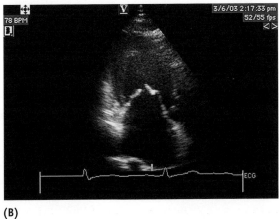

(B)

Fig. 12.8 Long axis echocardiogram of a patient with moderate mitral stenosis. Note the thickened mitral valve leaflets in systole (A) and the restricted leaflet opening in diastole (B).

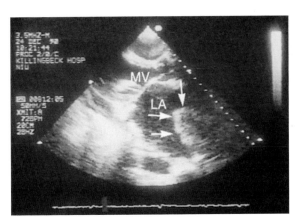

Fig. 12.9 Left atrial thrombus (arrowed) in a patient with severe mitral stenosis. Note the thickened mitral valve (MV) and dilated left atrium (LA).

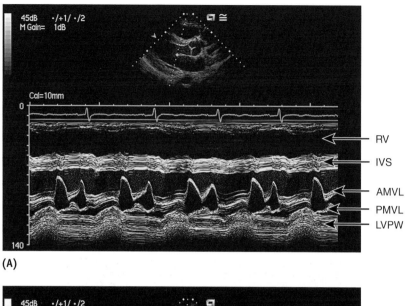

(A)

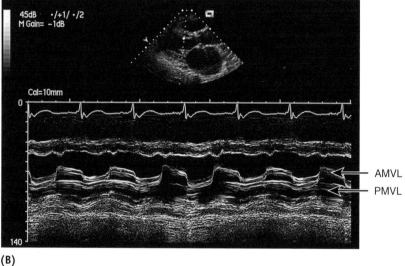

(B)

Fig. 12.10 M-mode echocardiogram of (A) a normal and (B) a stenotic mitral valve. In the normal valve, note the characteristic 'm' shape of movement of the anterior leaflet. The first upstroke is caused by passive filling of the left ventricle; this is followed by partial closure of the mitral valve as the pressures equilibrate. The second upstroke is caused by atrial contraction. In the stenotic valve, the diastolic closure rate is reduced (i.e. the slope becomes flatter) because the left ventricular and left atrial pressures do not equilibrate. The stenotic leaflets also show increased echogenicity.

the rate of decay of blood velocity (and thus driving pressure) throughout diastole can be estimated (Fig. 12.11). A measurement in common usage is the mitral valve pressure half-time, which is the time taken for the pressure gradient between the left atrium and left ventricle at the onset of diastole to decay to half of its initial value. In a normal mitral valve, the pressure half-time is no greater than 60 ms. The longer the pressure half-time, the more severe the mitral stenosis (see Table 12.1). A mitral pressure

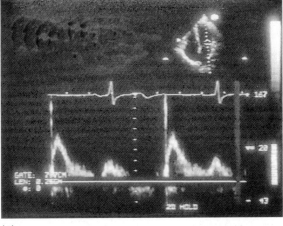

(A)

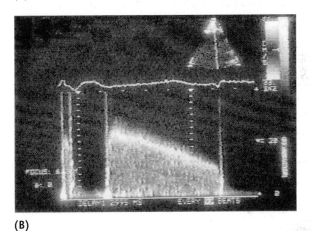

(B)

Fig. 12.11 Doppler examination of flow in diastole through (A) a normal and (B) a stenotic mitral valve. The 'flatter' the slope of decline in velocity, the more severe is the stenosis (see text for details).

Table 12.1 Mitral valve pressure half-time and stenosis

Pressure half-time (ms)	Stenosis
< 60	Normal
60–100	Mild
100–200	Moderate
> 200	Severe

half-time of 220 ms is equivalent to a mitral valve area of 1 cm² and represents severe stenosis.

- *Cardiac catheterization.* This investigation is seldom required for diagnostic purposes, but may be helpful in assessing the severity of the stenosis. This is most accurately done by simultaneously measuring the pressure on either side of the mitral valve and estimating the cardiac output. Angiocardiography is mainly of value in assessing the severity of any associated mitral or aortic regurgitation, and in assessing the coronary arteries prior to surgery.

Combined valve disease

Mitral stenosis is frequently complicated by disease of the other cardiac valves. The combination of rheumatic aortic regurgitation with mitral stenosis is a common one; in most cases the aortic regurgitation is the less important defect. The severity of the aortic regurgitation can be judged with reasonable assurance by the pulse volume, and by the diastolic pressure, which in severe cases is usually less than 60 mmHg. The combination of severe mitral stenosis and aortic stenosis is unusual but important, because one may mask the presence of the other.

Severe tricuspid stenosis complicates about 3% of cases of mitral stenosis and often obscures its signs.

Tricuspid regurgitation is common in advanced mitral stenosis because the tricuspid valve ring dilates with right ventricular enlargement. The associated pansystolic murmur may be heard not only at the left sternal edge but as far out as the apex. This may lead to the erroneous diagnosis of mitral regurgitation. Systolic venous pulsation in the neck, the increase in the murmur on inspiration, and the lack of transmission of the murmur to the axilla serve to identify its tricuspid origin.

Differential diagnosis

The presence of mitral stenosis can often be suspected from a history of rheumatic fever combined with progressive dyspnoea, a small and irregular pulse, and a mitral facies. Echocardiography is used to confirm the diagnosis, to estimate the severity of the stenosis and to assess suitability for balloon valvuloplasty or surgery. Echocardiography can also diagnose the very rare conditions that may mimic mitral stenosis; these include:

* left atrial myxoma
* left atrial ball valve thrombus
* cor triatriatum.

Course and prognosis

The characteristic physical signs of mitral stenosis, which can be present within a year of acute rheumatic fever, may precede the development of symptoms by 10–20 years. Breathlessness, usually the first complaint, is most likely to start between the ages of 20 and 30 years, but may be delayed much longer. In those in whom complications do not develop, the course is slowly but steadily downhill over a number of years. However, in Western countries, patients with signs of rheumatic mitral valve disease are now mainly seen in middle or old age, whereas in parts of Asia and Africa it is predominantly found in adolescents and young adults.

Sooner or later, some complication usually arises which leads to temporary or permanent deterioration. In young women, pregnancy is often responsible for the onset or aggravation of breathlessness; in the patient with severe stenosis, parturition may lead to pulmonary oedema and death. Once right-sided heart failure has developed, the prognosis without direct intervention on the valve is poor.

Medical treatment

Surgery or balloon valvuloplasty are eventually required in most cases, but it is usually necessary to prepare the patient for these procedures by appropriate medical therapy. Even after relief of the stenosis, treatment is often needed for the control of arrhythmias and the prevention of emboli.

Patients with mitral stenosis should be encouraged to live reasonably normal lives. They should be advised against being overweight, and discouraged from smoking. Infections must be treated promptly with appropriate antibiotics. Diuretics (usually furosemide [frusemide] or bumetanide) are effective in relieving pulmonary venous congestion and improving breathlessness. Anticoagulants should be used in all patients with atrial fibrillation unless there are exceptional circumstances. Even patients in sinus rhythm who have mitral stenosis are at risk of embolic events including stroke; anticoagulation should be considered in these patients. Careful supervision is required during pregnancy.

Digitalis is required for atrial fibrillation, but is of no value in pure stenosis in sinus rhythm. Cardiac failure is otherwise treated by the usual means (see Ch. 10). An attempt to restore sinus rhythm should be made after mitral valve surgery in patients with atrial fibrillation, particularly if this is known to be of recent onset.

Interventional treatment (mitral valvuloplasty)

In this procedure, carried out under local anaesthetic, a balloon is passed from the right femoral vein through the atrial septum into the left atrium using the trans-septal technique, and the balloon dilated within the valve (Fig. 12.12). This technique has been made very much more effective following the development of the Inoue balloon. This is a single balloon which which has three segments of differing thickness. As the balloon is inflated, so

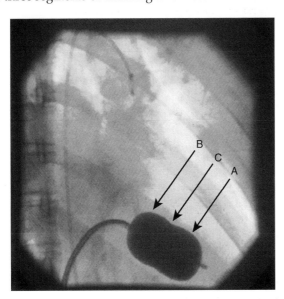

Fig. 12.12 Angiogram showing inflated Inoue balloon during mitral valvuloplasty. (A: distal portion of balloon in left ventricle; B: proximal portion of balloon in left atrium; C: central portion of balloon in mitral valve.)

the distal, then the proximal and finally the middle segments dilate. The technique involves passing the balloon through the mitral valve and into the left ventricle. The distal portion of the balloon is then dilated and the balloon pulled back against the mitral valve. As the operator continues to inflate the balloon, the proximal portion fills and fixes the central portion in the area of the valve leaflets. The operator then fully inflates the balloon and the central portion dilates the valve. The intention is to cause controlled tearing of the adhesions that are holding the valve leaflets together at the commissures. The entire inflation should take no more than 20–30 s since full inflation, by obstructing the mitral valve, effectively causes circulatory arrest. The main complications of the procedure are:

- complications related to trans-septal puncture including cardiac tamponade
- tearing of the mitral valve leaflets resulting in severe mitral regurgitation requiring mitral valve replacement surgery
- embolic complications (stroke, etc.)
- restenosis. This may occur after several years. 'Early' restenosis within 1 to 2 years usually reflects inadequate dilatation.

Transoesophageal echocardiography is essential in assessing whether or not balloon valvuloplasty is likely to be successful. Ideally, the valve leaflets should be pliant and mobile, there should be minimal calcification, particularly along the commissures, and the stenosis should be valvar without extensive thickening of the subvalvar apparatus. Significant mitral regugitation and the presence of left atrial thrombus (which might be dislodged during the trans-septal puncture) are absolute contraindications to mitral valvuloplasty, while rigid, immobile or calified mitral leaflets are a relative contraindication.

Mitral valve surgery

In patients unsuitable for percutaneous mitral vulvuloplasty, mitral valve surgery should be considered:

- Closed mitral valvotomy – this is now rarely performed. It comprises dilatation of the valve using a metal dilator without cardiopulmonary bypass.
- Open mitral valvotomy – carried out under cardiopulmonary bypass to allow the surgeon to inspect and repair the valve under direct vision.
- Mitral valve replacement – this is the most common operation.

The mortality of mitral valve surgery depends on the severity of the disease and the presence of complications. If the patient is in reasonably good health before the operation, and free of severe pulmonary hypertension and mitral regurgitation, the mortality rate should be less than 5% and, in the most favourable cases, less than 1%. Where there is advanced pulmonary hypertension or right-sided failure, the mortality rate may rise to 10% or more.

Operation should be avoided in the presence of rheumatic activity. Surgery should also be deferred until cardiac failure has been brought under control or when there has been recent pulmonary or systemic embolism. 'Prophylactic' intervention (either by valvuloplasty or by surgery) should be considered in young women with moderate or severe symptoms to avoid operation during pregnancy.

Mitral regurgitation

A number of different conditions may lead to mitral regurgitation by different mechanisms:

- *Rheumatic endocarditis* is the major cause in areas where rheumatic fever is prevalent, and is often accompanied by mitral stenosis. The valve cusps are usually rigid and deformed and the chordae tendineae fused and shortened. Calcification is common. Regurgitation may develop at the time of rheumatic fever, especially if this is severe, but does not usually produce major haemodynamic effects for several years because the progression of valve damage is slow.
- *Mitral valve prolapse.* Prolapse of the mitral valve is a common condition which may be associated with rare diseases of connective tissue such as Marfan's syndrome, pseudoxanthoma elasticum and osteogenesis elasticum. Usually, however, there is no other disease process; in such cases, there is a myxomatous change of the valve leaflets, which are voluminous and redundant. This most commonly involves the posterior mitral valve leaflet but may include the anterior or both leaflets. It is important to distinguish between billowing and prolapsing leaflets. Leaflets may billow into the left atrium but the line of coaption between the two leaflets may still be in the normal position and there may be no mitral regurgitation. Prolapse implies displacement towards the left atrium of the commissural surfaces of a leaflet and is usually accompanied by regurgitation. The usual auscultatory finding is a mid-systolic click and/or a late apical systolic murmur, but the click and murmur may occur at other times during systole. In any individual, the auscultatory features may vary considerably from time to time, and can be made to do so by standing, sitting and straining in the Valsalva manoeuvre. Most patients are asymptomatic, but some complain of left-sided chest pain or palpitations. The ECG may show minor ST abnormalities. Echocardiography, which has demonstrated this abnormality in some 5% of normal young people, characteristically reveals a mid-systolic 'buckling' of one or both leaflets into the left atrium. Most of these patients have trivial mitral regurgitation which will not progress. Some, however, will develop haemodynamically significant mitral regurgitation and will require mitral valve surgery. All patients with mitral valve prolapse should receive antibiotic prophylaxis against infective endocarditis.
- *Infective endocarditis* may produce destruction or perforation of the cusps, or rupture of chordae tendineae.
- *Congenital mitral regurgitation* occurs with or without other congenital abnormalities such as atrial septal defect.
- Spontaneous rupture of chordae tendineae may occur.
- *Papillary muscle malfunction* or rupture may result from myocardial infarction (usually inferior infarction).
- *Left ventricular dilatation* from any cause, such as hypertension, coronary artery disease, cardiomyopathy and aortic valve disease, may lead to

dilatation of the valve ring. The mitral regurgitation so produced leads to further enlargement of the left ventricle, and therefore further dilatation of the valve ring, with the development of a vicious circle.

Pathophysiology

The severity of mitral regurgitation depends on a number of factors:

- the size of the mitral valve orifice during ventricular systole. Although this can be of fixed size, as it is when the valve is calcified, it may be variable, depending on the degree of left ventricular dilatation
- the pressure relationships between the left ventricle, aorta and left atrium
- the left ventricular output.

Any factor which augments left ventricular output or raises aortic impedance increases mitral regurgitation. The degree of mitral regurgitation is limited by the distensibility of the left atrium and pulmonary veins. However, the pressure in the left atrium is much lower than that in the aorta; with a large valve orifice, therefore, as much blood may regurgitate into the left atrium during systole as is ejected into the aorta. A feature of chronic severe mitral regurgitation is that the left atrium is much larger than is usual in mitral stenosis.

During systole, the pressure in the left atrium may rise to a high 'v' peak, but will not do so if the regurgitated blood is readily accommodated in a voluminous left atrium. When mitral regurgitation develops abruptly, as with the rupture of papillary muscles or chordae tendineae, the left atrium is often small and the 'v' wave tall (see Fig. 5.1).

In diastole, there is a large flow from left atrium to left ventricle, consisting of the blood received from the pulmonary circulation combined with that which regurgitated during the preceding systole. At this time the pressure in the left atrium falls rapidly to the ventricular level. Therefore, although there may be a high 'v' wave, the mean left atrial pressure is often not greatly raised, and the pulmonary capillary pressure is seldom as high as that encountered in mitral stenosis. Eventually, however, with the development of left ventricular failure, the pulmonary capillary pressure rises and, with it, the pulmonary arterial pressure. Severe pulmonary hypertension and right-sided cardiac failure are unusual unless there is also an appreciable degree of mitral stenosis.

Complications

The complications are similar to those of mitral stenosis. Atrial fibrillation is frequent when mitral regurgitation is of rheumatic origin but less so when other disease processes are responsible. Infective endocarditis is more common than in mitral stenosis.

Symptoms

In cases of rheumatic origin, the physical signs precede symptoms by many years. When symptoms do occur, they usually increase slowly. Fatigue, perhaps attributable to the low cardiac output, may be the first complaint, but eventually dyspnoea on exertion, orthopnoea and, rarely, paroxysmal nocturnal dyspnoea develop.

When mitral regurgitation is due to perforation of a cusp, or to rupture of chordae tendineae or papillary muscles, the onset of symptoms is abrupt; the patient may present with acute pulmonary oedema.

Physical signs

The pulse is usually of normal volume; irregularity due to atrial fibrillation is common. The venous pressure is normal except when there is right-sided cardiac failure. The apex beat, which may be displaced downwards and outwards, often has the vigorous thrusting character of left ventricular hypertrophy and dilatation, and there is sometimes a systolic thrill.

The first sound is usually soft and introduces an apical pansystolic murmur which radiates to the axilla. The murmur may be of the same intensity throughout systole, but often increases towards the end of this period. When the regurgitation is due to papillary muscle malfunction or prolapse of a mitral cusp, the murmur may be exclusively in late systole. Rarely, it may radiate to the left sternal edge rather than to the axilla and may be mistaken for aortic stenosis. The intensity of the murmur bears some relation to the severity of the regurgitation, but is not a reliable guide. In most severe cases there is a third heart sound, sometimes followed by a short mid-diastolic murmur due to rapid filling of the left ventricle.

Investigations

- *ECG*. The ECG may be normal but P mitrale is often present if atrial fibrillation has not supervened. Left ventricular hypertrophy occurs in severe and chronic mitral regurgitation, often with a left ventricular strain pattern; if there is significant stenosis there may be evidence of biventricular hypertrophy.
- *Radiography*. Radiologically, the most conspicuous feature is the marked enlargement of the left atrium, but there may also be left ventricular enlargement. Calcification of the mitral valve is often visible in rheumatic cases. Evidence of pulmonary vein dilatation and pulmonary oedema develops when there is left ventricular failure.

  When mitral regurgitation is of acute onset due to malfunction or rupture of valve cusps, papillary muscles or chordae tendineae, the heart size may be normal because there has been insufficient time for the left atrium or the left ventricle to dilate. The lung fields, however, would normally show changes of pulmonary oedema.
- *Echocardiography*. Two-dimensional echocardiography allows examination of the mitral valve leaflets and may reveal thickening in rheumatic disease or prolapse of the anterior or posterior (Fig. 12.13) leaflets, or of both leaflets together. Echocardiography may also demonstrate the flail leaflet caused by ruptured chordae or papillary muscles. If the degree of regurgitation is haemodynamically significant, the left atrium will be dilated. Doppler examination and colour flow mapping are very sensitive techniques for detecting mitral regurgitation. Indeed, colour flow mapping will often demonstrate a small jet of mitral regurgitation in normal valves. Assessing the severity of mitral regurgitation by echo is more difficult but it is usually possible to differentiate mild, moderate and severe mitral

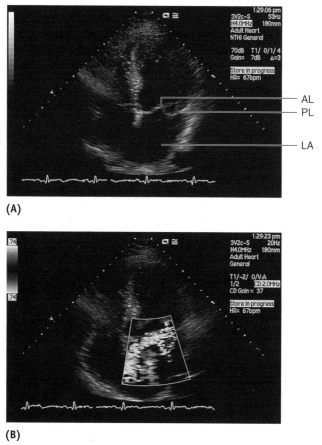

AL
PL

LA

(A)

(B)

Fig. 12.13 (A) Four-chamber echocardiogram demonstrating prolapse of the posterior mitral valve leaflet (PL). (B) The regurgitant jet is directed behind the anterior leaflet (AL) towards the inter-atrial septum.

regurgitation, particularly if the transoesophageal approach is used. Transoesophageal echocardiography is also useful in analysing the mechanism of mitral regurgitation. This may demonstrate such diverse causes of regurgitation as prolapse of a leaflet, tethering of a leaflet, perforation of a leaflet (usually a consequence of endocarditis) or structurally normal leaflets which fail to meet at the commissure because of dilatation of the mitral valve ring. This information is particularly useful to the surgeon if mitral valve repair is being considered.

- *Cardiac catheterization and angiography.* These procedures are seldom used for diagnosis, but the severity of regurgitation can be assessed by injecting radio-opaque contrast medium into the left ventricle. The presence of left ventricular failure may be confirmed by finding a high left ventricular end-diastolic pressure. A tall 'v' wave in the left atrial or pulmonary arterial wedge pressure tracing is suggestive of, but not diagnostic of, mitral regurgitation. In patients being considered for mitral valve surgery, it is normal practice to carry out coronary angiography in areas where the prevalence of coronary artery disease is high, because unsuspected coronary artery disease might lead to serious complications at the time of cardiac surgery.

Differential diagnosis

The diagnosis is usually based on the finding of an apical pansystolic murmur radiating to the axilla. The pansystolic murmur of tricuspid regurgitation may reach the apex, but does not radiate further and is usually increased on inspiration. The systolic murmur of aortic stenosis may be heard best at the apex, but is mid-systolic and does not radiate to the axilla. The murmur of ventricular septal defect is heard best at the lower left sternal edge.

It may be difficult to differentiate mitral regurgitation from a benign systolic murmur, but benign murmurs are never pansystolic, are seldom of grade 3 or greater intensity and tend to vary with posture and respiration.

Suggestive evidence of mitral regurgitation is provided by left atrial and left ventricular enlargement on the chest radiograph, and by P mitrale and left ventricular hypertrophy on the ECG. The definitive diagnosis is usually made by echocardiography or by ventriculography.

In mitral regurgitation of non-rheumatic origin, the diagnosis may be suggested by the sudden appearance of a loud apical systolic murmur accompanied by left ventricular failure.

Course and prognosis

The course of patients with mitral regurgitation is very variable. Those with mild regurgitation and without cardiomegaly may live a normal life span, although exposed to the risk of infective endocarditis. In rheumatic mitral regurgitation of moderate severity, the course is one of slow deterioration over 10–20 years with gradually increasing heart size until left ventricular failure develops. Unless this has been precipitated by a complication that can be corrected, the prognosis is then poor and death is likely to occur within a few years. When mitral regurgitation has been due to ruptured chordae tendineae, papillary muscles or cusps, the prognosis is generally poor, although the regurgitation is occasionally slight and well tolerated.

Medical treatment

Patients with mitral regurgitation should be advised to have antibiotic prophylaxis to cover surgical and major dental procedures. If the degree of regurgitation is mild, then no other medication is required. If the patient is symptomatic, or if there is left ventricular dilatation, then patients should receive the usual heart failure treatment including a loop diuretic and an angiotensin-converting enzyme (ACE) inhibitor. The patient should be anticoagulated when atrial fibrillation supervenes.

Mitral valve surgery

Until recently, the most commonly performed operation for patients with severe mitral regurgitation was mitral valve replacement. However, surgeons are increasingly attempting to preserve and repair the mitral valve if at all possible. This requires precise knowledge of the mechanism of regurgitation, which is usually gained from transoesophageal echocardiography. The efficacy of the repair procedure is then usually tested by transoesophageal echocardiography in the operating theatre. The repair technique employed depends on the mechanism of regurgitation and can include one or more of the following:

- resection of part of a prolapsing leaflet
- insertion of a mitral valve ring
- transposition of chordae from one leaflet to another
- insertion of prosthetic chordae
- suturing of the central portions of the anterior and posterior leaflets together to create a double orifice valve.

The most common, and most successful, repair procedure is to resect a quadrangular area in the central part of a prolapsing posterior leaflet. The two remaining edges are then sutured together and the mitral valve anulus is plicated. This is often combined with insertion of a ring around the mitral valve anulus, which prevents further dilation of the mitral valve anulus. If the mitral regurgitation is caused by anular dilation resulting in failure of coaption of otherwise normal leaflets, then insertion of a ring may be the only intervention required. Repair of a prolapsing anterior leaflet is technically more difficult than repair of a posterior leaflet and a number of different repair techniques have been tried (chordal transposition, prosthetic chordae, suturing of the central portions of the two leaflets together).

Timing of surgical treatment

In the past, mitral valve surgery was carried out only when patients had severe symptoms. As the risks of surgical treatment have fallen, so there has been a tendency to operate earlier in the disease process. Serial echocardiography is a useful investigation to detect progressive left ventricular dilatation, which may be an indication for surgery even when symptoms are mild or absent. Indeed, it has recently been suggested that asymptomatic patients should be considered for mitral valve repair even before the left ventricle starts to dilate. The reason for this is that the left ventricle 'off-loads' into a dilated left atrium in patients with established mitral regurgitation. The left ventricular contractility, therefore, may appear normal on echocardiography or left ventricular angiography when there is already dysfunction present. This dysfunction will become obvious only when the valve is repaired or replaced. For this reason, consideration for mitral valve surgery is recommended when the left ventricular end-systolic diameter (measured at echo) exceeds 3.5 cm. In contrast, surgery for aortic regurgitation (see below) is only recommended when the end-systolic diameter exceeds 4.5 cm.

AORTIC VALVE DISEASE

The normal aortic valve consists of three semilunar cusps attached to a fibrous valve ring. Immediately above the insertion of the valve cusps are the sinuses of Valsalva, from two of which the coronary arteries arise. In about 1% of individuals the aortic valve has only two cusps.

The aortic valve and adjacent structures may be involved in congenital, rheumatic, bacterial, syphilitic and atherosclerotic changes. Both stenosis and regurgitation may occur as isolated lesions but are often combined.

Calcification of the cusps is an important factor in the development of aortic valve disease and is often responsible for the stenosis that occurs in those with congenitally bicuspid valves.

Aortic stenosis

Aortic stenosis is most commonly the result of disease of the aortic valve cusps, but may also be due to narrowing in the outflow tract of the left ventricle below the cusps (subvalvar) and, very rarely, a constriction in the first part of the aorta (supravalvar stenosis).

Aetiology and pathology

Aortic valve stenosis may be congenital, rheumatic or sclerotic. Most instances of aortic stenosis occur in middle-aged or elderly patients, in whom there is no evidence of involvement of other valves. Calcification of the valve is usually severe and largely responsible for the stenosis. Even at necropsy it may be impossible to determine the aetiology, but many have congenitally bicuspid valves. Rheumatic aortic stenosis results from adherence of adjacent cusps with thickening, fibrosis and subsequent calcification.

Subvalvar aortic stenosis may result from a congenital membrane or from fibrous tissue situated in the outflow tract of the left ventricle. This may be combined with valve stenosis, and thus form a tunnel in the outflow tract. A distinctive form of subvalvar stenosis is caused by hypertrophy of the muscle of the outflow tract of the left ventricle, particularly affecting the interventricular septum. This disorder has received a large variety of names including 'idiopathic hypertrophic subvalvular aortic stenosis' and 'hypertrophic obstructive cardiomyopathy' (see also p. 226).

Supravalvar aortic stenosis is usually congenital and may be associated with a distinctive facial appearance ('elfin' facies) and mental disability (Williams' syndrome). It can also occur as part of the rubella syndrome or in association with hypervitaminosis D and hypercalcaemia.

Aortic stenosis is commonly associated with regurgitation. This is especially so in rheumatic and congenital valve stenosis and in congenital subvalvar stenosis. It is seldom severe in the calcific stenosis of the elderly and almost unknown in hypertrophic subaortic stenosis. Mitral valve disease usually predominates over aortic stenosis in rheumatic valve disease.

The left ventricle hypertrophies in response to the pressure load imposed upon it. The weight of the heart is often doubled in severe cases. There is usually little ventricular dilatation unless there is associated aortic regurgitation. Coronary artery disease may coexist with aortic stenosis, but commonly the coronary arteries are larger than normal. In aortic valve stenosis, there is poststenotic dilatation of the ascending aorta (an effect of the jet of blood which is propelled through the valve).

Pathophysiology

A minor degree of stenosis has little or no effect upon the function of the heart; only when the area of the valve orifice is reduced to a quarter of the normal are there serious consequences. The left ventricle responds to the pressure load by contracting more forcibly, and the left ventricular systolic pressure increases (see Fig. 12.14). A systolic pressure difference develops between the left ventricle and aorta (Fig. 12.15). The magnitude of this difference in pressure depends on the size of the orifice and the flow of blood through it. The obstruction delays emptying of the left ventricle, so that the phase of ejection becomes prolonged. The cardiac output is usually maintained within the normal range but at the expense of a considerable increase in left ventricular work. In consequence, left ventricular hypertrophy increases progressively as the valve orifice narrows. Although the hypertrophy is a compensatory phenomenon, it eventually contributes to the burden on the heart. The thickened ventricle is less compliant and is therefore less

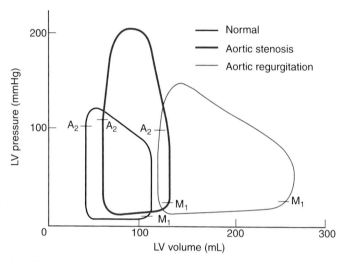

Fig. 12.14 Relationships between left ventricular volume and pressure in the normal heart, in aortic stenosis and in aortic regurgitation. M_1 = mitral valve closure. A_2 = aortic valve closure. Note high pressure generated in aortic stenosis and large end-diastolic volume (at M_1), with increased stroke volume in aortic regurgitation.

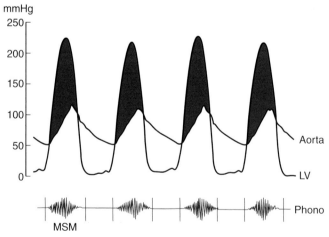

Fig. 12.15 Simultaneous pressure recordings and phonocardiographic appearances in aortic stenosis. Note the systolic pressure difference ('gradient') between the left ventricle and aorta, and the corresponding midsystolic murmur (MSM).

easily filled during diastole; atrial contraction contributes more and more to the filling process. The hypertrophied muscle increasingly outstrips the ability of the coronary arteries to supply it with blood, resulting in ischaemia.

Symptoms

There is a characteristic triad of symptoms:

- breathlessness
- syncope on exertion
- angina pectoris.

To these may be added the liability to sudden death.

Breathlessness on exertion is the earliest symptom in most cases. Later, orthopnoea and paroxysmal nocturnal dyspnoea may occur. Eventually, right-sided heart failure with peripheral oedema may develop.

Syncope is much commoner in aortic stenosis than in other types of valvar heart disease and its relationship to exertion is of diagnostic value. Its mechanism is uncertain, but it may be due to the inability of the heart to increase its output sufficiently, or to reflex vasodilatation, or to arrhythmias.

Like syncope, anginal pain is much commoner in aortic stenosis than in other valve lesions. It does not differ in character from that seen in coronary artery disease.

Death is often sudden and may not be preceded by any symptoms. However, it is particularly likely to occur in those who have experienced syncope or angina pectoris. It is believed that ventricular fibrillation is usually responsible.

Physical signs

An aortic systolic murmur is the first abnormality to appear and may be present for decades before evidence of severe stenosis develops.

The pulse is abnormal in most severe cases. Characteristically it is small in volume, rises slowly to its peak, and takes an unusually long time to pass the finger. The pulse pressure is correspondingly small. When there is an appreciable degree of aortic regurgitation as well, the pulse pressure may be normal or large, and the pulse may take on a 'bisferiens' quality in which a double pulse is felt.

The apex beat may be in the normal position or displaced downwards and to the left. It has a slow heaving quality. A systolic thrill can often be felt in the second right intercostal space, and also in the carotid arteries and along the left edge of the sternum.

There is a midsystolic murmur, which is usually loud and harsh. This may be best heard in the second right interspace, along the left sternal edge, or even at the apex. It is often audible over the carotid arteries. It is accompanied by an early systolic ('ejection') click in those cases in which there is aortic valve stenosis without heavy calcification. This sign is probably due to sudden tensioning of the valve cusps at the time of opening. Other signs may include a fourth (atrial) heart sound over the left ventricle and reversed splitting of the second heart sound. This latter sign is due to delay in left ventricular emptying and aortic valve closure. The aortic component of the second heart sound may not be audible if there is calcification.

Investigations

- *ECG.* The ECG usually shows left ventricular hypertrophy, the extent of which roughly parallels the severity of the stenosis. Other abnormalities which sometimes occur include asymmetrical inversion of T waves and left bundle branch block.
- *Chest X-ray.* The chest X-ray in aortic stenosis may be normal, but the ascending aorta is usually dilated in aortic valve stenosis. Left ventricular enlargement may be evident (Fig. 12.16).
- *Echocardiography.* Echocardiography is the principal investigation in aortic stenosis. Two-dimensional echocardiography will demonstrate the thickened aortic valve leaflets with restricted opening (Fig. 12.17). The left ventricular cavity is usually small with marked hypertrophy of the walls. Doppler examination can be used to estimate the severity of aortic

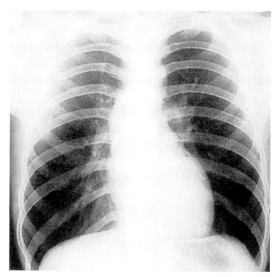

Fig. 12.16 Aortic stenosis. The rounded configuration of the left ventricular outline suggests left ventricular hypertrophy. The ascending aorta shows post-stenotic dilatation.

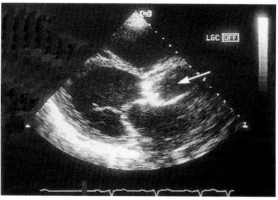

Fig. 12.17 Thickened and stenotic aortic valve producing dense echoes (arrowed).

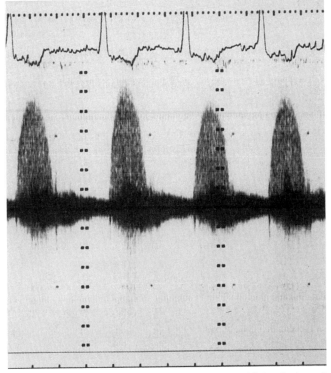

Fig. 12.18 Continuous wave Doppler recording in a patient with aortic stenosis and atrial fibrillation. The height of the signal varies with the velocity of the jet and in this case varies from cycle to cycle depending on the preceding cycle length. The maximum velocity is 6 metres per second which calculates out at a gradient of 144 mmHg.

stenosis. Using the Bernoulli equation (p. 48), the blood velocity through the stenotic aortic valve can be measured and the aortic valve gradient estimated (Fig. 12.18). This requires considerable patience and skill. In heavily disorganized valves, the aortic jet is often eccentric; multiple transducer positions will be required to align the Doppler signal with the aortic jet and so record the maximum gradient. Failure to do so may result in a serious underestimation of the aortic valve gradient. The advent of Doppler examination has, in many cases, obviated the need for cardiac catheterization to establish a diagnosis of aortic stenosis.

- *Cardiac catheterization.* The systolic pressure difference across the stenosis is measured with catheters in the left ventricle and aorta or by the withdrawal of a catheter from left ventricle to aorta (Fig. 12.19). If the stenosis is severe, the left ventricular systolic pressure exceeds that in the aorta by more than 50 mmHg. For technical reasons, the gradient recorded at catheterization is usually lower than that recorded at echocardiography (instantaneous vs. peak-to-peak gradient, see Ch. 5). In advanced cases of aortic stenosis with left ventricular dysfunction, the gradient, both at catheterization and by echo, may be low despite the presence of severe stenosis. A reported gradient of 30–40 mmHg should be interpreted with caution, therefore, if the left ventricular function is poor, since this may represent severe stenosis requiring early surgery.

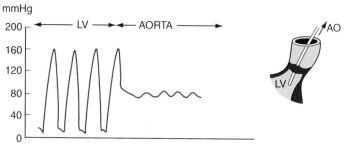

Fig. 12.19 Pressure tracing recorded as catheter is withdrawn from left ventricle to aorta in aortic valve stenosis. Note sudden fall in systolic pressure as the catheter tip enters the aorta.

Complications

The most frequent cause of death is cardiac failure, but there is considerable risk of sudden death. Infective endocarditis may occur and, by eroding the cusps, cause severe aortic regurgitation.

Diagnosis and differential diagnosis

The diagnosis is often suggested by the triad of symptoms (dyspnoea, angina, syncope on exertion), or by the finding of the typical murmur associated with a thrill and a small pulse. Hypertrophic subaortic stenosis can be differentiated from other varieties by the pulse, which rises rapidly rather than slowly, and by the absence of an ejection click, valve calcification and aortic regurgitation; the diagnosis is established by echocardiography.

Prognosis

Cases of mild aortic stenosis have a good prognosis; if there is no appreciable degree of left ventricular hypertrophy, the patient is likely to survive for many years. Once the symptoms of breathlessness, angina or syncope have developed, death is likely to occur suddenly at any time, or within 5 years from heart failure.

Treatment

Little or no benefit can be expected from medical treatment. When symptoms have developed, strenuous activity should be avoided and the conventional treatment of heart failure and angina pectoris employed. Surgery is indicated in nearly all symptomatic patients and usually takes the form of aortic valve replacement. The mortality rate associated with aortic valve replacement is generally less than 5%. Mortality, however, is higher if the patient also requires coronary bypass surgery or has co-existent renal, hepatic or respiratory disease. This risk must be weighed against the grave prognosis in those with advanced symptoms. Balloon valvuloplasty of the aortic valve has been attempted but probably has no place in current practice.

In children and young adults, an alternative surgical approach is the Ross procedure. In this operation, the normal pulmonary valve is transplanted into the aortic position and a homograft is used for the excised pulmonary valve. The operative mortality is higher than for aortic valve replacement but the long-term results are good and life-long anticoagulation is not required.

Increasingly, adults are being identified with moderate aortic stenosis but no symptoms. It is now generally agreed that these patients do not require surgery but that they should be considered for early surgery as soon as symptoms occur. If these patients are followed at an out-patient clinic, then the approximate rate of progression is that the echo Doppler aortic valve gradient increases by 5–10 mmHg per annum.

Aortic regurgitation

Aetiology

Aortic regurgitation is commonly due to rheumatic heart disease. It can also be of congenital origin, in which case it is usually of less importance than the lesions that accompany it, such as aortic and subaortic stenosis and ventricular septal defect. Other causes include bicuspid valves, hypertension, infective endocarditis, Marfan syndrome, dissecting aneurysm, syphilitic aortitis, ankylosing spondylitis and Reiter's disease. In a substantial proportion of cases no cause can be found, i.e. they are 'idiopathic'.

Pathology

Aortic regurgitation can result either from damage to the cusps or from dilatation of the aorta and the valve ring. In rheumatic heart disease, the cusps are thickened and shortened and there may be some fusion of commissures. Varying degrees of stenosis and regurgitation occur. Calcification of the valve, which is usually severe in aortic stenosis, is seldom of importance in pure aortic regurgitation.

Syphilitic aortitis leads to aortic regurgitation as a result of dilatation of the aorta and the valve ring; stenosis is not a feature.

Infective endocarditis can cause erosion or perforation of the cusps, which have usually had some pre-existing abnormality.

Pathophysiology

In aortic regurgitation, a large volume of blood is regurgitated into the left ventricle in each diastole. The left ventricular output may be more than doubled. The increased stroke volume necessary to achieve this is associated with dilatation of the left ventricle. The regurgitant flow is greatest in early diastole when the difference in pressure between the aorta and left ventricle is maximal. The amount of blood that regurgitates is largely determined by the severity of the aortic valve disease but is also influenced by the compliance of the left ventricle and the systemic vascular resistance.

The dilated left ventricle contracts more powerfully in accordance with Starling's law, but there is an increased tension in the myocardium and increased oxygen consumption. The initial dilatation thus leads eventually to hypertrophy.

The diastolic pressure in the aorta is abnormally low, partly due to the leak and partly to peripheral vasodilatation. The left ventricular end-diastolic pressure is normal in the milder case but rises when cardiac failure supervenes.

Clinical features

Rheumatic aortic regurgitation usually develops at the time of acute rheumatic carditis and persists subsequently. Many years may elapse between the appearance of the murmur and the onset of symptoms.

Almost invariably, the first complaint is that of dyspnoea on exertion, although fatigue is also frequent. Other minor symptoms include dizziness and an awareness of the vigorous heart action.

The dyspnoea progresses slowly; eventually orthopnoea and paroxysmal dyspnoea may develop. Typical angina pectoris is infrequent except when the regurgitation is severe. In the advanced case, signs of right-sided failure complicate those of left-sided failure.

The arterial pulse in aortic regurgitation, often called 'collapsing' or 'water-hammer', rises rapidly and falls abruptly. This is most easily appreciated by placing the palm of one's hand on the anterior aspect of the patient's forearm (the arm being held vertically upright) because by this means, one may accentuate the backflow of blood during diastole. Sometimes the pulse is of bisferiens type, i.e. is felt to have two equally prominent waves, particularly if the regurgitation is accompanied by stenosis. The cardiac rhythm is usually normal unless there is associated mitral valve disease. The systolic pressure is often abnormally high and the diastolic low. In a severe case the systolic pressure may be 250–300 mmHg and the diastolic 30–50 mmHg. Vigorous arterial pulsation is often visible in the neck.

If the regurgitation is substantial, the apex beat is displaced outwards and downwards and is overactive and heaving. The essential feature on auscultation is an early diastolic murmur, usually best heard over the midsternal region or at the lower left sternal edge. In some cases, particularly in syphilitic aortitis, it is loudest in the second right intercostal space. There is often an accompanying systolic murmur; this does not necessarily indicate coexistent aortic stenosis but may be due to the increased stroke volume. The early (or 'immediate') diastolic murmur is often difficult to hear, and is frequently overlooked by the inexperienced. It must be specifically sought, with the stethoscope diaphragm placed at the lower left sternal edge, with the patient sitting up, the breath held in expiration.

In some patients with advanced aortic regurgitation, a mid-diastolic murmur may be heard even in the absence of mitral stenosis. This murmur (known as the Austin Flint murmur) has been attributed to the effect of the regurgitant jet on the anterior leaflet of the mitral valve which is interposed between the mitral and aortic valve orifices (see Fig. 12.2). One should hesitate to diagnose an Austin Flint murmur in rheumatic heart disease because concomitant mitral stenosis is likely, particularly if there is a loud first sound or opening snap.

Investigations

- *ECG.* The ECG shows increasing evidence of left ventricular hypertrophy as the disease process advances. There may also be a left ventricular strain pattern (ST segment depression and/or T wave inversion in the lateral chest leads). This is generally a sign that surgery should be considered.
- *Chest X-ray.* On the chest X-ray, there is usually left ventricular enlargement, with an elongated heart shadow and dilatation of the ascending aorta.

- *Echocardiography*. Two-dimensional echocardiography may show thickened aortic valve leaflets although the leaflets can appear normal even in severe regurgitation. If the regurgitation is haemodynamically significant, the left ventricle will be dilated and there may be early closure of the mitral valve. Before the advent of colour flow mapping, the fine oscillation of the anterior mitral valve leaflet was an important echocardiographic sign of aortic regurgitation. This movement was caused by the regurgitant jet striking the anterior leaflet. With the advent of colour flow mapping, the regurgitant jet or jets can now be seen easily (Fig. 12.20). Factors such as the width of the regurgitant jet and the distance into which it penetrates the left ventricle can provide a semi-quantitative estimate of severity.

- *Cardiac catheterization*. Gross aortic regurgitation is so readily recognized clinically and by non-invasive methods that cardiac catheterization is seldom required for diagnostic purposes. This investigation is, however, necessary when the degree of severity is in doubt; it is of particular value in evaluating the significance of an aortic diastolic murmur in a patient needing surgery for concomitant mitral valve disease. The cineangiographic

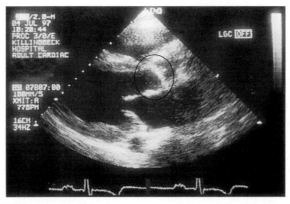

(A)

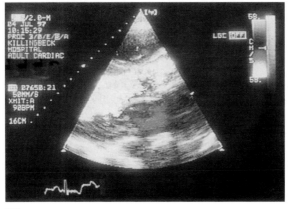

(B)

Fig. 12.20 (A) Grossly thickened aortic valve (circled). (B) Colour flow Doppler examination demonstrates severe regurgitation through the valve and into the left ventricular cavity.

demonstration of the regurgitation of contrast medium injected into the aorta provides a reasonable estimate of severity:

- *Grade 1* – minor regurgitation
- *Grade 2* – contrast just filling the whole of the left ventricle
- *Grade 3* – contrast filling the whole of the left ventricle, but cleared during each systole
- *Grade 4* – contrast filling the whole of the left ventricle, but not cleared during each systole

Cardiac catheterization is also necessary to assess the coronary arteries prior to any surgical intervention.

Differential diagnosis

The clinical diagnosis of aortic regurgitation is usually not difficult if it is moderate or severe. A large pulse pressure is also observed in other conditions, such as persistent ductus arteriosus, arteriovenous fistulae, pregnancy, anaemia and thyrotoxicosis. The early diastolic murmur may be confused with that of pulmonary regurgitation, but this rare lesion is seldom found in the absence of severe pulmonary hypertension.

In determining the aetiology of aortic regurgitation, it is important to look for other valve lesions and for evidence of disease in other systems. The signs of mitral stenosis or regurgitation suggest a rheumatic origin. Syphilis should be suspected particularly when there is aneurysmal dilatation of the aorta or calcification of the ascending aorta. Congenital aortic regurgitation is usually overshadowed by aortic or subaortic stenosis.

Clinical course and prognosis

Minor degrees of aortic regurgitation are compatible with freedom from symptoms and a normal life span although the risk of infective endocarditis is ever present. In the moderate to severe case, symptoms and signs develop slowly, and it is usually not until the fourth or fifth decade that disability sets in. The severity of aortic regurgitation can be judged, to a large extent, by the pulse pressure and the size of the left ventricle. Increasing dyspnoea and an enlarging heart are signs that the patient is unlikely to survive for more than a few years. Sudden death is unusual in asymptomatic patients but may occur when an advanced stage has been reached.

Treatment

Medical treatment (diuretics and ACE inhibitors) should be given to most patients with regurgitation. If the patient is still symptomatic, then surgical treatment (aortic valve replacement) should be considered. Aortic valve replacement should also be considered in asymptomatic patients with progressive dilatation of the left ventricle in the hope of preventing permanent damage to the left ventricle. Serial echocardiography is useful in detecting such dilatation. Recent American Heart Association guidelines have suggested referral for surgery when the end-systolic left ventricular diameter exceeds 4.5 cm in aortic regurgitation (compared with 3.5 cm for patients with mitral regurgitation).

In good hands, the results of aortic valve replacement, either by artificial valves or bioprostheses, are low, but there is an operative mortality rate of about 2%. Artificial prostheses necessitate anticoagulant therapy; bioprostheses do not but are less durable and may require replacement within 5–10 years. Successful surgery is accompanied by a diminution in heart size, although not necessarily to normal. Symptoms are relieved, but medical measures may still be required.

Combined aortic stenosis and regurgitation

Aortic stenosis and regurgitation are often combined. When the lesion is congenital, atherosclerotic or calcific, the stenosis is usually the more important. In rheumatic heart disease, all gradations between the two can occur. In deciding which is dominant, the character of the pulse and the pulse pressure are of great value. A collapsing pulse is incompatible with severe stenosis; a small pulse makes major regurgitation unlikely. The murmurs can be deceptive as loud aortic systolic murmurs are not uncommon in aortic regurgitation even when stenosis is slight or absent. Likewise, the intensity of an aortic diastolic murmur is an unreliable guide to the severity of regurgitation. Echocardiography and, if necessary, cardiac catheterization and angiography permit adequate assessment of the relative contribution of each lesion.

TRICUSPID VALVE DISEASE

The structure of the tricuspid valve is similar to that of the mitral valve, except for the presence of three cusps. It may be affected by either stenosis or regurgitation. Tricuspid stenosis is nearly always rheumatic in origin and is rarely the dominant cardiac lesion. Some degree of tricuspid stenosis occurs in about 10% of cases of rheumatic heart disease, but is of significance in only about 3%. Organic tricuspid regurgitation, which is uncommon, is usually due to rheumatic heart disease. Functional tricuspid regurgitation is a frequent complication of right ventricular failure whatever the cause. Endocarditis of the tricuspid valve is being seen increasingly in intravenous drug abusers. Ebstein's anomaly, a congenital form of tricuspid valve dysplasia, is discussed in Chapter 13.

When tricuspid valve lesions are due to rheumatic heart disease, the pathological appearances are similar to those seen in the mitral valve. The valve cusps are thickened and the chordae may be adherent and shortened. Dilatation of the tricuspid valve ring is a major factor in regurgitation and occurs as a result of either dilatation of the right ventricle or the rheumatic process.

Tricuspid stenosis

The narrowed valve obstructs flow from the right atrium to the right ventricle during ventricular diastole. As a consequence, right atrial pressure rises, cardiac output falls, and the right atrium and venae cavae dilate. Atrial contraction becomes increasingly forceful and produces large 'a' waves in the venous pulse if sinus rhythm is preserved, as it usually is. Hepatic engorgement follows and ascites and peripheral oedema eventually develop.

In most cases of tricuspid stenosis, mitral stenosis is also present and dominates the clinical picture. For this reason, breathlessness is the commonest symptom, but because tricuspid stenosis restricts right ventricular throughput, pulmonary congestion is often less severe than it is in isolated mitral stenosis. The patient with mitral stenosis may become less breathless as tricuspid stenosis progresses, but at the expense of right-sided cardiac failure.

Large flicking venous 'a' waves may be seen even in early cases. When the lesion is more advanced, the venous pressure as a whole is elevated. The 'a' wave disappears when atrial fibrillation develops. The flow of blood from the atrium into the ventricle during diastole is slow and the 'y' descent of the venous pulse is therefore prolonged. The liver is enlarged and may exhibit presystolic pulsation corresponding with the large 'a' waves. On auscultation, mid-diastolic and presystolic murmurs may be heard at the lower left sternal edge which are similar in timing to those of mitral stenosis but of a rather more scratchy quality. The murmurs are accentuated by inspiration, because of increased venous return to the right atrium at this time. The signs of mitral stenosis may be masked.

On the ECG, the only characteristic feature is the presence of the tall P waves of right atrial enlargement. The chest radiograph shows enlargement of the right atrium and superior vena cava; the features of mitral stenosis are also usually present. The lung fields are often relatively clear. Echocardiography may demonstrate thickening and reduced movement of the tricuspid valve leaflets. As in the assessment of mitral stenosis, it is possible to measure a tricuspid pressure half-time which will be prolonged in patients with tricuspid stenosis.

On cardiac catheterization, a diastolic pressure difference can be demonstrated between right atrium and right ventricle, and there is usually a large 'a' wave in the right atrial pulse.

The prognosis of patients with tricuspid stenosis is often relatively good. However, if the lesion is severe, progressive signs of right-sided cardiac failure develop; ascites, jaundice and cachexia are characteristic.

In the majority of patients with tricuspid stenosis, the lesion is insufficiently severe to warrant surgery, which should be undertaken only if the stenosis is responsible for major symptoms. Valvotomy seldom restores normal valve function; replacement by a prosthesis is usually necessary.

Tricuspid regurgitation

Functional tricuspid regurgitation is a common complication of right ventricular failure and pulmonary hypertension. Since most patients with this condition have evidence of rheumatic heart disease, it is often difficult to be certain whether or not there is organic tricuspid disease as well.

The features of tricuspid regurgitation are the consequence of a large volume of blood being regurgitated through the valve from the right ventricle. As a result, the forward flow into the pulmonary circuit is reduced and the right ventricle has to cope with a large volume load. When regurgitation is severe, large systolic ('cv') waves develop in the right atrium, which are transmitted to the peripheral veins and liver. There is a high flow of blood through the tricuspid valve during diastole, as both the regurgitated and the forward flow must be transported at this time. Both diastolic and systolic flow through the valve are increased on inspiration as an increased volume of blood is drawn into the heart.

Coexistent mitral valve disease usually dominates the clinical picture and dyspnoea is the major symptom. Tricuspid regurgitation may reduce the effects of the mitral valve disease on the lungs at the expense of producing right-sided heart failure. As the disease progresses, there is an increase in venous pressure, hepatic enlargement, ascites and peripheral oedema. Large systolic waves are present in the jugular veins; systolic pulsation of the liver may be felt. A systolic murmur is heard at the lower left sternal edge; this is usually increased on inspiration. There may also be a tricuspid diastolic murmur due either to concomitant tricuspid stenosis or to high flow through the orifice during this phase.

There are no specific ECG features of tricuspid regurgitation; the chest radiograph usually shows right atrial enlargement. If the tricuspid regurgitation is secondary to mitral valve disease and pulmonary hypertension, the characteristic radiological features of these lesions will be present. On echocardiography, the right ventricle and right atrium will usually be dilated and colour flow mapping will show a broad jet of tricuspid regurgitation.

At cardiac catheterization, the chief feature is the large systolic venous wave of the right atrial pulse. The finding of severe pulmonary hypertension suggests the regurgitation is functional. A near normal pulmonary artery pressure is an indication that the tricuspid disease is organic.

It is often difficult to differentiate mitral regurgitation from tricuspid regurgitation, or to determine whether there is a combination of the two. Mitral regurgitation is suggested by radiation of the murmur to the axilla and by left ventricular enlargement, tricuspid regurgitation by systolic venous pulsation and by inspiratory accentuation of the murmur. Tricuspid regurgitation is often tolerated for a long time, but sooner or later the features of advanced right-sided cardiac failure become disabling, often with jaundice and cachexia. Severe oedema and ascites develop and are progressively less responsive to treatment.

If the tricuspid regurgitation is functional, there may be striking improvement with digitalis and diuretic therapy. Usually, surgery for associated mitral valve disease is required, and, if successful, leads to the disappearance of the tricuspid leak. Often the surgeon will inspect and repair the tricuspid valve at the time of mitral valve surgery. Occasionally replacement by a prosthesis is necessary.

PULMONARY VALVE DISEASE

Pulmonary valve disease is relatively uncommon. Pulmonary stenosis is usually of congenital origin and is discussed in Chapter 13. Other causes of pulmonary stenosis include rheumatic heart disease and malignant carcinoid. Obstruction of the outflow tract of the right ventricle may occur in hypertrophic cardiomyopathy and mediastinal tumours.

Pulmonary regurgitation is usually secondary to pulmonary hypertension, but occasionally occurs as a consequence of infective endocarditis, as a complication of the surgical relief of pulmonary stenosis, and as a congenital anomaly. It is nearly always overshadowed by the heart disease to which it is secondary. In most cases, there are signs of pulmonary hypertension, and the only feature which suggests the diagnosis is an early diastolic murmur (the Graham Steell murmur) in the second or third left intercostal spaces which becomes louder on inspiration. It is often difficult to decide whether a murmur in this position is due to pulmonary or aortic regurgitation. Pulmonary regurgitation is unlikely in the absence of signs of pulmonary hypertension and right ventricular hypertrophy. Aortic regurgitation is suggested by a collapsing pulse and the signs of left ventricular hypertrophy, although these signs may be absent if the regurgitation is slight. The diagnosis may be confirmed by echocardiography and Doppler examination.

INFECTIVE ENDOCARDITIS

The term *infective endocarditis* is now preferred to older terms such as subacute bacterial endocarditis. This is a relatively uncommon condition with around 1500 cases per annum in the UK. It most commonly occurs in patients with pre-existing mitral or aortic valve disease although the pre-existing valve abnormality may be minor and of no haemodynamic consequence. Two new forms of endocarditis have emerged over the last 20 years; these are prosthetic valve endocarditis in patients with artificial valves and tricuspid valve endocarditis in intravenous drug abusers. Despite advances in surgery and the development of new antibiotics, the mortality of this condition remains high at 20–40%.

Types of endocarditis

Native valve endocarditis
The majority of patients have a predisposing cardiac lesion. The pattern of underlying cardiac disease has been changing, reflecting the decline in the incidence of rheumatic heart disease. Currently the commonest acquired underlying lesions, in decreasing frequency, are mitral valve prolapse, degenerative aortic and mitral lesions, and rheumatic heart disease. The most common congenital lesions predisposing to endocarditis in the adult are bicuspid aortic valve, ventricular septal defect, coarctation of the aorta and pulmonary stenosis. Endocarditis can occur on a previously normal valve but this is rare.

Endocarditis in intravenous drug abusers
Endocarditis in the absence of underlying cardiac disease is common amongst intravenous drug abusers. The tricuspid valve is the focus of infection in about 50% of cases, with the mitral and aortic valves each accounting for about 20% of cases. Pulmonary valve endocarditis also occurs but is rare.

The presentation of right-sided endocarditis differs from left-sided. Typically, patients may present with pneumonia or multiple septic pulmonary emboli.

Prosthetic valve endocarditis

Prosthetic valve endocarditis is divided into 'early' and 'late'. By definition, endocarditis is early when symptoms occur within 60 days of valve implantation and late if they occur after this time. Early infection is generally due to contamination in the perioperative period, from sources such as intravenous cannulae, central lines or urinary catheters. The majority of cases are due to staphylococcal infection. The bacteriology of late prosthetic valve endocarditis more closely resembles native valve endocarditis.

Pathology

The pathogenesis of endocarditis is thought to involve a high pressure jet passing into a lower pressure chamber. The jet causes physical trauma to the endocardial surface on which bacteria then settle. Because a high pressure jet is important, endocarditis is more likely to occur in association with a ventricular septal defect (VSD) than an atrial septal defect (ASD) and is rare in patients with pure mitral stenosis.

A large number of different organisms may cause bacterial endocarditis. Common organisms include:

- *Streptococcus viridans.* An oral commensal of several varieties, this is the organism most frequently responsible for endocarditis, accounting for some 50–70% of cases. Most are highly sensitive to penicillin.
- *Streptococcus faecalis.* These organisms normally inhabit the gastrointestinal tract. They are generally resistant to penicillin. High doses must be used and an aminoglycoside added to achieve a bactericidal effect.
- *Streptococcus bovis.* This organism is frequently associated with the presence of colonic polyps or colonic malignancy. It is highly sensitive to penicillin.
- *Staphylococcus aureus.* This skin organism accounts for about 25% of cases of native valve endocarditis. It is the commonest cause of endocarditis amongst intravenous drug abusers, in whom it is responsible for some 60% of cases. The majority of organisms are highly resistant to penicillin. Multiple metastatic abscesses are common.
- *Staphylococcus epidermidis.* This organism is a relatively rare cause of native valve endocarditis, but a common cause of prosthetic valve endocarditis. Different strains vary in their sensitivity to penicillin.
- Other rare causes of endocarditis include *Neisseria gonorrhoeae, Coxiella burnetii* (Q fever), *Chlamydia psittaci* (psittacosis), anaerobic Gram-negative bacilli and the HACEK group of Gram-negative bacilli.

Infection leads to the formation of friable vegetations which have necrotic tissue, platelets, fibrin, white cells and red cells in their base, with superficial layers of fibrin and microorganisms. Ulceration may lead to erosion or perforation of the valve cusps or of a sinus of Valsalva. The location of the endocarditis depends upon the underlying lesion. In aortic regurgitation, endocarditis affects the ventricular surface of the valve; in mitral regurgitation it involves the atrial surface of the mitral valve. In a ventricular septal defect, the vegetations may form around the defect itself but are often located either on the tricuspid valve or where the jet impinges on the right ventricular wall. Invasion of the adjacent myocardium is common and may proceed to abscess formation, and to pericardial involvement.

Embolization from the vegetations is frequent and is responsible for many of the clinical features of the disease. Large emboli may cause occlusion of the cerebral, renal or splenic arteries. Microemboli affect nearly all parts of the body and, in particular, lead to skin lesions and a glomerulonephritis. Pulmonary emboli develop when the right side of the heart is involved, as it is when there is a ventricular septal defect or persistent ductus arteriosus.

Several of the manifestations of the disease, including arthritis and glomerulitis, are thought to be due to immune complex deposition.

Clinical features

In the majority of patients, the portal of entry of the infective agent is not known. A history of dental treatment (usually fillings or dental extraction) may be elicited and in a small proportion there has been preceding urethral, pelvic or cardiac surgery. *Strep. bovis* usually gains entry via the colon and patients with this strain of endocarditis should be screened for carcinoma of the colon. Occasionally, patients who are already in hospital may develop endocarditis as a result of infected vascular cannulation sites or central venous pressure lines. The organism is usually staphylococcal and is likely to be penicillin-resistant.

The onset is often insidious, with malaise and feverishness being the earliest complaints. The symptoms often mimic those of influenza. If left untreated, a characteristic clinical picture develops which was common in the days before antibiotic therapy. The complete syndrome of fever, anaemia, petechiae in the skin, clubbing, splenomegaly, a cardiac murmur and microscopic haematuria is seldom seen nowadays.

Abnormal clinical features in patients with endocarditis include:

- *heart murmurs*. The appearance of a new murmur or change in character of an existing murmur is suggestive of endocarditis.
- *petechiae*. These may develop on any part of the body. They may be embolic or vasculitic. They should be sought particularly in the conjunctivae, in the mouth and in the ocular fundi (Roth's spots are small oval, retinal haemorrhages with a pale centre). Haemorrhagic lesions on the palms and soles are termed Janeway lesions
- *splinter haemorrhages*. These are small linear streaks in the nailbeds of fingers and toes
- *Osler's nodes*. These are small tender nodules in the tips of the fingers and toes
- *clubbing*. This arises only if the disease is present for several months
- *splenomegaly*. This too takes several months to develop and is a feature of long-standing disease
- *proteinuria and microscopic haematuria*
- *neurological complications* are common and are due to embolic occlusion of cerebral vessels or to mycotic aneurysms.

Investigations

Most patients with infective endocarditis have a normochromic normocytic anaemia. The C-reactive protein (CRP) level will be raised, although this is not a specific abnormality for infective endocarditis. Chest radiography and ECG are of little value except in the diagnosis and assessment of the underlying cardiac abnormality. Confirmation of the diagnosis depends on obtaining a positive blood culture, which is possible in some 90% of cases. At least six specimens of blood should be obtained over a period of 1–2 days. The blood should be incubated aerobically and anaerobically, and special cultures should be set up for fungi. If the patient has received penicillin previously, penicillinase should be incorporated in the culture medium. Complement fixation tests must be undertaken for the diagnosis of *Coxiella* and *Chlamydia* infection.

Echocardiography is an important investigation of this disorder, both because of its ability to demonstrate vegetations and because it can help in the assessment of the severity of valvar involvement. Vegetations are seen in only 60% of cases by the cross-sectional technique. The absence of vegetations on echocardiography, therefore, does not exclude endocarditis. Transoesophageal echocardiography can achieve higher success rates, and can identify the presence of vegetations in some 90% of patients with endocarditis.

Diagnostic criteria

The currently used criteria for the diagnosis of endocarditis are those devised by Durack in 1994. The diagnosis is made when two major, or one major and three minor, or five minor criteria are fulfilled. The criteria are as follows:

Major criteria:

- positive blood cultures (two or more with the same organism)
- evidence of endocardial involvement – vegetations on echocardiography, abscess formation, etc.

Minor criteria:

- fever greater than 38°C
- known predisposition to endocarditis
- vascular phenomena – arterial emboli
- immune phenomena – Roth spots, glomerulonephritis
- further echo evidence – progressive valve regurgitation
- further microbiology – serolgy, etc.

These criteria have been criticized on the grounds that they are not sensitive for the diagnosis of prosthetic valve endocarditis or Q fever endocarditis. Newer criteria are being devised by the European Society of Cardiology.

Treatment

It is important that the responsible organism should be identified without delay, so that the appropriate antibiotics can be given. However, 'best guess' therapy should be started immediately after the blood cultures have been taken and adjusted once the culture results are available. Bactericidal agents should be employed, because bacteriostatic drugs produce only temporary suppression of the infection. Following isolation and identification of an organism, careful discussion with the microbiology department is advisable to guide antibiotic selection. Intravenous administration is essential; peripheral venous canulae can be used but should be changed every 72 h to prevent thrombosis of the peripheral veins. Central lines are preferred if treatment is likely to be for several weeks. Standard central lines puncture the skin and then the vein (usually internal jugular or subclavian) immediately below the skin; venous thrombosis is unlikely but infection at the puncture site can occur. With a 'tunnelled' central line ('Hickman line'), the line passes subcutaneously for several centimetres before entering the vein. A tunnelled line is much less likely to become infected and should last for the full duration of treatment, even if this is 6 weeks.

Antibiotic selection
- When the organism is penicillin sensitive (e.g. *Strep. viridans* or *Strep. bovis*), a combination of penicillin and gentamicin is given. Administration must be intravenous, at least for the first 2 weeks. Standard dosage would be penicillin G, 1.2 megaunits (MU) every 4 h and gentamicin 80–120 mg every 12 h according to renal function and blood levels. A change to oral therapy may be possible later, given a good response.
- Some streptococci, such as *Strep. faecalis*, may be more resistant to penicillin. They are usually treated with amoxicillin or ampicillin 2 g i.v. every 4 h plus gentamicin 80 mg i.v. every 12 h for at least 4 weeks.
- Penicillin-sensitive staphylococci will respond to penicillin, but the more common penicillin-resistant strains demand large doses of penicillinase-resistant drugs (e.g. flucloxacillin 2 g i.v. every 4 h). Gentamicin is usually added for possible synergistic benefit. Coagulase-negative staphylococci such as *Staph. epidermidis* are frequently methicillin-resistant and resistant to all beta-lactam antibiotics. In cases of methicillin resistance, vancomycin should be substituted for flucloxacillin, with the addition of gentamicin. Oral rifampicin is also of value in the management of penicillin-resistant staphylococci.
- The treatment of other rarer causes of endocarditis, such as Gram-negative organisms, *Coxiella*, Q fever and fungi should be discussed with the microbiology department.

A minimum of 4 weeks' therapy is thought necessary in all cases. Antibiotic therapy is constantly changing as new drugs become available and as organisms become resistant to those in current use.

The temperature usually falls to normal within 3 days of the start of effective antibiotic therapy. If pyrexia recurs, there are several possible explanations:

- emergence of resistant organisms
- superinfection with another organism
- development of a reaction to the antibiotic
- development of an abscess.

Culture-negative endocarditis
In around 10% of patients, no organism may be identified after the initial sets of blood cultures. There are several possible explanations for this:

- *Previous antibiotic therapy.* Even a single dose of antibiotics prior to blood being taken for culture reduces the chance of successfully identifying the infecting organism. If the patient has recently been treated with penicillin, then the blood can be cultured with penicillinase.

- *Fastidious or cell-dependant organisms.* Q fever and *Chlamydia* are usually diagnosed by serological tests rather by culture.
- *Fungal infection.* This should be considered in patients who are immuno-compromised, patients who have had prolonged treatment with broad-spectrum antibiotics and patients with prosthetic valves.
- *Incorrect diagnosis.* If cultures are repeatedly negative, consider other diagnoses such as left atrial myxoma, malignancy and connective tissue diseases.

Treatment monitoring

Because the complications listed above are common, the patient with endocarditis still requires close monitoring even when a correct diagnosis has been made and an appropriate antiobiotic regimen commenced. This monitoring should include:

- CRP measurement at least twice per week. Failure of the CRP to fall suggests inappropriate antibiotic selection, superinfection with a second organism or abscess development.
- Monitoring of renal function at least twice per week. Deterioration in renal fuction is commonly due to gentamicin toxicity and is an indication to reduce the dose.
- Where appropriate, monitoring of antibiotic levels. This is mandatory with gentamicin which, in addition to causing renal failure, causes oto-toxicity. If the peak level is too high, then the dose should be reduced. If the trough level is too high, then the time interval between doses should be extended.
- Echocardiography once per week.

Complications

Complications are a common occurrence in patients with endocarditis:

- *Congestive heart failure* may occur due to progressive valve destruction.
- *Systemic emboli* are a particular concern, and may result in stroke or myocardial infarction.
- *Mycotic aneurysm formation* may lead to occlusion of vessels or to haemorrhage. Neurological complications may be due either to emboli or to the presence of a mycotic aneurysm.
- *Renal failure.* This may arise due to immune complex deposition causing glomerulonephritis or because of antibiotic (usually gentamicin) toxicity.
- *Intracardiac abscess formation.* Aortic root abscess formation is a serious complication and an indication for surgical intervention. It should be suspected in patients with persistent or recurrent pyrexia. Septal extension from an abscess may cause widening of the PR interval and heart block. Abscess cavities can usually be seen on transoesophageal echocardiography.

Surgical treatment

In most cases it is appropriate to undertake medical management and first to attempt to control and cure the infection. Even in patients in whom surgery is inevitable, a short period of antibiotic treatment to try to control sepsis seems reasonable. Surgery is clearly indicated in patients with:

- heart failure due to progressive valvar regurgitation
- inability to control infection with antibiotics
- multiple embolic episodes.

Other possible indications for surgery:

- paravalvar abscess, usually in relation to aortic endocarditis. These patients are all likely to require surgery but the timing of surgery is controversial. Some people advocate early surgery (i.e. within 48 h of diagnosis) for all patients with aortic abscesses, while other surgeons prefer to treat with antibiotics for 2 or more weeks provided the CRP is falling and the patient is not haemodynamically compromised
- patients with large and friable vegetations visible on echo – this is also controversial. There is some evidence that larger vegetations (1–2 cm in diameter) are more likely to embolize and that these patients should be considered for early surgery
- prosthetic valve endocarditis – in these patients, cure with antibiotics alone is unlikely and the threshold for surgical intervention should be correspondingly lower.

Anticoagulation in endocarditis

The use of anticoagulants in the management of endocarditis is problematic. On the one hand, embolic phenomena are common. On the other, anticoagulation will not necessarily reduce the incidence of emboli and increases the potential risk of bleeding from a mycotic aneurysm. In general, if a patient is already on anticoagulant therapy (e.g. for a mechanical valve prosthesis), this should be continued, but anticoagulants should not be commenced de novo unless very clear-cut indications exist.

Prognosis

Recovery from infective endocarditis is rare unless effective and prolonged antiobiotic therapy is given. Death, which may be due to heart failure, emboli or renal failure, often does not occur until several months after the onset. Even with modern antibiotic treatment, the mortality rate is still in the region of 40%.

Prevention of endocarditis

Although endocarditis may occur in the absence of any obvious cause and in patients without known heart disease, in other cases the risk can be identified and many cases are preventable. A number of medical or dental procedures may provoke bacteraemia and place predisposed individuals at risk of endocarditis. In practice, the most commonly encountered risk arises with dental treatment. Antibiotic prophylaxis should be considered in any individual at risk of endocarditis undergoing any dental procedure likely to provoke gingival or mucosal bleeding. These include cleaning and scaling, but exclude simple fillings above the gum line. Careful attention to oral hygiene may be as important as antibiotic prophylaxis in safeguarding against orally acquired infection. Antibiotic prophylaxis is also advisable in at-risk individuals for many gastrointestinal, urological, gynaecological or obstetric procedures.

<table>
<tr><td>

Box 12.1

</td><td>

Patients at risk of endocarditis

Relatively high risk
Previous infective endocarditis
Prosthetic heart valves
Cyanotic congenital heart disease
Patent ductus arteriosus
Aortic regurgitation or stenosis
Mitral regurgitation
Ventricular septal defect
Aortic coarctation
Surgically repaired congenital heart disease with residual haemodynamic
  abnormality

Intermediate risk
Mitral valve prolapse with a mitral regurgitant murmur
Pure mitral stenosis
Tricuspid valve disease
Pulmonary stenosis
Hypertrophic cardiomyopathy
Bicuspid or calcified aortic valve
Surgically repaired intracardiac disease with no haemodynamic abnormality within
  6 months of surgery

Very low or negligible risk
Mitral prolapse without a regurgitant murmur
Trivial valve regurgitation or echo without structural abnormality
Isolated secundum atrial septal defect
Cardiac pacemaker or defibrillator

</td></tr>
</table>

Patients can be divided into groups at relatively high risk, intermediate risk and very low or negligible risk (Box 12.1). Antibiotic prophylaxis is indicated before bacteraemia-producing procedures in individuals at high and intermediate risk, but not in those at low risk. The standard prophylactic regimen for dental procedures is 3 g amoxicillin orally, given 1 h before the procedure. If the patient is allergic to penicillin or has had amoxicillin within the past month, then either clindamycin 600 mg as a single oral dose 1 hour before the procedure or erythromycin (1.5 g orally before and 0.5 g 6 h later) is recommended.

For procedures under general anaesthetic, ampicillin 1 g i.v. is given at the time of the premedication followed by 0.5 g 6 h later. For patients allergic to penicillin, vancomycin, teicoplanin or clindamycin can be used.

FURTHER READING

Carabello, B.A. & Crawford, F.A. (1997) Valvular heart diseases. *New England Journal of Medicine* **337**:32–41.
Bonow, R.O., Carabello, B., De Leon, A.C. et al (1998) AHA/ACC guidelines for the management of patients with valvular heart disease: a report of the American College of Cardiology/American Heart Association task force on Practice guidelines (committee on management of patients with valvular heart disease). *Journal of the American College of Cardiology* **32**:1486–1588.

Congenital heart disease

J.D.R. Thomson

A congenital anomaly of the heart is present in nearly one in every hundred babies born. Thirty years ago, many lesions carried a poor prognosis with little prospect of survival beyond the first few years of life. As surgeons have become more daring, the outlook for the majority of patients with congenital heart defects has been transformed. Survival into adulthood and beyond is now very much the norm in all but a handful of severe lesions. Consequently, there are ever growing numbers of older patients with structurally abnormal hearts and for many lesions (and patients) an entirely new natural history has had to be learnt. The practice of congenital heart disease can no longer be viewed as an entirely paediatric subspecialty. Diagnosis and management of patients with congenital heart disease starts in fetal life, and continues through childhood and into adult life, when most patients with congenital heart defects will require continued attention.

VARIETIES OF CONGENITAL HEART DISEASE

Congenital heart disease can be divided into four types:

- *Communications between the systemic and pulmonary circulations, e.g. ventricular septal defect, atrial septal defect, patent ductus arteriosus.* The impedance to flow is normally lower on the right side of the heart and in the pulmonary artery than it is on the left side of the heart and in the aorta. Consequently, the intracardiac pressures are relatively low on the right side. When the two sides of the heart are in communication, provided there is no other abnormality, there is a shunt of blood from left to right through the defect and an increased blood flow through the lungs. In patients with ventricular septal defects and persistent ducti, the volume load falls predominantly on the left ventricle, which enlarges accordingly. In an atrial septal defect, the load falls on the right ventricle.

  Increased pulmonary blood flow frequently leads to a moderate elevation of pulmonary arterial pressure. In most cases, the resistance of the pulmonary arteries is normal but, sometimes, changes take place in the arterial walls which cause a high pulmonary vascular resistance. Severe and irreversible pulmonary hypertension may then ensue and, eventually, lead to reversal of the shunt (see pulmonary vascular disease).

- *Cyanotic cardiac lesions, e.g. tetralogy of Fallot, transposition of the great arteries.* The mechanisms for cyanosis in these conditions are dealt with in their respective sections. Generally for cyanosis to occur in a patient with congenital heart disease, there must be obstruction to the right ventricular outflow tract and the substrate for a shunt. Although tetralogy of Fallot is the most well known example, other lesions such as severe pulmonary stenosis and even the Eisenmenger syndrome (in which the right ventricular outflow tract obstruction can be thought of at a very distal level) cause cyanosis by the same mechanism. A few relatively rare lesions (e.g. total anomalous pulmonary venous drainage and truncus arteriosus) cause a combination of cyanosis and breathlessness due to high pulmonary blood flow with abnormal mixing of the pulmonary and systemic circulations.
- *Obstructive lesions, e.g. coarctation of the aorta, aortic and pulmonary stenosis.* When isolated these lesions impose a pressure load on their respective ventricle which if severe can lead to cardiac failure or even ductal dependency. Obstructive lesions often coexist with other abnormalities such as a pulmonary stenosis with a ventricular septal defect (tetralogy of Fallot) or coarctation, aortic and mitral stenosis (so called Shones syndrome).
- *Complex lesions.* Many complex congenital cardiac abnormalities, both of form and position, exist. Presentation, diagnosis and management cannot necessarily be generalized (see tricuspid atresia). Descriptions of individual lesions are beyond the scope of this chapter.

COMMUNICATIONS

Atrial septal defects (ASDs)

Defects of the atrial septum are relatively common, frequently occurring in isolation (Fig. 13.1). Types of defects include:

- *Patent foramen ovale (PFO).* This is a remnant of the normal fetal circulation rather than a true atrial septal defect. A potential gap (the so called 'probe patent' foramen) exists between the normal primum and secundum portions of the atrial septum in approximately 25% of the population. The main clinical relevance of a PFO is the association with unexplained thrombotic stroke in young adults. This is caused by paradoxical embolization of clot from the deep veins of the leg through the PFO and into the arterial circulation hence causing a stroke. The identification of a PFO in a young patient with an unexplained stroke may be an indication for its closure, which can be achieved surgically or increasingly through the percutaneous delivery of a closure device.
- *Secundum atrial septal defects (Fig. 13.2).* Defects of the fossa ovalis of the atrial septum are the most common variety of ASD. Secundum ASDs are usually central. They vary markedly in their size and anatomical margins but do not encroach upon the atrioventricular valves.
- *Primum atrial septal defects (Fig. 13.2).* These are a form of defect 'low down' in the atrial septum. Primum ASDs are atrioventricular septal defects (AVSDs). Unlike any other defect of the atrial septum, primum ASDs have an abnormality of the atrioventricular junction and a common atrioven-

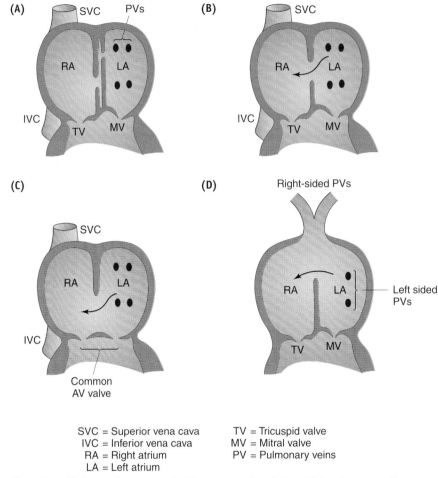

(A) SVC PVs
RA LA
IVC
TV MV

(B) SVC
RA LA
IVC
TV MV

(C) SVC
RA LA
IVC
Common
AV valve

(D) Right-sided PVs
RA LA — Left sided PVs
TV MV

SVC = Superior vena cava   TV = Tricuspid valve
IVC = Inferior vena cava   MV = Mitral valve
RA = Right atrium   PV = Pulmonary veins
LA = Left atrium

Fig. 13.1 (A) Patent foramen ovale. The construction of the atrial septum normally prevents shunting form left to right. (B) Ostium secundum atrial septal defect. The atrioventricular valves are unaffected. (C) Primum ASD with common atrioventricular valve (note the lack of offset of the left and right AV valve components). (D) Sinus venous atrial septal defect with anomalous drainage of the right pulmonary veins.

tricular valve. Although the valve is separated into two portions by the anchorage of the ventricular septum, the valve morphology is fundamentally different to that of the normal heart, with separate tricuspid and mitral valves. Such valves are sometimes stenotic, often regurgitant and frequently require surgical attention in their own right.

- *Sinus venosus atrial septal defects.* These are rare defects accounting for 5–10% of all ASDs. They occur in the upper part of the atrial septum outside of the confines of the fossa ovalis, usually adjacent to the superior vena cava. Sinus venosus ASDs are almost always associated with anomalous pulmonary venous drainage. Surgery is required, often with the construction of a baffle to redirect pulmonary venous flow into the left atrium.

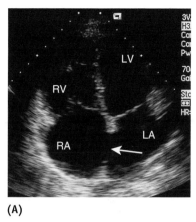

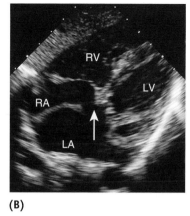

(A)   **(B)**

Fig. 13.2 (A) Secundum atrial septal defect. Echocardiogram shows a defect in the central portion of the atrial septum (arrowed). ECG typically shows an rsR pattern, with right axis deviation. (B) Primum atrial septal defect. Echocardiogram shows a defect low in the atrial septum (arrowed) with a common atrioventricular valve. ECG shows a rsR pattern, but there is left axis deviation. (LA: left atrium; LV: left ventricle; RA: right atrium; RV: right ventricle)

Physiology

The right ventricle is normally thinner and more distensible than the left and, at a given pressure level, more easily filled with blood. Therefore when both atria are in communication, blood flows preferentially into the right ventricle from both atria and the shunt through the defect which is primarily in diastole is almost exclusively from left to right. Pulmonary blood flow is usually two or three times the aortic blood flow, but the distensibility of pulmonary arterioles is such that they can readily accommodate this with little or no increase in pulmonary arterial pressure. The increase in pulmonary blood flow maintained over many years very occasionally leads to changes in the small pulmonary vessels which increase pulmonary vascular resistance and can cause severe pulmonary hypertension. Significantly elevated pulmonary vascular resistance is a contraindication to ASD closure.

Symptoms

The secundum type of defect seldom gives rise to disabling symptoms before the third decade of life, but breathlessness and fatigue can develop before the age of 40. Symptoms are often progressive and are exacerbated when atrial arrhythmias develop, as they commonly do.

Clinical signs

The arterial pulse is relatively small; the venous pressure is usually normal. The right ventricle is strikingly overactive. Splitting of the second sound is wide, and varies little with respiration ('fixed' splitting of the second sound). This is due to relatively late closure of the pulmonary valve as a consequence of delayed emptying of the overburdened right ventricle. A systolic murmur in the second left interspace due to high flow across the pulmonary valve is almost invariable. Larger defects cause mid-diastolic murmur at the lower left sternal edge, accentuated by inspiration, and produced by increased flow through the tricuspid valve. In primum ASDs, left-sided atrioventricular valve regurgitation is often present which is indistinguishable clinically from mitral regurgitation, often leading to clinical signs suggestive of left ventricular enlargement.

Investigation

- The *electrocardiogram (ECG)* nearly always shows the features of partial right bundle branch block. In the common ostium secundum type, there is frequently right axis deviation, whilst in the ostium primum type of ASD there is usually left axis deviation. This feature is of importance in differentiating the two types of defect (Fig. 13.2).

- On the *chest radiograph*, the heart is usually slightly enlarged, and the pulmonary artery and its branches prominent, as are the right atrium and the right ventricle. The aorta is small and may not be visible. In patients with primum ASDs and significant left-sided atrioventricular valve regurgitation, overall cardiomegaly may be present in addition to left atrial enlargement.

- *Echocardiography*, in a significant ostium secundum defect, demonstrates right ventricular volume loading (Fig. 13.2). As a result, 'paradoxical' motion of the interventricular septum, in which the septum moves towards the right ventricle in systole instead of its usual movement towards the posterior left ventricular wall, is often seen. In ostium primum defects, a common valve is present which can be visualized on short axis echocardiographic cuts. Colour flow Doppler will demonstrate regurgitation through the left-sided portion of the common valve and will also demonstrate stenosis or rarer abnormalities such as a double orifice valve.

- *Cross-sectional echocardiography* reliably demonstrates all forms of ASD and differentiates easily between them. *Transoesphageal echocardiography* can be required to demonstrate a patent foramen ovale or the exact anatomy of a sinus venosus defect. *Doppler ultrasonography* provides supporting evidence but is less reliable in calculating the pulmonary to systemic shunt. In any event, more useful is echocardiographic right ventricular volume loading, which if present confirms a haemodynamically important shunt.

Clinical and echocardiographic features are generally sufficient for accurate diagnosis. Routine confirmation by cardiac catheterization is not required unless associated lesions are suspected.

Treatment

Closure of a secundum defect is advisable in all patients with evidence of right ventricular volume loading on transthoracic echocardiogram. Although closure in the hands of a skilled surgeon carries a low mortality, increasingly, suitable defects are closed percutaneously using a number of different devices (Fig. 13.3). Percutaneous ASD closure is only suitable for patients with a secundum ASD and is limited to those defects under 4 cm in size with good margins all the way around the defect for device anchorage.

Correction of an ostium primum type of defect is always surgical and is more difficult with a higher mortality rate. Surgery is usually undertaken if there are symptoms or when the shunt is large. Occasionally, patients present during adult life without evidence of a significant shunt or important atri-

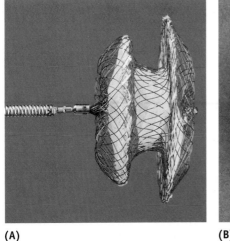 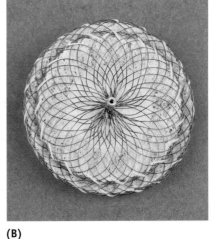

(A)   (B)

Fig. 13.3   Amplatzer atrial septal occluder. (A) Lateral view attached to delivery cable. (B) En face, posterior aspect.

oventricular valve regurgitation and they can be left alone, but the majority require surgery during childhood. Because of the the common nature of the atrioventricular valve, the difficulty is fashioning a 'neo mitral valve' that functions normally after surgery, and it is the norm for such valves to leak – subsequent valve replacement is then likely.

Ventricular septal defects (VSDs)

Excluding biscuspid aortic valves, ventricular septal defects (VSDs) are the most common congenital cardiac lesion, occurring in isolation or in association with other congenital cardiac defects.

The ventricular septum is divided into four components, the trabecular or muscular septum extending to the apex, the inlet (posterior) septum between the atrioventricular valves, the outlet septum which subtends the great arteries and the membranous septum which lies under the aortic root. Defects can arise in any position but the membranous septum is most commonly affected.

Physiology

Defects of the ventricular septum, which may be large in relation to the size of the heart at birth, tend to become smaller or to close in early childhood. If closure is insufficient to prevent a large shunt, the small pulmonary vessels may be damaged by being exposed to the ejectile force and pressure of left ventricular contraction. Irreversible pulmonary hypertension may be produced (see Pulmonary Vascular Disease in this chapter).

The effect of a ventricular septal defect (VSD) depends upon its size and upon the impedance to blood flow imposed by the pulmonary arterial vessels. If the defect is small, the jet of blood from the high pressure left ventricle to the low-pressure right ventricle has little haemodynamic effect. If the defect is large and the impedance of the pulmonary vessels low, a large shunt develops and the pulmonary blood flow becomes substantially more than systemic. If, on the other hand, there is a high pulmonary vascular resistance, the pulmonary blood flow is little or no more than the systemic and the pressure in both circuits is similar. If the pulmonary vascular resistance is very high, the shunt reverses (the so called Eisenmenger complex).

Symptoms

In the patient with a small defect, there are no symptoms, but there is a loud 'tearing' pansystolic murmur often accompanied by a thrill, maximal to the left side of the lower sternum.

Newborn infants have a high pulmonary vascular resistance which falls to normal levels in the first 3 months of life. At this point, a large defect at ventricular level is liable to produce cardiac failure and require treatment.

Clinical signs

Cardiac failure is usually obvious in the infant or small child with a significant left-to-right shunt through a large VSD. In the presence of a large left-to-right shunt, the pulse is usually small and the venous pressure normal, unless there is right heart failure. Both left and right ventricles may be hyperdynamic and with a large shunt, a soft pansystolic murmur is heard at the lower left sternal edge, usually accompanied by a mid-diastolic murmur at the apex due to high flow through the mitral valve.

Although there are some patients in whom large defects get smaller and become restrictive to flow, most, if untreated will ultimately progress to irreversible pulmonary hypertension as a result of pulmonary vascular disease. The development of pulmonary vascular disease is often heralded by an improvement in the symptoms of cardiac failure as the resistance to flow through the lungs decreases flow (a worrying sign in a patient with a large VSD). In patients who develop pulmonary vascular disease the signs of the ventricular septal defect are less obvious, although there may still be a systolic murmur between the apex and the left sternal edge. Right ventricular hypertrophy is evident; the pulmonary second sound may be accentuated and followed by the early diastolic murmur of pulmonary regurgitation.

Investigation

- The *ECG* in small defects is normal. When the left-to-right shunt is large, there is usually evidence of biventricular enlargement, manifested by abnormally deep but narrow Q waves and tall R waves in the left chest leads. In cases with pulmonary vascular disease, the ECG pattern of isolated right ventricular hypertrophy develops.
- The *chest radiograph* is normal with a small defect, but with a large left-to-right shunt there is some enlargement of the heart and, more specifically, prominence of the pulmonary vessels, left atrium and both ventricles.
- *Echocardiography*. Tiny defects will sometimes only be detectable with the stethoscope, even with the aid of modern colour Doppler echocardiography. With larger defects, left ventricular volume loading is present and

the defect can be visualized and its exact location in the septum established using 2D echocardiography. Doppler studies allow an assessment of the degree of resistance to flow between the two ventricles and therefore an indication of the overall size and haemodynamic importance of a particular defect. A high velocity Doppler signal indicates a defect that is restrictive to flow and hence likely to be haemodynamically unimportant. Care must be taken with children in the first 3 months of life, as falling pulmonary vascular resistance means that Doppler velocities can change over this period.

Correlation of these features usually provides sufficient evidence for accurate clinical diagnosis in spite of the various forms that defects of the ventricular septum may take. Further investigation is rarely indicated for patients with isolated VSDs and surgery can be safely undertaken on the basis of the clinical and echocardiographic findings alone. *Cardiac catheterization* may be indicated in complex cases: in the rare equivocal case in which the echocardiographic data is unclear or for quantification of the pulmonary vascular resistance in patients presenting late to determine if surgery is advisable or not. At catheter, the pulmonary artery saturation will be high in the patient with a left-to-right shunt and injection of radio-opaque contrast medium into the left ventricle will demonstrate the defect. In a small defect or if there are equal pressures in the systemic and pulmonary circulations, no shunt of oxygenated blood may be demonstrable.

Treatment

In deciding the appropriate therapy for a patient with VSD, the expected prognosis must be taken into account. This depends upon the age of the patient, the size of the defect, and the pulmonary vascular changes. Left untended, large VSDs are an important cause of death in the infant. Failure to thrive due to heart failure should prompt surgical closure of the defect. Infants with significant VSDs but with acceptable weight gain can be carefully watched in the hope that the defect will get smaller, with a low threshold for surgical intervention before the onset of pulmonary vascular disease. After the first year, few affected children die. A group of patients with modest defects, too small to threaten pulmonary vascular disease or cause significant symptoms, but large enough to put the left ventricle under a volume load due to a moderate shunt, may eventually come to intervention. There has been some early success with transcatheter delivered devices with these defects (Fig. 13.4). By the time patients with small VSDs reach adulthood, it is unlikely that the defect will spontaneously close. Such patients have a normal life span, but are exposed to the risk of infective endocarditis for which antibiotic prophylaxis, where appropriate, is always indicated. Long-term follow-up is required, particularly for those with high membranous VSDs in which there is a risk of aortic regurgitation due to prolapse of a valve leaflet caused by blood flow through an adjacent defect.

When the pulmonary vascular resistance is high, surgery is usually contraindicated as it cannot correct and may, indeed, worsen the pulmonary hypertension.

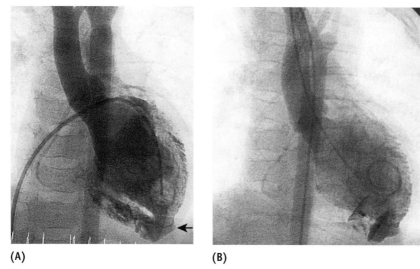

(A)   **(B)**

Fig. 13.4 Left ventricular angiograms showing apical muscular ventricular septal defect (arrowed) (A) after defect closure with a transcatheter delivered device (B).

Persistent ductus arteriosus (PDA) (Fig. 13.5)

During fetal life, the ductus arteriosus permits blood to flow from the pulmonary artery into the aorta. Within days after birth, it narrows and then closes.

Physiology and symptoms

In a few term infants and a sizeable proportion of premature neonates, the ductus arteriosus remains open and permits a flow of blood from the high-pressure aorta to the low-pressure pulmonary artery. This may cause heart failure in the first few weeks of life. More commonly, the ductus arteriosus undergoes partial closure and the shunt from aorta to pulmonary artery is relatively small. This gives rise to no symptoms during the first few years of life and is usually detected at a routine physical examination. A persistent ductus arteriosus may eventually become harmful for three reasons. First, it may act as a focus for infective endarteritis. Second, the leak of blood from the aorta to the pulmonary artery and the consequent high pulmonary blood flow may lead to cardiac failure in adolescence or adult life. Thirdly, but rarely, severe pulmonary hypertension may develop.

Clinical signs

The pulse may be of normal volume if the duct is small, but if it is large, the diastolic leak from the aorta causes a collapsing pulse. Correspondingly, the diastolic blood pressure may be low. The heart may be of normal size, or the left ventricle enlarged. The most characteristic feature of the condition is the 'continuous murmur', situated in the second left intercostal space by the sternal edge but often loudest 5–7.5 cm above or to the left of this. This murmur continues from systole into diastole and is maximal about the time of the second sound. In a few instances, particularly in infants, it may occur as a crescendo in late systole only. The murmur is due to flow of blood from the aorta through the persistent ductus arteriosus into the pulmonary artery in both phases of the

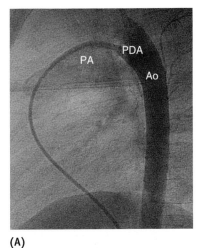

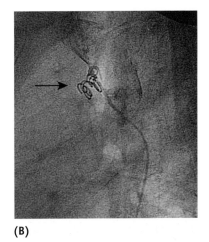

(B)

(A)

Fig. 13.5 (A) Angiogram in the descending aorta in the lateral projection in a patient with a persistent ductus arteriosus (PDA); the catheter is crossing from the pulmonary artery (PA) across the ductus arteriosus and into the descending aorta (Ao). (B) Occlusion of the ductus with embolisation coils (arrowed).

cardiac cycle. If the shunt is large, the increased venous return from the lungs causes a mid-diastolic murmur at the apex as it crosses the mitral valve.

The clinical diagnosis is usually easy because of the characteristic continuous murmur. Special investigation is seldom required even prior to surgical treatment. Care, however, is necessary to avoid confusion with the venous hum which is common in normal children. The hum is usually maximal to the right of the sternum below the right clavicle, diminishes or disappears when the child lies flat and can usually be abolished by compression of the jugular veins on the right side. Continuous murmurs due to other causes are rare and their maximum intensity is usually below and medial to the pulmonary area.

Investigation
- The *ECG* is usually normal but may show left ventricular hypertrophy.
- The *chest radiograph* may show enlargement of the left ventricle, aorta and pulmonary artery, and the features of increased pulmonary blood flow.
- *Echocardiography*. The duct can almost always be visualized by cross-sectional and colour Doppler echocardiography. With a significant shunt, volume loading of the left side of the heart is observed. Doppler echocardiography will establish the presence or absence of a pressure gradient between the aorta and pulmonary artery. It is important to remember, however that even with a pressure drop between the two, a significant shunt can still occur.

Special investigation beyond echocardiography is rarely necessary. Occasionally *magnetic resonance imaging (MRI)* can be helpful in delineating exact ductal anatomy in an adult. Cardiac catheterization is not required for diagnosis, and haemodynamic shunt calculations in this setting are inaccurate.

Treatment

The majority of PDAs are small and can be closed percutanously at cardiac catheterization (Fig. 13.5). Closure of small PDAs is undertaken in a clinically evident ductus to avoid the risk of endarteritis in later life. A number of percutaneously delivered devices are available to this end, and selection depends on the anatomy of the ductus (usually determined angiographically at the time of closure). Surgical treatment is reserved for the very large ductus causing heart failure in infants and premature neonates who remain a technical challenge beyond therapeutic catheterization. After surgery, a small number recannalize and require further attention (usually closure with a device) at a later date.

In symptomatic low birth weight premature infants, the ductus may cause life-threatening cardiac decompensation. Administration of indomethacin, a prostaglandin inhibitor, can induce duct closure medically.

Pulmonary vascular disease (Fig. 13.6)

Pulmonary vascular disease refers to changes in the small vessels of the distal pulmonary bed leading to pulmonary hypertension. As well as being irreversible, the condition is progressive and eventually fatal. The original description was in a patient with a ventricular septal defect with central cyanosis in the absence of proximal pulmonary stenosis (Eisenmenger syndrome) (Fig. 13.6). In this and most other cases, the cause of the damage to the pulmonary arterioles was a large and untreated left-to-right shunt.

Physiology and symptoms

Irreversible pulmonary arterial changes can develop at any time during childhood or adolescence. Symptoms are extremely variable; some patients develop them during childhood but many remain relatively symptom-free well into adulthood. Dyspnoea and fatigue are commonly reported. Other

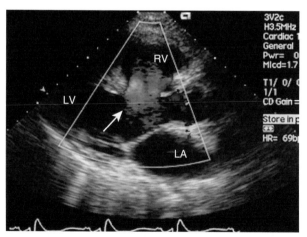

Fig. 13.6 Echocardiogram (parasternal long axis view) in a patient with Eisenmenger syndrome due to a large ventricular septal defect (arrowed). (LA: left atrium; LV: left ventricle; RV: right ventricle).

complaints include syncope, angina and haemoptysis, which are usually the result of the rupture of prominent bronchial vessels and generally self-limiting.

Clinical signs

On examination, the patient is cyanosed. When the shunt is through a ductus arteriosus, the venous blood is directed into the descending aorta and only the lower limbs become cyanosed ('differential cyanosis').

The arterial pulse is usually small, due to a low stroke volume; a large 'a' wave may be present in the venous pulse, due to forceful atrial contraction in the face of right ventricular hypertrophy. On palpation, one can detect right ventricular hypertrophy. On auscultation, the signs are mainly those of pulmonary hypertension: a loud second heart sound, a right ventricular fourth heart sound, a pulmonary early systolic ('ejection') click and, occasionally, the early diastolic murmur of pulmonary regurgitation and the pansystolic murmur of functional tricuspid regurgitation. In VSD, there is a single second sound, because the pressure in both ventricles is identical. In persistent ductus arteriosus, there is normal splitting of the second heart sound.

Investigation

- The *ECG* shows right atrial and right ventricular hypertrophy.
- On the *chest radiograph* there are large main pulmonary arteries but small peripheral arteries ('pruning'), together with right ventricular and right atrial enlargement.
- *Echocardiography* demonstrates features of pulmonary hypertension – right ventricular hypertrophy and high velocity tricuspid, and pulmonary regurgitation reflecting the raised right-sided pressures. Echocardiography will show the causative lesion as well.
- *Cardiac catheterization* allows further confirmation of the underlying anatomy but should not be undertaken lightly; injection of contrast into the pulmonary arteries in these patients can lead to sudden death. Catheterization allows a study of pulmonary vascular reversibility when challenged with a number of agents and this data is important in assessing suitability for treatment.

The diagnosis is suggested by the combination of central cyanosis and pulmonary hypertension in an adolescent or young adult. The Eisenmenger syndrome differs from tetralogy of Fallot (the commonest cardiac cause of central cyanosis in this age group) both in terms of physical signs (no pulmonary systolic thrill or murmur), and differences in the chest radiograph and echocardiogram.

Natural history

The progress of the Eisenmenger syndrome is usually slowly downhill, death commonly occurring between the ages of 20 and 40. The main causes of death are right heart failure (whose clinical features are a late sign), arrhythmias and, less often, infective endocarditis. Pregnancy is particularly hazardous in these patients and should be avoided.

Treatment

There is no conventional surgical treatment, other than heart–lung transplantation. Recent advances in the treatment of primary pulmonary hypertension with pulmonary vasodilators delivered by a number of routes may offer hope for the future. Temporary benefit can result from the conventional treatment of cardiac failure.

CYANOTIC LESIONS

Tetralogy of Fallot (Fig. 13.7)

Physiology

The fundamental anatomical abnormalities in tetralogy of Fallot are pulmonary stenosis with a VSD. Right ventricular hypertrophy and and dextroposition of the aorta (overriding the VSD) are the other components of the association (Fig. 13.7). The VSD is always unrestrictive so the physiology depends on the degree of right ventricular outflow tract obstruction. If the stenosis is slight, shunting will occur exclusively from left to right. In most cases however, pulmonary stenosis is severe enough that there is a right-to-left shunt. Generally, right ventricular outflow tract obstruction occurs in the infundibular area of the right ventricle, due to anterior deviation of the outlet septum but pulmonary valve stenosis and abnormalities of the distal pulmonary artery tree can occur as well. Infundibular stenosis tends to become more severe with advancing age and in most cases there is a progressive increase in the proportion of blood shunted from right to left. At the extreme end of the anatomical spectrum, infundibular stenosis can be so severe that the pulmonary artery is detached from the right ventricle (pulmonary atresia with ventricular septal defect). An infant presenting with this combination of abnormalities will be dependant on other sources (either the ductus arteriosus or collateral vessels) to maintain flow into the distal pulmonary tree and may therefore be ductus dependant (see Ductal Dependency later in this chapter).

Symptoms

Symptoms depend on the degree of pulmonary stenosis. It is not uncommon for an infant early in life with tetralogy of Fallot to behave like a child with a large VSD (breathlessness, failure to thrive, etc.) until sufficient pulmonary

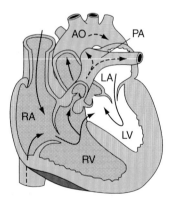

Fig. 13.7 Tetralogy of Fallot. Note infundibular pulmonary stenosis and ventricular septal defect, with right-to-left shunt at ventricular level.

stenosis develops to reverse the shunt. It is not until this occurs that the child displays central desaturation.

PRACTICE GUIDELINES

Hypercyanotic spells

Some children with tetralogy of Fallot are liable to sudden attacks of intense cyanosis known as hypercyanotic spells. Muscular spasm of the infundibulum of the right ventricle is responsible. In severe cases, these can be associated with syncope.

Hypercyanotic attacks should always be taken seriously. Generally admission to hospital is necessary and treatment with beta-blockade is usually required. In the child with severe or frequent spells, oxygen and morphine should be given. Sometimes medical therapy will not control a spelling child, and a cycle of desaturation, acidosis and deterioration develops. In this situation there may be no alternative but to place a surgical shunt as an emergency.

Clinical signs

The child is often small and may be dysmorphic. Recognition and management of associated problems is an important element of care of these children. Central cyanosis with finger clubbing are present in classical cases. The arterial pulses are small and venous pulses normal. There is a loud systolic murmur often accompanied by a thrill in the second or third left intercostal space, unless the stenosis is so severe that virtually no blood traverses it. The second heart sound is often single because the pulmonary valve component is inaudible.

Investigations

- The *ECG* shows right ventricular hypertrophy.
- The *chest radiograph* characteristically shows a 'boot-shaped' heart with a concavity on the left border in the place where the pulmonary artery is normally seen, and a prominent and elevated apex (Fig. 13.8). The pulmonary vascularity is decreased.
- Diagnosis is easily confirmed on *echocardiogram*, which shows a large aorta overriding the septum, the normal continuity between the anterior aortic wall and septum being lost. Using echocardiography, the proximal pulmonary artery anatomy can almost always be delineated. The distal pulmonary artery anatomy is less reliably delineated on echocardiogram, particularly in severe cases in which little or no (in the case of pulmonary atresia) blood flow passes through the proximal right ventricular outflow tract.

Tetralogy of Fallot is the most common cardiac lesion in children with central cyanosis after the first weeks of life. This frequency and the characteristic clinical, electrocardiographic, radiological and echocardiographic features usually make the diagnosis easy.

Although many units operate on children with less severe variants of tetralogy of Fallot on the evidence of the echocardiogram alone, *cardiac catheterization* is still frequently required. *Angiography* demonstrates distal pulmonary artery abnormalities which are often difficult to visualize on echocardiogram

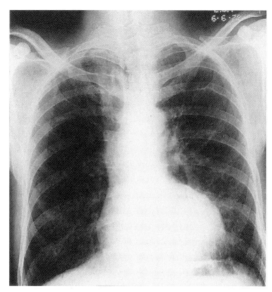

Fig. 13.8 Tetralogy of Fallot. The heart shadow is typically 'boot-shaped' with a concavity of the left heart border, instead of the normal pulmonary artery shadow. The apex is high and rounded. The lung fields are oligaemic.

and that may require surgical attention, and reliably rules out abnormal coronary artery anatomy which occurs in a significant proportion and which can complicate repair. At catheter, a systolic pressure drop can be demonstrated between the body and the outflow tract of the right ventricle. Pressures in the right and left ventricles are identical. Injection of contrast medium into the right ventricle delineates the region of stenosis and demonstrates the shunt through the VSD.

Treatment

Without surgery many patients with tetralogy of Fallot will die during childhood. Death in the unrepaired patient may result from hypercyanotic spells, from cerebrovascular accidents as a result of thrombosis promoted by polycythaemia, from infective endocarditis and from cerebral abscesses. The type of surgery depends upon the severity and exact anatomical details of the lesion and the patient age. The abnormality is corrected by relief of the pulmonary stenosis and by closure of the VSD. With improvements in neonatal surgical techniques, surgeons are now prepared to repair tetralogy of Fallot at an earlier age. In most centres, patients with uncomplicated tetralogy of Fallot will be surgically repaired before 3 years of age. In severely affected infants, particularly those with pulmonary atresia there may be no choice but to perform a palliative procedure first, usually the creation of a shunt by anastomozing the subclavian artery directly or a Goretex tube to the pulmonary artery. This increases the proportion of blood going through the lungs and increases oxygenation. The child can be given several years of comparatively good health and growth before the corrective procedure is performed.

Transposition of the great arteries (Figs 13.9 and 13.10)

Physiology

In transposition of the great arteries, the aorta arises from the right ventricle and the pulmonary artery from the left. As a consequence, there are separate systemic and pulmonary circulations; life cannot be sustained unless there is some communication between them (Fig. 13.9). Usually there is one or more of the following:

- patent foramen ovale
- atrial septal defect
- ventricular septal defect
- persistent ductus arteriosus.

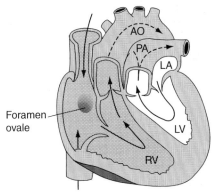

Fig. 13.9 Transposition of the great arteries. The aorta rises from the right ventricle and the pulmonary artery from the left. Life can be sustained only if communications exist between systemic and pulmonary circulations.

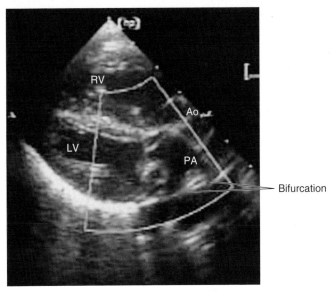

Fig. 13.10 Echocardiogram (parasternal long axis view) in a patient with transposition of the great arteries. Connected to the left ventricle is the pulmonary artery which bifurcates. (LV: left ventricle; RV: right ventricle; Ao: aorta; PA: pulmonary artery.)

CHAPTER

13

Congenital heart disease

Clinical signs

The infant is characteristically of normal size. Cyanosis develops at birth or shortly thereafter. Often, save for cyanosis, the clinical examination will be relatively normal.

Investigations

- The *chest radiograph* may show little abnormality at birth, but within a few days the heart becomes enlarged and the vascularity of the lung fields increased.
- The ECG shows little more than the right ventricular dominance, normal for this age group.
- *Echocardiography* is an invaluable diagnostic tool. It shows the aorta, arising from the right ventricle and lying anterior to the pulmonary artery (Fig. 13.10), and also allows detection of other defects.

Transposition of the great arteries is the most common cardiac cause of cyanosis in the first week of life. Accurate diagnosis at this stage is urgent, as without rapid treatment infants can deteriorate and die.

Treatment

Once the diagnosis is made on echocardiogram, it is necessary to proceed to balloon septostomy which can be carried out either in the cardiac catheterization laboratory or at the bedside under echocardiographic guidance. The procedure is performed by introducing a catheter with a deflated balloon at its tip into the femoral vein and advancing it via the right atrium and foramen ovale into the left atrium. The balloon is then inflated and withdrawn abruptly so as to tear the atrial septum. This procedure is almost always effective in the early neonatal period, but is more difficult in those presenting later in life. The purpose of the septostomy is to mix enough blood at atrial level to maintain systemic oxygenation – the child will, however remain cyanosed. Although this form of palliation will allow an infant to survive up to and beyond the first birthday, surgery is usually carried out in the first few weeks.

Over the last 15–20 years, the arterial switch has completely replaced atrial rerouting of the circulation (Mustard or Senning procedures – see Adult Congenital Heart Disease later in this chapter). The great vessels are divided above the level of the semilunar valves and anastomosed to the opposite outflow tract. The pulmonary artery must be brought in front of the new aorta so it lies anteriorly and this can lead to supravalvar pulmonary stenosis in the long term. The coronary arteries are translocated on a button of arterial wall and reanastomosed into the new aorta. Procedural mortality in the best hands is less than 5%. Reported results so far have been excellent but for the longer term, only time will tell.

OBSTRUCTIVE LESIONS

Coarctation of the aorta (Fig. 13.11)

Coarctation of the aorta represents a spectrum from the typical discrete aortic narrowing ('adult type'), usually just beyond the origin of the left subclavian

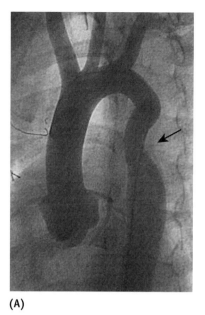
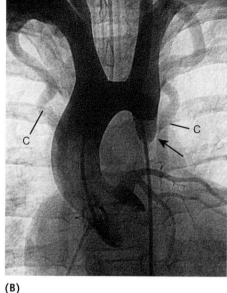

(A)　　　　　　　　　　　　**(B)**

Fig. 13.11　Coarctation of the aorta. (A) Ascending aortic angiogram showing a mild discrete coarctation (arrowed). Note the lack of collateral vessels. (B) Ascending aortic angiogram in a patient with severe coarctation (almost atresia) (arrowed) with significant collateral vessel formation (C).

artery, to the diffusely hypoplastic aortic arch of the neonate, which forms the interface with the hypoplastic left heart syndrome.

Physiology, symptoms and signs

Only a small volume of blood flows through the narrowed segment. In a patient with a significant coarctation, the obstruction is eventually bypassed by collateral vessels which can attain great size. The blood pressure in the lower half of the body is lower than that in the upper half and the pulse wave takes longer to arrive. Femoral pulsation is therefore delayed or absent.

In adults, collateral vessels may be seen and felt along the borders of the scapulae and over the posterior chest wall (Fig. 13.11). The left ventricle is often enlarged. A systolic murmur is almost invariably heard over the area of the coarctation at about the level of the fourth intercostal space posteriorly, and tends to be louder than a systolic murmur which is often audible in the second intercostal spaces close to the sternum. A more continuous murmur may be heard over collaterals. Upper limb hypertension may not be obvious in early childhood. Abnormalities of vascular function leading to abnormal blood pressure responses can be demonstrated even after a good repair, particularly if surgery is performed later in life. Hypertension leading to accelerated coronary artery disease is an important cause of attrition in patients after repair of coarctation; other risks include infection of the coarctation or of a bicuspid aortic valve, rupture or dissection of the ascending aorta, and cerebral haemorrhage. Cystic medial necrosis of the aortic wall, which is present in only a few patients with coarctation, is the deciding factor in rupture. Rupture of an intracranial aneurysm is the usual cause of the relatively rare complication of subarachnoid haemorrhage.

Coarctation may produce no symptoms and is often suspected during a routine medical examination when a systolic murmur is heard or hypertension detected.

Investigations

- The *ECG* is usually normal; left ventricular hypertrophy is uncommon before adult years.
- The *chest radiograph* is seldom abnormal in childhood, but characteristically shows an abnormal aortic knuckle with an enlarged left subclavian artery and poststenotic dilatation of the aorta in adults. Another feature is notching of the undersides of the ribs due to the erosion by enlarged intercostal arteries.
- The diagnosis is usually made without difficulty on clinical grounds and it can be confirmed *echocardiographically*. It is usually possible to visualize the stenosed segment from the suprasternal notch in children, but this can be more difficult in adults. *Doppler echocardiography* in a patient with discrete coarctation will almost always demonstrate a gradient across the coarctation site in addition to prolongation of the systolic flow well into diastole (Fig. 13.12). In adults, *MRI* or *angiography* may be necessary to fully delineate the anatomy.

Treatment

Treatment for native coarctation is surgery. A number of techniques including resection of the coarctation and restoration of the aorta by end-to-end anastomosis, subclavian flap augmentation (in younger patients) or, if necessary, the insertion of an interposition graft, all have their place depending on the preference of individual surgeons and the exact anatomy of the aortic arch. Repair should be performed as early as possible as there is evidence that long-term outcome worsens with age at repair.

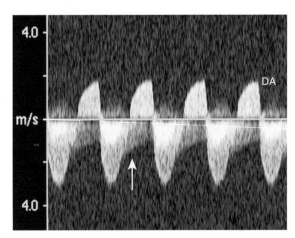

Fig. 13.12 Doppler trace from the suprasternal notch in a patient with coarctation of the aorta showing raised velocity (pressure drop across the stenosis of 50 mmHg) and prolongation of systolic flow into diastole (arrowed). Flow in the opposite direction is across a small patent ductus arteriosus (DA).

Balloon angioplasty and stent implantation have been used with varying success in the treatment of coarctation; the role of both in native coarctation is still uncertain but angioplasty is particularly effective in the 5–10% of patients who have a recurrence of the coarctation after surgery.

Neonatal coarctation

Coarctation in the neonate is an altogether more complex problem. Invariably there is some degree of transverse arch hypoplasia in addition to any discrete narrowing. Associated intracardiac lesions are frequent as are other left-sided abnormalities, such as mitral stenosis, aortic valve dysplasia and left ventricular hypoplasia.

In severe neonatal coarctation, the ductus bypasses the narrowed area and its closure often precipitates cardiovascular collapse. Signs at presentation very much depend on the clinical state of the infant and the presence of absence of associated cardiac lesions. The right ventricular impulse is prominent and the femoral pulses are usually absent, even in those patients in whom the ductus remains open. Hepatomegaly and other signs of cardiac failure may be clinically detectable. ECG and chest X-ray are not discriminatory in this setting; echocardiography provides the diagnosis – angiography is rarely required. Critical in decision-making is demonstration of a left side of the heart that is viable.

Reopening of the ductus arteriosus with intravenous prostaglandin allows stabilization and resuscitation of the patient. Often, radical arch surgery is required to resect the stenosis and enlarge a significant portion of the aorta. If necessary, associated intracardiac lesions can be surgically addressed at the same time.

Neonatal cardiology

Recognition and initial management (including safe transfer to another unit when necessary) of an infant with possible congenital heart disease is the responsibility of the general paediatrician. It is not always possible to make an exact anatomical diagnosis but by recognition of important clinical signs, appropriate triage and a safe initial management plan can be devised.

The definitive diagnosis is usually made by an expert in neonatal cardiology. Echocardiography is the primary diagnostic modality – it is rare to require urgent diagnostic catheterization.

Important symptoms and signs in the neonate are:

- *Cyanosis* in a newborn infant is always a serious finding (see section on transposition of the great arteries). If there is no response to a high concentration of inspired oxygen, an urgent referral for cardiac assessment should be made.
- *Signs of heart failure* are tachypnoea, tachycardia, liver enlargement and most importantly in a young infant, poor feeding. Lung crepitations and peripheral oedema, although important clinical signs in adults, are rarely seen in infants. Many lesions from VSDs to hypoplastic left heart syndrome can present with signs of heart failure. Recognition of

infants in whom serious lesions are suspected is important, particularly those who are likely to be ductus dependant.

- *Absence of the femoral pulses* is a very important sign in the neonate, with suspected congenital heart disease often occurring in babies with important left heart obstruction (see Neonatal Coarctation above and Hypoplastic Left Heart below). Urgent cardiac assessment is required.

Ductal dependency

Many severe congenital cardiac lesions that present in the neonatal period are dependant on the patency of the ductus arteriosus to bypass the lesion (see sections on Hypoplastic Left Heart, Neonatal Coarctation and Tetralogy of Fallot in this chapter). Closure of the ductus arteriosus (which usually occurs in the days or early weeks after birth) precipitates cardiovascular collapse, quickly followed by death.

Of the many advances in the care of infants with congenital heart disease over the last 3 decades, perhaps the most important has been prostaglandin E2. Intravenous administration will reopen the ductus arteriosus, maintain ductal patency and allow stabilization and resuscitation of the infant.

The presence of a ductus dependant cardiac lesion should always be considered in a collapsed neonate and treatment with a prostaglandin infusion given until an important cardiac lesion can be ruled out. Prostaglandin E2 has few serious side-effects although it can induce apnoea, in which case, facilities for mechanical ventilation are required.

Hypoplastic left heart (Fig. 13.13)

This term describes a number of lesions in which the fundamental problem is a left side of heart which is too small to support the systemic circulation.

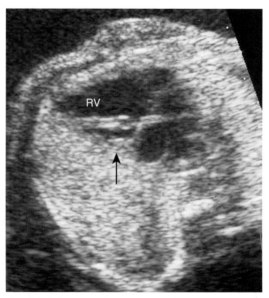

Fig. 13.13 Hypoplastic left heart syndrome (small left ventricle arrowed) in a fetus at 18 weeks gestation (RV: right ventricle.)

Clinical characteristics are not consistent, although hypoplastic left heart syndrome will almost always become apparent within the first days of life when the ductus arteriosus closes. This precipitates cardiovascular collapse and if untreated, death. At presentation, babies with this condition are often confused with other ductus dependant cardiac lesions, in particular, other forms of left heart obstruction (see Neonatal Coarctation above). Diagnosis is made with echocardiography.

The outlook for infants with hypoplastic left heart has been transformed since the description of staged palliation, as described by William Norwood, an American surgeon. This series of operative procedures now offers some hope, allowing affected children to survive into adolescence or young adulthood. Ultimately, failure of the single ventricle and cardiac transplantation becomes inevitable. Despite improving results, the surgical protocol (at least three operations) is a formidable undertaking and significant complications (intractable atrial arrhythmias, etc.) are common. Parents of a child with hypoplastic left heart have a slightly increased risk of having another affected child.

Fetal echocardiography

Diagnosis of structural heart disease is possible in utero. Scanning is generally performed between 18–20 weeks gestation. The indications for fetal echocardiography have expanded over the years but the primary aim is still the identification of major congenital heart disease, such as the hypoplastic left heart syndrome, enabling counselling of affected parents. Many decide to terminate the pregnancy; in those who continue, plans for delivery and management of a ductus dependant baby can be made in advance.

Pulmonary stenosis

Pulmonary stenosis is almost invariably of congenital origin. Obstruction to the right ventricular outflow tract can occur at a number of levels. Infundibular (subvalvar) or supravalvar obstruction is less common than valvar stenosis but multilevel obstruction is frequent and establishing the anatomy of the whole right ventricular outflow tract is important for planning treatment. In valvar pulmonary stenosis, the leaflets are thickened and dysplastic. These may be fused to form a cone-shaped structure with a narrow orifice.

Physiology and symptoms

Obstruction to right ventricular emptying leads to a high right ventricular systolic pressure and a systolic pressure drop across the pulmonary valve. In severe cases, right ventricular failure develops. If the foramen ovale is unsealed, or if there is an atrial septal defect, a right-to-left shunt with central cyanosis may develop as the right atrial pressure rises. Severe pulmonary stenosis with a right-to-left atrial shunt is part of the differential diagnosis in the cyanosed neonate. It is rare for pulmonary stenosis to cause right ventricular failure in the first few weeks of life, although some infants are dependant on the patency of the ductus arteriosus to bypass a severe obstruction. Cardiovascular collapse can occur if the ductus arteriosus is allowed to close. Given a well-formed right ventricle, survival into late adult life is normal. Often the lesion is first detected on routine clinical examination in asymptomatic individuals, but some patients present with fatigue, breathlessness or syncope.

Clinical signs

The arterial pulse is usually normal. The jugular venous pulse is usually normal, but in severe grades, it exhibits a large 'a' wave as the right atrium contracts forcibly in the face of the non-compliant hypertrophied right ventricle. On palpation, there is often a systolic thrill in the second left intercostal space; the left parasternal heave of right ventricular hypertrophy can sometimes be felt. The first heart sound is normal, but it is often followed by an early systolic 'ejection' click and a loud midsystolic murmur, best heard in the second left intercostal space. The second sound is normal in the mild case, but in the more severe, it is split abnormally wide and the second (pulmonary) element is soft.

Investigations

- The *ECG* is often an indicator of the severity of the pulmonary valve stenosis. Older patients with significant stenosis will have ECG features of right ventricular hypertrophy.
- The *chest radiograph* may show poststenotic dilatation of the pulmonary artery. In severe cases, right ventricular hypertrophy and diminution in the pulmonary vascular markings may be detected. An accurate diagnosis can usually be made clinically.
- The mainstay of investigation is the *echocardiogram* which will reliably give the diagnosis, provide anatomical information about the level and degree of obstruction and identify associated lesions.
- *Cardiac catheterization* is rarely required as a diagnostic procedure.

Treatment

A minor degree of pulmonary stenosis is compatible with a normal life span. When the stenosis is severe and untreated, death is likely to ensue sooner or later from right ventricular failure; relief of the stenosis should not be delayed too long as irreversible fibrotic changes take place in the hypertrophied right ventricle. Although surgical valvotomy is a low risk technique, balloon valvoplasty is firmly established as an effective and safe method of enlarging the valve orifice, with good long-term results (Fig. 13.14). It should be viewed as the procedure of choice except in patients with infundibular and supravalvar stenosis, in which surgical enlargement is required.

COMPLEX CONDITIONS

Single ventricle physiology

Although it is almost always possible to identify a hypoplastic second ventricle, there are a number of complex cardiac lesions in which the heart functions physiologically as a single chamber. Of all the morphological variants, the most common lesion of this kind is tricuspid atresia. The prognosis and management strategy for all patients with single ventricle physiology depends

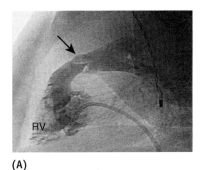 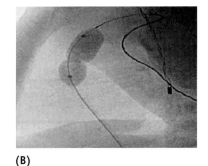

(A)   (B)

Fig. 13.14 (A) Right ventricular angiogram in the lateral projection showing a thickened and dysplastic pulmonary valve (arrowed). (B) Balloon positioned and inflated across the pulmonary valve, note the presence of a waist at the site of stenosis. (RV: right ventricle)

on the exact anatomical details; here, tricuspid atresia is used to illustrate these principles.

Tricuspid atresia

In tricuspid atresia, there is absence of the normal atrioventricular connection on the right and the right ventricular cavity is usually small. For life to be sustained after birth, an ASD and a VSD must be present. Frequently, there is associated pulmonary stenosis or pulmonary atresia and, more rarely, transposition of the great arteries. Blood flows into the right ventricle and its connecting great artery via the VSD. The presentation of these infants depends on the exact anatomy:

• Babies with tricuspid atresia, normally connected great arteries and no pulmonary stenosis, present with breathlessness rather like a patient with a large VSD.
• Those with pulmonary stenosis may shunt right to left across the VSD in the manner of tetralogy of Fallot and hence be cyanosed. Transposition of the great arteries in this context can lead to aortic obstruction at a number of levels.

The intracardiac anatomy is frequently uncorrectable in infants with complex lesions and treatment is therefore palliative – aimed at prolonging life as long as possible. When unrestricted pulmonary blood flow is present, as a primary procedure, a pulmonary artery band is necessary to surgically induce pulmonary stenosis and protect the pulmonary vasculature from the effects of a large shunt. Babies with pre-existing pulmonary stenosis may become severely cyanosed and the primary procedure in this situation will be a surgically placed arterial shunt. Ultimately, if the pulmonary vasculature is protected from a large shunt and remains under low pressure, the long-term management strategy is a venous shunt procedure (e.g. a Glenn shunt). Later, a Fontan circuit is created, in which the systemic venous return (both superior and inferior caval blood flow) is directed back into the pulmonary circulation.

Although this sort of management protocol will ensure the single ventricle works for as long as possible, heart failure is inevitable and ultimately, all of these patients will die early or require cardiac transplantation.

Adult congenital heart disease

Since 80–85% of children now survive, adult patients with congenital heart defects are increasingly common – in the UK these patients will numerically out-number children within a decade or so. Adults with congenital heart defects have different problems to children and it is wrong to view them as paediatric cases. Most deaths from congenital heart disease now occur in adults and important complications such as arrhythmias and heart failure are relatively prevalent. Minor lesions often do not require specialist follow-up but effective care of patients with significant congenital heart disease needs to be undertaken by trained staff in dedicated clinics. The spectrum of adult congenital heart disease is wide and a full review is beyond the scope of this chapter, but a few of the commoner issues are presented.

Tetralogy of Fallot

Patients surviving into adult life are frequently left with important pulmonary regurgitation after the original operation to address right ventricular outflow tract obstruction. As a consequence, the right ventricle becomes dilated and after many years, may fail (Fig. 13.15). Both atrial and ventricular arrhythmias occur in this patient group, often reflecting residual haemodynamic problems. Further intervention may be required, particularly valve replacement to address severe pulmonary incompetence or balloon dilation of distal pulmonary artery stenoses.

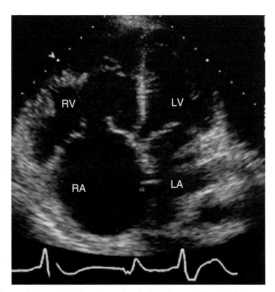

Fig. 13.15 Echocardiogram (4 chamber view) showing a dilated right ventricle as a consequence of free pulmonary incompetence in an adult, 20 years after repair of tetralogy of Fallot (LA: left atrium; LV: left ventricle; RA: right atrium; RV: right ventricle.)

Mustard or Senning repair for transposition of the great arteries

Prior to the arterial switch procedure, patients with transposition of the great arteries underwent rerouting of the circulation at atrial level. The inevitable consequence of this procedure (and the stimulus for the development of the arterial switch) was a morphological right ventricle pumping in the systemic position. In later life, failure of this ventricle is common as are atrial arrhythmias and bradycardia resulting from extensive atrial surgery.

Conventional surgical options for a patient with systemic (right) ventricular failure in this setting are limited and often transplantation is the only option.

Increasing numbers of patients after the arterial switch operation will be seen in the future and concerns after this procedure are pulmonary stenosis (due to stretching of the vessel at the operation) and the translocated coronary arteries in which problems may occur during later life.

Coarctation of the aorta

Although native coarctation is still diagnosed, the majority of adult patients will have had surgical repair. Reintervention may be required for restenosis and aneurysm formation at the site of the operation. Longer term issues are hypertension and accelerated coronary artery disease both of which are major causes of mortality. Imaging the aortic arch in adults is often difficult with echocardiography and so MRI or angiography can be required.

Fontan circulation

The end point of surgical management strategy for patients with single ventricle physiology (see Tricuspid Atresia above) is a Fontan circulation. There are many variations of the procedure, all of which redirect venous effluent (both superior and inferior vena cava) directly back to the pulmonary arteries. Frequently, these patients suffer atrial arrhythmias (which in this context can be very dehabilitating) and ventricular dysfunction. Although some success has been reported treating complications with conventional surgery, often combined with aggressive treatment of the arrhythmia, ultimately, these patients will come to transplantation.

Pregnancy

Contraception, pregnancy and genetic counselling are important elements of the care of women with congenital heart disease. Many patients will cope well with the haemodynamic stresses of pregnancy with little risk of cardiac deterioration. Others require specific management to optimize outcome and a small number, for example those with pulmonary vascular disease, should avoid pregnancy altogether. Effective management of these patients requires a multidisciplinary approach with particular cooperation between cardiologists and expert obstetric services.

Endocarditis

Most, but not all patients with congenital heart disease require life-long antibiotic prophylaxis against bacterial endocarditis in circumstances where they are at risk. Education of patients and carers is important as endocarditis in congenital heart disease can have a high mortality. Intracardiac infection can occur in any region of the heart in structural heart disease and typical vegetations are not always seen on echocardiogram.

FURTHER READING

Anderson, R.H., Macartney, F. J., Shinebourne, E.A. et al (1987) *Paediatric Cardiology*, 2nd edn. Edinburgh: Churchill Livingstone.

Garson, A. Jnr, Bricker, J.T., Fischer, D.J. et al (1990) *The Science and Practice of Pediatric Cardiology*, 2nd edn. Baltimore: Williams and Wilkins.

Perloff, J.K. & Child, J.S. (1988) *Congenital Heart Disease in Adults*. Philadelphia: Saunders.

14

Hypertension and heart disease

Hypertension is a major risk factor for cardiovascular morbidity and mortality. It accelerates the process of atherosclerosis in the coronary, cerebral and renal arteries, as well as increasing the workload of the heart. As a result, the hypertensive patient is at risk of developing myocardial infarction, stroke, renal failure and congestive cardiac failure. In total, hypertension is probably directly or indirectly responsible for 10–20% of all deaths.

For reasons that will become apparent, it is impossible to define hypertension. For practical purposes, the blood pressure may be regarded as abnormally high if it persistently exceeds 150/95 mmHg in a quietly resting individual. This does not imply that individuals with raised pressure necessarily require treatment. The presence of other risk factors and evidence of target organ damage from hypertension must be taken into account before initiating treatment that is likely to be life-long.

THE CONCEPT OF NORMAL BLOOD PRESSURE

Within populations, blood pressure, like height and weight, is normally distributed (Fig. 14.1). There is, therefore, no clear separation between hypertension and normotension. Within individuals, the level of arterial pressure

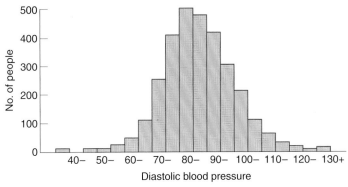

Fig. 14.1 Diastolic blood pressure at screening in a normal population. (After Hawthorne et al, 1974, with permission from the BMJ Publishing Group.)

is determined by the cardiac output and peripheral vascular resistance, two factors that vary widely from individual to individual, and within one individual at different times. Marked variations have been observed in individuals in whom the blood pressure is continuously monitored throughout the day. The mean pressure during sleep may be 30 mmHg lower than it is in the waking state. Factors that transiently increase pressure include anxiety and cold. Exercise leads to a brisk rise in systolic pressure but little change in the diastolic pressure. A transient doubling of systolic pressure may occur at the climax of coitus.

Certain identifiable factors are associated with persistently high blood pressure. Thus, at least in Western societies, both diastolic and systolic pressure increase with age. The blood pressure averages about 80/60 mmHg at birth and rises slowly throughout childhood. The resting blood pressure in the adolescent is often in the region of 120/70 mmHg, whilst in middle age 140/80 mmHg is more common. The systolic pressure often continues to rise into old age as the aorta becomes increasingly rigid. However, in many individuals and throughout some societies (e.g. in some Pacific islands) hypertension is virtually non-existent and there is no rise with age. In the younger age groups, males, on average, have higher pressures than females, but this tendency is reversed after the age of 45. Obese individuals tend to have pressures higher than can be accounted for by recording errors due to increased arm circumference.

The variability of arterial pressures within one individual and between individuals makes it impossible to define normality. It has been established, however, that the higher the pressure even within the 'normal' range, whether systolic or diastolic, the more likely the individual is to develop life-threatening cardiovascular disease processes including coronary artery disease, cerebrovascular disease and renal disease (Fig. 14.2).

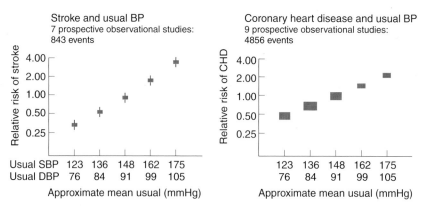

Fig. 14.2 The relationships between blood pressure and risk. The relative risk of stroke and of coronary artery disease rises as the blood pressure rises. These graphs are derived from multiple prolonged prospective observational studies. Note that the relationship between hypertension and stroke is stronger than the relationship between hypertension and coronary disease as reflected by the steeper slope of the graph. (From MacMahon, S. et al, 1990, with permission.)

Blood pressure is usually measured in the arm. The usual method involves a 'cuff' which is wrapped around the upper arm. The cuff contains an inflatable rubber bladder. The cuff is then inflated with air until the pressure from the cuff occludes the brachial artery. The cuff is then slowly deflated and the pressure in the cuff is continuously measured using either a mercury manometer or an aneroid manometer. At the same time as the operator regulates the deflation of the cuff, he or she listens with a stethoscope over the brachial artery immediately distal to the cuff. As the cuff is deflating, the pressure at which regular sounds first appear over the brachial artery is taken as the systolic blood pressure. As the pressure continues to fall, the sounds become muffled and then disappear. The pressure at which the sounds disappear completely is the diastolic pressure.

Classification of hypertension (Box 14.1)

Normal adult blood pressure has been defined as a systolic blood pressure equal to or below 140 mmHg together with a diastolic (fifth Korotkoff phase) equal to or below 90 mmHg.

Hypertension may be regarded as 'mild' if the diastolic pressure is between 90 and 104 mmHg, 'moderate' if between 105 and 114 mmHg, and 'severe' if above this. Hypertension is said to be in the *malignant* or accelerated phase if there is widespread arterial fibrinoid necrosis. The diastolic pressure is very high (often above 130 mmHg) with retinal haemorrhages and exudates and frequently papilloedema.

Although the unqualified term 'hypertension' generally refers to elevation of the diastolic blood pressure, it is also possible to define systolic hypertension. A systolic pressure above 160 mmHg is regarded as abnormal, even when the diastolic pressure is within normal limits.

AETIOLOGY OF HYPERTENSION

In 95% of patients with high blood pressure, no specific cause can be identified. This condition is termed 'essential' or 'primary' hypertension. In

---

Box 14.1

Definitions of hypertension

Diastolic pressure (mmHg)
<85	Normal
85–90	High normal
90–104	Mild hypertension
105–114	Moderate hypertension
>115	Severe hypertension

Systolic pressure (mmHg)
<140	Normal
140–159	Borderline isolated systolic hypertension
>160	Isolated systolic hypertension (diastolic < 90 mmHg)

approximately 5% of hypertensive patients, a specific cause can be identified and the hypertension is termed 'secondary'. Although secondary hypertension accounts for a small minority of all hypertensive patients, it is important to identify this condition because specific and potentially curative treatment may be available.

Essential hypertension

Although no single cause has been identified for this condition, a number of factors have been shown to influence the development of essential hypertension:

Genetic influences

The influence of heredity is unquestioned, hypertension being many times more common in the families of hypertensive patients than in those of normotensive individuals. Although some have suggested that hypertension is due to a single dominant gene, most of the evidence points to the influence of many genes.

Dietary influences

There is an undoubted relationship between weight and blood pressure. Weight loss in the obese substantially lowers the blood pressure. Very low salt intake appears to protect against hypertension, but there is little evidence to incriminate excessive sodium chloride intake as a cause of high blood pressure. A high potassium intake may be protective. There is some evidence that a high intake of saturated fats may raise blood pressure. High alcohol consumption has been identified as a risk factor for hypertension, as has cigarette smoking, at least in regard to the malignant phase.

Physical activity

Physical exercise can reduce blood pressure in hypertensive subjects. This suggests that inactivity may play a role in the genesis of hypertension in some individuals.

Hormonal changes

Hormonal changes are implicated in a number of causes of secondary hypertension. The possibility that hormonal changes might also be involved in the pathogenesis of essential hypertension has attracted particular interest. Attention has concentrated on the adrenergic and renin–angiotensin systems, but there is as yet no clear evidence indicating a primary role for either system in the genesis of essential hypertension.

Haemodynamic changes

A slight sinus tachycardia and a high cardiac output may be found in early hypertensives before there is a rise in peripheral resistance. These features may result from an excessive adrenergic influence. There is good evidence that baroreceptors are reset in hypertension, as bradycardia is not induced by the rise in pressure.

The causes of secondary hypertension

Renal
    Acute glomerulonephritis
    Chronic glomerulonephritis
    Chronic pyelonephritis
    Polycystic kidneys
    Renal artery stenosis
    Diabetic nephropathy

Endocrine
    Adrenal
        Primary aldosteronism
        Cushing's syndrome
        Phaeochromocytoma
    Acromegaly
    Exogenous hormones
    Oral contraceptives
    Glucocorticoids
    Mineralocorticoids – liquorice

Coarctation of the aorta

Pregnancy

Neurological

Raised intracranial pressure

Secondary hypertension

The most common causes of secondary hypertension are renal disease, adrenal disease, coarctation of the aorta and drug-related hypertension (Box 14.2).

Renal disease

All forms of parenchymal renal disease can be associated with significant hypertension. These include acute and chronic glomerulonephritis, chronic pyelonephritis and polycystic kidney disease. Control of the blood pressure in all of these conditions is important and slows the progression of renal damage.

Renal artery stenosis as a cause of hypertension deserves special consideration. In this condition, the stenosis may be unilateral or bilateral and may take the form of a fibromuscular narrowing in young patients or atheromatous narrowing in older patients, who will often have evidence of atherosclerosis elsewhere. Renal artery stenosis results in ischaemia of the kidney with high circulating levels of angiotensin II. High levels of angiotensin II then lead to hypertension by two different mechanisms (Fig. 14.3). Hypertension in these patients is often relatively resistant to drug treatment. Angiotensin-converting enzyme (ACE) inhibitors, by preventing the release of angiotensin II, will lower the blood pressure markedly but should be avoided in

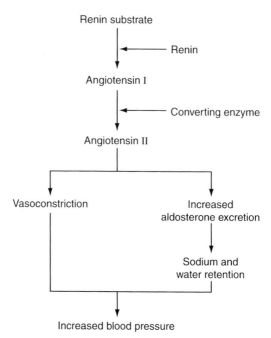

Fig. 14.3 The renin–angiotensin system.

patients suspected of having renal artery stenosis because they reduce renal perfusion and may result in renal infarction. If a patient has bilateral renal artery stenoses, the introduction of an ACE inhibitor can precipitate acute renal failure.

Investigation of suspected 'renal' hypertension

Abdominal ultrasonography provides a simple non-invasive means of assessing renal anatomy in patients with a suspected renal cause for hypertension. In patients with chronic nephritis, kidney size is reduced. In patients with pyelonephritis, there is likely to be dilatation of the calyceal system. In unilateral renal artery stenosis, kidney size is reduced on the side of the stenosis. If renal artery stenosis is suspected, then renal arteriography remains the investigation of choice although the diagnosis can now often be made using either spiral computed tomography (CT) or magnetic resonance imaging (MRI). If the patient is shown to have either unilateral or bilateral renal artery stenosis, then renal revascularization either by renal artery angioplasty or by a surgical approach should be considered. If there is doubt as to whether a renal artery lesion is the cause of hypertension, bilateral renal vein sampling of plasma renin activity may be helpful; high levels of renin activity coming from the affected side would suggest that the stenosis is significant and that revascularization would probably improve blood pressure control.

Endocrine disease

Cushing's syndrome

This results from cortisol excess and may be due to hyperplasia of the adrenal cortex, adrenal tumours, or to the excessive administration of glucocorticoids or adrenocorticotrophic hormone (ACTH). Adrenal hyperplasia is often the result of increased ACTH production by a pituitary microadenoma.

Hypertension, which occurs in more than 50% of cases, may be severe and may proceed to the malignant phase. Other features of the syndrome are muscle weakness, osteoporosis, purple cutaneous striae, obesity of the trunk, a 'buffalo' hump, a 'moon' facies and diabetes mellitus. There may also be hirsutism, amenorrhoea, a liability to spontaneous bruising, and dependent oedema.

Diagnosis. The diagnosis should be suggested by the combination of hypertension, diabetes and truncal obesity. Investigations include:

- excessive 24-h urinary free cortisol excretion
- failure to suppress plasma cortisol levels following dexamethasone administration
- the ACTH levels are valuable in determining the cause, being high with pituitary tumours and low if the adrenal is responsible
- CT or MRI imaging of the adrenal glands.

Management. Treatment depends upon the aetiology of the condition. Surgical removal of one or both adrenal glands or of a pituitary tumour may be necessary.

Primary aldosteronism

Aldosterone, which is secreted by the zona glomerulosa of the adrenal cortex, promotes sodium reabsorption and potassium excretion in the distal tubules of the kidney. Normally, aldosterone secretion is largely regulated by angiotensin, but in primary aldosteronism there is an overproduction of aldosterone as a result of an adrenal cortical adenoma (Conn's syndrome) or bilateral hyperplasia; angiotensin and, therefore, plasma renin levels are abnormally low. The condition occurs most often in young and middle-aged females. Because of the mode of action of aldosterone, the symptoms and signs are related to sodium retention, hypokalaemia and hypertension. Frequently, the patient presents with mild to moderate hypertension, but the predominant complaints are those of muscle weakness, headache, thirst and polyuria. The hypertension is seldom severe and malignant changes are rare. There is usually hypokalaemia, with a serum potassium level of less than 3.0 mmol/L and a serum sodium concentration that is normal or high. Characteristically, there is a metabolic alkalosis and a low serum chloride level. The diagnosis should be suspected in patients with hypertension and hypokalaemia, particularly if this is associated with hypernatraemia. However, hypokalaemia is not uncommon in other hypertensive patients, particularly if they have been treated with diuretics. Furthermore, patients with malignant hypertension develop 'secondary aldosteronism' with low serum potassium. These patients usually do not have a high serum sodium.

Diagnosis. The diagnosis is suggested by:

- hypokalaemia, persisting after stopping diuretic therapy
- excessive urinary potassium loss
- elevated plasma aldosterone levels

- suppressed renin levels which fail to rise on assumption of an upright posture
- CT or MRI imaging is now the investigation of choice in establishing the presence of an adenoma and differentiating this from hyperplasia.

Management. Adenomas should be removed surgically. Patients with hyperplasia should be treated medically with spironolactone or amiloride, which antagonize the actions of aldosterone.

Phaeochromocytoma

Phaeochromocytoma arises in chromaffin tissue, usually in the adrenal gland. It is sometimes described as the '10% tumour'. This is because 10% are said to arise outwith the adrenal gland, 10% are malignant and 10% are bilateral. The tumours usually secrete noradrenaline (norepinephrine), but adrenaline (epinephrine) may predominate.

Phaeochromocytomas may produce either paroxysmal or persistent hypertension. The paroxysms are associated with the sudden onset of bilateral headache, and with perspiration, palpitations and pallor (features often regarded as neurotic). The attacks usually last from a few minutes to an hour. If the hypertension is persistent, the clinical picture is that of severe hypertension, often of the malignant variety. Because of the hypermetabolic state induced by the phaeochromocytoma, the patients are rarely obese.

Diagnosis. The diagnosis should be suspected in any severe case of hypertension, particularly if the hypertension is paroxysmal. The diagnosis is confirmed by:

- excessive excretion of the catecholamine metabolite vanilmandelic acid (VMA) in the urine is a useful screening test
- urine and plasma catecholamine levels
- CT scanning to localize the tumour.

Management. Phaeochromocytomas should be removed surgically. This is a potentially hazardous procedure and requires close control of the blood pressure and careful anaesthesia. Beta-adrenergic blocking drugs should not be used alone because unopposed alpha-adrenergic activation may aggravate hypertension and lead to serious complications such as stroke. This can be avoided by the initial use of an alpha-adrenergic blocking drug. The non-competitive alpha-antagonist phenoxybenzamine is frequently chosen. Once alpha-adrenergic blockade is fully established, beta-blockade can be added.

Coarctation of the aorta

This is a congenital condition associated with a narrowing of the lumen of the aorta just beyond the origin of the left subclavian artery. It is described in more detail in Chapter 13.

Drug-related causes

The oral contraceptive pill may lead to a small rise in arterial pressure but this is now much less common than 30 years ago when higher doses of oestrogen were used. It is wise, however, to check the blood pressure within a few months of starting the oral contraceptive pill. Other drugs that may be associated with hypertension include steroids (see under Cushing's Syndrome above), carbenoxolone and liquorice.

PATHOPHYSIOLOGY OF HYPERTENSION

The high blood pressure in essential hypertension is due to increased peripheral vascular resistance as a result of widespread constriction of the arterioles and small arteries. The cardiac output and the viscosity of the blood are normal. In the earlier stages, the hypertension is largely explicable on the basis of increased arteriolar muscle tone, but subsequently, structural alterations take place in the arterioles. These changes may account for the fact that hypertension tends to beget further hypertension, and the removal of the cause of hypertension does not necessarily lead to a fall in the blood pressure to normal.

In the heart, there are two major consequences of sustained hypertension. The increased work of the heart imposed by the higher resistance results in hypertrophy of the myocardial cells. As this process progresses, the myocardial hypertrophy may outstrip the coronary blood supply; this occurs particularly in the subendocardial layers which are the most vulnerable to ischaemia. Just as in the peripheral vessels, fibrous tissue is then deposited in the subendocardium leading to reduced ventricular compliance and, ultimately, to heart failure. The second effect of hypertension is to accelerate the development of atherosclerosis. This occurs not only in the coronary arteries but also in the cerebral arteries, particularly those of the basal ganglia, and in the renal arteries. The mechanism of this action is less clear but may be related to long-standing mechanical stresses; in experimental situations, hypertension, like cigarette smoking and hypercholesterolaemia, has been shown to induce dysfunction of the endothelial layer of the coronary arteries which, in turn, is thought to herald the development of atherosclerosis.

There are racial differences in the pathophysiological effects of hypertension on the heart. In black patients, 'pressure' effects with the development of severe left ventricular hypertrophy and subsequent left ventricular failure are more common while white patients are more likely to present with the clinical consequences of atherosclerosis.

EXAMINATION AND INVESTIGATION OF THE HYPERTENSIVE PATIENT

Most patients with hypertension are asymptomatic, the high blood pressure usually having been noted during an incidental clinical examination. A proportion will present with a major complication of hypertension such as stroke or myocardial infarction, but only a small number will present with symptoms directly attributable to hypertension such as breathlessness or headache.

Examination and investigation should be directed towards the detection of an underlying cause of hypertension (see secondary hypertension) and the assessment of end-organ damage, which may influence the decision to treat the patient. Blood pressure levels should be recorded after the patient has been lying quietly for 5 min.

Examination of the hypertensive patient

Clinical examination should take note of:

Signs suggestive of secondary hypertension
- Features of endocrine abnormalities, particularly Cushing's syndrome
- Multiple neurofibromatoma – present in 5% of patients with phaeochromocytoma
- Inappropriate tachycardia, suggesting catecholamine excess
- Abdominal or loin bruits, suggesting renal artery stenosis
- Renal enlargement (suggestive of polycystic kidney disease)
- Radiofemoral delay, due to coarctation of the aorta.

Signs suggestive of end-organ damage
- A forcible and displaced apex beat due to left ventricular hypertrophy
- Accentuation of the aortic component of the second heart sound
- Added heart sounds. A fourth sound may be audible, reflecting decreased ventricular compliance. As failure develops a third sound may occur
- Fundal examination to detect hypertensive retinopathy.

Fundoscopy
Examination of the optic fundus is of great importance in the evaluation of patients with hypertension, for it is only in the retina that the state of the arterioles can be directly observed. The grading introduced by Keith, Wagener and Barker is widely used:

- *grade 1* – increased tortuosity of the retinal arteries with increased reflectiveness, termed silver wiring
- *grade 2* – grade 1 with the addition of compression of the veins at arteriovenous crossings (AV nipping)
- *grade 3* – grade 2 with the addition of flame-shaped haemorrhages and 'cotton wool' exudates
- *grade 4* – grade 3 with the addition of papilloedema – the optic disc is pink with blurred edges and the optic cup is obliterated.

Investigation of the hypertensive patient

Routine investigation of all hypertensive patients should include:

- *ECG.* This is usually normal in patients with mild hypertension but may show evidence of left ventricular hypertrophy. This is characterized by tall R waves in the lateral chest leads and deep S waves in the anteroseptal leads. There are many ECG criteria for left ventricular hypertrophy. In the most commonly used criteria, LVH is said to be present if the sum of the S wave in V1 and the R wave in V5 or V6 exceeds 35 mm. In severe hypertrophy, or if there is accompanying ischaemic heart disease, the T waves in the lateral chest leads become flattened and then inverted, and the ST segment may show down-sloping depression in the same leads. This is the so-called 'left ventricular hypertrophy and strain' pattern (Fig. 14.4) which carries a high risk of major events including sudden

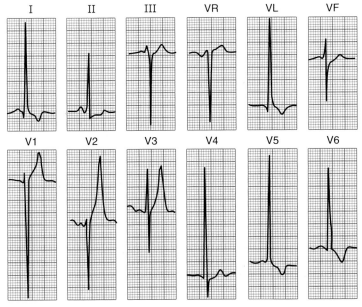

Fig. 14.4 ECG showing left ventricular hypertrophy and 'strain' in a patient with severe hypertension. This pattern is characterized by large voltages in the chest leads and the presence of ST segment depression and T wave inversion in leads V5 and V6.

death (30–40% 5-year mortality rate). These voltage criteria can only be applied to individuals over 35 years of age. They have high specificity but low sensitivity.

- *Urinalysis.* Proteinuria, hyaline and granular casts may be found when there is renal disease or malignant hypertension. There is little or no protein in the urine of patients with benign essential hypertension.
- *Urea and electrolytes.* A raised level of urea suggests renal impairment, which may be the cause or an effect of hypertension. A low serum potassium concentration in the absence of diuretic therapy might suggest Conn's or Cushing's syndrome.
- *Lipids.* Although not directly related to the blood pressure, an increased level of cholesterol is a risk factor for cardiovascular events, which may require specific treatment and which should be monitored in all hypertensive patients.

The following additional investigations may also be helpful:

- *24-h ambulatory blood pressure monitoring.* In this technique, the patient wears a sphygmomanometer cuff for a period of 24 h while going about their normal activities. The cuff is connected to an automatic inflation device and to a recorder which records the blood pressure at regular intervals, usually every 15–30 min. Blood pressure levels are generally lower during ambulatory recordings than during single clinic visits. The finding of high clinic readings and substantially lower ambulatory readings is sometimes used to reassure patients that they do not have 'sustained' hypertension, and the phrase 'white coat hypertension' has been coined. Although white coat hypertension is a real entity, the term should only be applied to those patients without evidence of target organ damage. Patients with left ventricular hypertrophy, or with abnormal renal function, should be treated even if their blood pressure levels are borderline.

- *Echocardiography*. Echocardiography is much more sensitive than the ECG for the detection of left ventricular hypertrophy. In patients with borderline hypertension, therefore, the finding of echocardiographic left ventricular hypertrophy, which is associated with an increased risk of cardiovascular events, will influence the clinician towards starting the patient on antihypertensive medication.
- *Detailed investigation of suspected secondary hypertension*. This may involve CT or MRI of the adrenal glands, MRI renal angiography and 24-h urine collections for catecholamines.

It is impractical to screen all hypertensive patients for secondary causes of hypertension. Selection of patient groups for further investigation is arbitrary, but investigation is particularly appropriate in the following groups:

- young patients under 40 years of age
- patients with malignant hypertension
- patients resistant to antihypertensive therapy
- patients with unusual symptoms (such as sweating attacks or weakness) which might suggest an underlying cause
- patients with abnormal renal function, proteinuria or haematuria
- patients with hypokalaemia off diuretic therapy.

The nature and scale of further investigations will be determined by the index of suspicion of a secondary cause for hypertension.

THE DECISION TO TREAT

Almost all patients with untreated malignant hypertension die within 1 year. Death is usually due to uraemia but heart failure and cerebrovascular accidents are common. In these patients, and in those with moderate to severe hypertension, there is clear evidence that treatment prolongs life.

The situation in patients with mild essential hypertension is more complicated. If the diastolic blood pressure is greater than 100 mmHg on multiple readings over a period of 3–4 months, then treatment is probably indicated. If the diastolic pressure is in the range of 95–100 mmHg, treatment should be started if there is evidence of end-organ damage. This might include left ventricular hypertrophy by electrocardiogram (ECG) or echocardiographic criteria, evidence on blood testing of renal dysfunction, or clear-cut changes on fundoscopy. In the absence of evidence of structural change, it is reasonable to keep the blood pressure under review. The current guidelines for the initiation of antihypertensive treatment are summarized in Figure 14.5.

Other risk factors should also be taken into account when deciding whether to initiate therapy. Factors such as age, sex, hypercholesterolaemia, cigarette smoking and diabetes are not simply additive but multiplicative

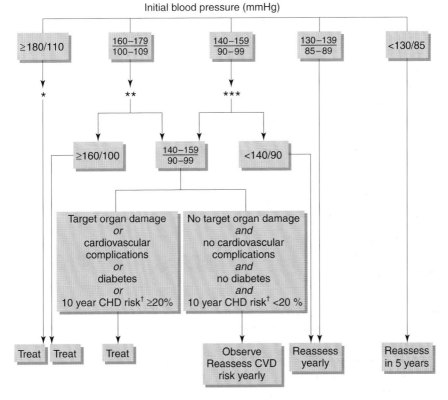

Initial blood pressure (mmHg)

≥180/110 | 160–179 / 100–109 | 140–159 / 90–99 | 130–139 / 85–89 | <130/85

* | ** | ***

≥160/100 | 140–159 / 90–99 | <140/90

Target organ damage
or
cardiovascular
complications
or
diabetes
or
10 year CHD risk† ≥20%

No target organ damage
and
no cardiovascular
complications
and
no diabetes
and
10 year CHD risk† <20 %

Treat | Treat | Treat | Observe Reassess CVD risk yearly | Reassess yearly | Reassess in 5 years

* Unless malignant phase, of hypertensive emergency, confirm over 1–2 weeks, then treat

** If cardiovascular complications, target organ damage, or diabetes is present, confirm over 3–4 weeks, then treat; if absent, remeasure weekly and teat if BP persists at these levels over 4–12 weeks

*** If cardiovascular complications, target organ damage, or diabetes is present, confirm over 12 weeks, then treat; if absent remeasure monthly and treat if these levels are maintained and if estimated 10 year CVD risk is ≥20%

† Assessed with Cardiac Risk Assessor computer program or coronary heart disease risk chart

Fig. 14.5 Thresholds for initiating drug treatment in patients with hypertension. (British Hypertension Society, 1999.)

in terms of the risk to the individual. Patients with multiple risk factors, therefore, are more likely to benefit from antihypertensive treatment than those with the same level of blood pressure but no other risk factors.

In deciding when to initiate treatment, two patient groups require specific mention. These are the elderly (patients over 70 years of age) and those with isolated systolic hypertension (systolic blood pressure greater than 160 mmHg and diastolic blood pressure less than 95 mmHg). In the past, these groups of patients were thought not to benefit from antihypertensive therapy. However, recent studies have demonstrated that both elderly patients and those with isolated systolic hypertension (who are also likely to be elderly) derive very considerable benefit from treatment. Indeed, recent studies have demonstrated not only a reduction in stroke risk, but also a significant reduction in cardiac death in elderly patients. This is possibly because the absolute number of events (strokes, myocardial infarctions and deaths) is much higher in the elderly than in younger hypertensive patients.

In patients with mild to moderate hypertension, treatment has effectively eliminated death from cardiac failure and has reduced the incidence of fatal and non-fatal strokes by around 35–40%. These benefits are seen up to the age of 80 and in patients with isolated systolic hypertension. Early studies were disappointing in terms of reduction of the risk of myocardial infarction; however, pooled data from a number of studies show a reduction in myocardial infarction risk of around 15–20%. Although the percentage reduction in myocardial infarction is less than that in stroke death, this nonetheless represents a large absolute number of lives saved, as myocardial infarction is a much commoner cause of death in hypertensive patients than stroke.

TREATMENT OF HYPERTENSION

Malignant hypertension, demonstrating retinal haemorrhages and exudates, requires urgent hospitalization and treatment. Patients with severe hypertension (diastolic > 120 mmHg) require early initiation of treatment. In most patients in whom there is evidence of target organ damage, early drug therapy will be required.

In all hypertensive patients, attention should be paid to non-pharmacological interventions that will reduce blood pressure and obviate the need for drug therapy in mild hypertensives, particularly if there is no evidence of end-organ damage. These include:

- weight reduction
- regular exercise
- reduction of alcohol consumption.

All hypertensive patients should be strongly advised against smoking and given dietary advice to reduce cholesterol intake and to reduce overall coronary risk.

Drugs used in the treatment of hypertension

There are a large number of drugs in current use for the treatment of hypertension, and new ones are continually being added. It is only possible to mention those which, at present, seem to be of greatest value. Every physician should be familiar with the use of four or five of these drugs as patients vary from one another in their response to therapy and no one drug can be regarded as superior in all respects to others.

Although the aim should be to make the blood pressure 'normal', it is not necessary to reduce the blood pressure rapidly in most patients and many drugs can take weeks or even months before the full hypotensive effect is seen. Too rapid a reduction in blood pressure may impair the circulation to the heart, brain or kidneys and precipitate myocardial infarction, stroke or renal failure.

An important consideration is the effect of treatment on the quality of life, particularly in patients with mild hypertension, only an unidentifiable minority of whom will gain benefit from antihypertensive drugs.

The principal classes of drugs used are described below.

Beta-adrenoceptor blocking drugs

Beta-blockers are effective antihypertensive drugs whose mode of action remains uncertain. They are more effective when combined with a diuretic or other antihypertensive drugs but are often sufficient on their own and produce no marked orthostatic effects. To improve patient compliance, it is best to use a preparation that needs to be given only once or twice per day (atenolol 50 mg once or twice daily, or bisoprolol 5 mg once daily). These drugs may exacerbate obstructive airway disease, heart failure and intermittent claudication, and should probably be avoided in patients with these conditions. Minor side-effects, such as fatigue and cold extremities, are relatively common and disappear on stopping the drug.

Thiazide diuretics

These drugs have been used widely in the treatment of essential hypertension for many years. Their mechanism of action remains unclear. Initially, plasma volume and cardiac output may be reduced, but these values later normalize. Much has been made of the undesirable metabolic effects of thiazides which include hypokalaemia, hyperuricaemia, hypercholesterolaemia and hyperglycaemia. With the currently used low doses of thiazides (e.g. bendroflumethiazide (bendrofluazide) 2.5 mg once daily or hydrochlorothiazide 25 mg once daily), these effects are small and of doubtful significance. In their favour, only the thiazides, along with the beta-blockers, have been shown to reduce stroke risk in patients with mild to moderate hypertension.

ACE inhibitors

This class includes captopril, enalapril, ramipril, lisinopril and perindopril. These drugs block the enzyme that converts angiotensin I to angiotensin II (see Fig. 14.1). They cause a fall in blood pressure by reducing systemic vascular resistance, without having any major effect on heart rate and cardiac output. The fall in systemic vascular resistance is probably mainly due to a reduction in plasma angiotensin II levels, but there is also a secondary fall in aldosterone concentration.

ACE inhibitors are effective alone in all grades and types of hypertension, but their action is potentiated by diuretics. A small rise in plasma urea and creatinine values is normal with ACE inhibitors but a marked increase may indicate unsuspected renal artery stenosis and is an indication for stopping the drug and considering renal angiography. Hyperkalaemia can occur because of the antialdosterone effects; therefore, concomitant use of ACE inhibitors and potassium-sparing diuretics is not recommended. Profound hypotension may occasionally be induced on first commencing treatment but this is usually seen only in patients who are already hypovolaemic as a result of high-dose diuretic therapy. This can be avoided by omitting diuretics on the day of starting the ACE inhibitor and also by starting with a small dose.

Cough is a particularly troublesome side-effect, occurring in some 5% of patients. Other side-effects include taste disorders, nausea, diarrhoea, rashes, neutropenia and proteinuria. Acute angioneurotic oedema is a rare but serious side-effect which occurs in 0.1–0.2% of patients and is more common in black patients.

Calcium-blocking drugs

These drugs have become increasingly used in the treatment of hypertension over the last 10–15 years. The dihydropyridine group, including nifedipine, nicardipine and amlodipine, all act predominantly by relaxing vascular smooth muscle and hence lowering peripheral vascular resistance. Side-effects with these agents include headache, flushing and ankle swelling.

The phenylalkylamine calcium channel blockers, such as verapamil and diltiazem, act more on the myocardium and conducting tissue. These are free from the vasodilator side-effects of the dihydropyridine class but do have negative inotropic effects and may potentiate heart failure.

Alpha-blockers

This class includes prazosin, terazosin and doxazosin. These drugs have marked arteriolar and venous vasodilating effects and the initial dose may produce profound postural hypotension. For this reason, the first dose should be taken on retiring to bed and the dosage gradually increased over a period of several weeks.

Angiotensin receptor antagonists

These include losartan, valsartan and candesartan. These agents act by blocking the angiotensin II receptor. They appear to be effective in lowering blood pressure and are relatively free from side-effects. Unlike the ACE inhibitors, they do not cause cough, possibly because they do not interfere with bradykinin degradation.

Other vasodilator agents

Drugs such as hydralazine and minoxidil are not now used as first-line therapy but may still be useful in combination with other agents when multiple drugs are required to control blood pressure. Diazoxide and nitroprusside are very effective vasodilators but are generally used only in hypertensive emergencies.

Choice of therapy for the individual patient

All drugs cause side-effects in some people. This is a particular problem in the treatment of hypertension where patients are usually asymptomatic before the commencement of medication. The unexpected development of side-effects will often cause the patient to stop taking the medication and it is generally better to warn patients that side-effects may occur. Finding a treatment regimen that is acceptable to both patient (in terms of side-effects) and doctor (in terms of blood pressure control) involves a degree of 'trial and error' and may take 6–12 months.

As a first choice, many clinicians would use either a thiazide diuretic, such as bendroflumethiazide (bendrofluazide) 2.5 mg once daily, or a long-acting beta-blocker, such as atenolol 50–100 mg once daily or bisoprolol 5 mg once daily. Thiazides and beta-blockers are favoured because both have been shown to reduce stroke risk in patients with mild to moderate hypertension. Other classes of drug, such as the ACE inhibitors and the alpha-blockers, have theoretical advantages over the more established drugs; thus alpha-blockers may have beneficial effects on lipid levels and the development of atherosclerosis, whereas ACE inhibitors may be more effective than other agents in producing regression of left ventricular hypertrophy.

The choice of medication is also determined by coexisting disease and the side-effect profile of a given agent. In patients with angina, for example, a beta-blocker would be a logical choice to treat both the angina and hypertension, whereas diuretics and ACE inhibitors would be preferable in patients with impaired left ventricular function. Beta-blockers should be avoided in patients with asthma or severe heart failure, and diuretics should be avoided in those patients with gout. ACE inhibitors should be used with caution in patients with impaired renal function.

If the response to a single drug is inadequate, a second agent should be added. Particularly useful combinations include:

- beta-blocker plus diuretic
- beta-blocker plus dihydropyridine calcium antagonist
- ACE inhibitor or angiotensin II antagonist plus diuretic.

If a two-drug regimen does not give adequate blood pressure control, a third or fourth agent can be added. If the patient has not already been investigated for secondary hypertension, this should be considered if the hypertension appears to be resistant to drug treatment. It is also important to remember that non-compliance is common in the treatment of hypertension, and this should be suspected if the blood pressure fails to fall despite the use of multiple drugs.

Other drugs used in the treatment of hypertensive patients

Lipid lowering agents
Recent studies of the HMG CoA reductase inhibitor drugs (or 'statins') have shown that these drugs reduce cardiovascular morbidity and mortality by around 30% regardless of the starting level of cholesterol. There is, therefore, an argument that these drugs should be prescribed to all patients who are at high risk of cardiovascular events. This would include many hypertensive patients. The current British Hypertension Society guidelines recommend that uncomplicated hypertensive patients should receive lipid-lowering drugs if their estimated 10 year coronary risk exceeds 30%.

Aspirin
Blood pressure treatment reduces cardiovascular risk by around 25% in those patients with an estimated coronary heart disease risk of > 15%. The addition of aspirin 75 mg once per day further reduces risk by around 15% and is recommended once the blood pressure has been brought under control. Starting aspirin when blood pressure is still high may increase the risk of intracranial bleeding.

A patient embarking on antihypertensive treatment should be aware that drug treatment is usually for life and that regular monitoring of the blood pressure will be required. Finally, the physician should bear in mind that the purpose of blood pressure reduction is to reduce the risk of a major vascular event. As hypertension is only one of a number of risk factors for cardiovascular disease, it follows that all risk factors should be addressed in the hypertensive patient; this may well include advice about diet, smoking, curbing excess alcohol consumption and regular exercise.

FURTHER READING

Beevers, G., Lip, G.Y.H., & O'Brien, E. (2001) *ABC of Hypertension*, 4th edn. London: British Medical Journal Books.

British Hypertension Society (1998) *Blood Pressure Measurement* (CD-ROM). London: *British Medical Journal Books.*

British Hypertension Society (1999) Blood pressure, stroke and coronary heart disease. Part 1. Prolonged differences in blood pressure; prospective observational studies corrected for the regression dilution bias. *Journal of Human Hypertension* **13**: 569–592.

British Cardiac Society, British Hyperlipidaemia Association, British Hypertension Society, British Diabetic Association. (2000) Joint British recommendations on prevention of coronary heart disease in clinical practice: summary. *British Medical Journal* **320**:705–708.

Hawthorne, V.M., Greaves, D.A. & Beevers, D.G. (1974) Blood pressure in a Scottish town (Renfrew Community Study). *British Medical Journal* **3**: 600–603.

MacMahon, S., Peto, R. & Cutler J. (1990) Blood pressure, Stroke and Coronary heart disease. *Lancet* **335**: 765–774.

Ramsay, L.E., Williams, B., Johnston, G.D. et al (1999) Guidelines for the management of hypertension: report of the third working party of the British Hypertension Society. *Journal of Human Hypertension* **13**:569–592.

CHAPTER 15

Diseases of the aorta

THE NORMAL AORTA

The normal aorta is composed of three layers:

- a thin endothelial lining or *intima*
- a thick middle layer, or *media* containing predominantly elastic tissue, but with some smooth muscle
- a thin, fibrous outer layer, the *adventitia*. This layer also contains the *vasa vasorum*, small blood vessels which nourish the outer part of the aortic wall including much of the media.

The strength of the aorta lies in the media. This layer is also responsible for the elasticity of the aortic wall. The elastic tissue is stretched during systole and subsequently recoils during diastole, thereby maintaining the forward circulation of blood throughout the cardiac cycle.

This elasticity of the aorta is crucial to its normal function. Even in normal and apparently healthy adults elasticity declines with age, contributing to the increase in pulse pressure observed in the elderly. A number of disease states, most particularly hypertension, hypercholesterolaemia and coronary disease, are associated with premature loss of aortic elasticity.

IMAGING OF THE AORTA

The aorta can be visualized in a number of ways:

- *Chest X-ray*. A chest X-ray is still a valuable simple means for aortic imaging, although it is likely that if an abnormality is suspected then other more definitive means of imaging will need to be considered.
- *Echocardiography*. Transthoracic and more especially, transoesophageal echocardiography are of value in imaging the aorta.
- *Computed tomography (CT)* and *magnetic resonance imaging (MRI)* scanning are of particular value.
- *Aortic angiography* is valuable in some situations.

The most appropriate choice of imaging modality depends on clinical circumstances and the problem or potential problem under investigation.

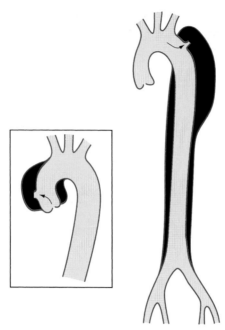

Fig. 15.1 Dissecting aneurysm of the aorta. This usually starts either a short distance above the aortic valve (left) or just below the origin of the left subclavian artery. (right).

DISSECTING ANEURYSM

A dissecting aneurysm (Fig. 15.1) results from the entry of blood into the media, either as a consequence of the rupture of vasa vasorum or from a tear of the aortic intima. No histological abnormality is seen in the media of most cases although cystic changes are sometimes present. Dissecting aneurysm is an important complication of Marfan's syndrome and of pregnancy, but the majority of cases occur in middle-aged or elderly men with systemic hypertension. The dissection usually starts either in the ascending aorta, a short distance above the aortic valve, or just beyond the origin of the left subclavian artery. The blood dissects a channel between the intima and the adventitia and usually advances distally. In so doing, it may occlude branches of the aortic arch and the descending aorta, including the renal and iliac arteries. If the dissection spreads proximally, the aortic valve may be involved, producing aortic regurgitation and, occasionally, occlusion of a coronary artery. The aneurysm usually ruptures externally into the pericardium, pleural cavity, mediastinum or retroperitoneal tissues, but sometimes it perforates the intima and the dissection 're-enters' the aortic lumen. Occasionally, the dissection becomes chronic without perforation.

Dissecting aneurysm is a particularly serious condition with a very high mortality. It usually presents with the sudden onset of a 'tearing' pain of extreme severity. The site of the pain depends upon the location of the dissection and moves as the dissection progresses. The pain may start in the anterior or posterior chest or in the abdomen, but nearly always affects the upper back at some stage. Intervals of freedom from pain may occur;

with recurrences, the pain may involve the neck, arms, chest, trunk or legs. Occasionally, the pain is slight; breathlessness or syncope may then be the presenting symptom.

Classification

The majority of aortic dissections originate in one of two locations, the ascending aorta a few centimetres above the aortic valve and the descending aorta just distal to the origin of the left subclavian artery. This distinction forms the basis of the classification of dissecting aneurysms into two types:

- *type A or proximal* – involvement of the ascending aorta with or without extension into the descending aorta
- *type B or distal* – involvement of the descending aorta without involvement of the ascending aorta.

Type A dissections account for about two-thirds of cases and type B for one-third. Distinction between the two types of dissection is important both for prognostic and therapeutic reasons.

Clinical features

- The patient appears pale and sweaty and has a tachycardia.
- Although there may be the appearance of shock, the blood pressure is usually within normal limits, having fallen from hypertensive levels.
- There may be evidence of *aortic regurgitation* or even cardiac tamponade if the dissection extends proximally. Occasionally, a coronary artery may be occluded resulting in myocardial infarction.
- *Pulse deficits* are common, due to occlusion of branches of the aorta. These most usually involve the femoral or left subclavian arteries. There may be a difference in blood pressure between the two arms.
- *Neurological manifestations* are common due to interference with the cerebral or spinal circulation.
- *Pleural effusion* is occasionally seen which may arise from a transient leak from the descending aorta. This may progress to haemothorax.

Investigations

- The *electrocardiogram (ECG)* is of little diagnostic value, but pre-existing hypertension may have caused left ventricular hypertrophy. The appearances of myocardial ischaemia or myocardial infarction may be present if there has been encroachment on a coronary artery.
- The *chest X-ray* may show an increase in the width of the mediastinum. However, it is important to realise that a normal chest X-ray does not exclude a diagnosis of dissection and if dissection is suspected on a basis of history, confirmation with other diagnostic techniques should be sought.
- *Transoesophageal echocardiography* (Fig 15.2) allows visualization of intimal flaps, the false lumen and the detection of flow in the false lumen. It is

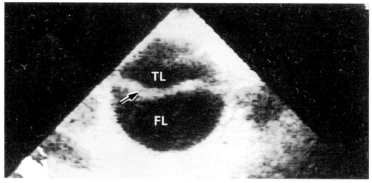

Fig. 15.2 Aortic dissection. Transoesophageal echocardiogram showing the descending aorta in cross-section. A flap is demonstrated (arrowed) separating the true lumen (TL) from the false lumen (FL).

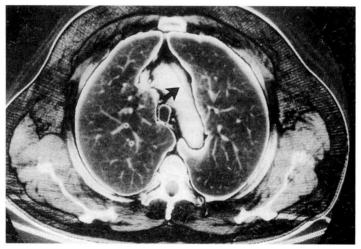

Fig. 15.3 Computed tomogram of an aortic dissection. The arrow points to detached flap in aorta.

frequently used because of its speed, wide availability and the fact that it can be performed at the patient's bedside. False negatives are few and generally arise with dissections involving the aortic arch, because this is difficult to visualize with transoesophageal echocardiography.

- *CT scanning* (Fig 15.3) allows visualization of intramural haematoma and, in about 70% of cases, the intimal flap.
- *MRI* is a very effective means of investigation of possible dissections, but has the drawback of being time-consuming and having limited out-of-hours availability in most institutions.
- *Aortic angiography* is generally not necessary but may be required in cases of doubt or if clear anatomical definition is required for management.

Each imaging method carries both advantages and disadvantages. Selection of an imaging modality depends on many factors including the availability of equipment and trained personnel and the length of time necessary to perform a particular procedure in addition to clinical considerations. In most institutions, CT scanning or transoesophageal echocardiography will be the investigations of choice.

Management

The value of the type A/type B classification (see above) lies in the differentiation of management between the two types of dissecting aneurysm. In general:

- *type A* dissections are best managed by early surgery
- *type B* dissections can be managed medically.

In *type A dissections*, there is a strong likelihood of further dissection and death unless surgical repair is undertaken. Patients should first be stabilized medically. Blood pressure should be lowered to reduce the strain on the aorta; beta-blockers are preferred for this purpose. Labetolol, which combines the properties of an alpha- and beta-blocker, is particularly useful in the management of aortic dissection. In occasional patients, a nitroprusside infusion may be required to control blood pressure.

The choice of surgical procedure depends on the extent of dissection. If the dissection involves the aortic root, it may be necessary to insert a Dacron tube graft with resuspension or replacement of the aortic valve and reimplantation of the coronary arteries.

In *type B dissections*, the risks of surgery are generally considered to exceed the risks of medical management. Treatment is directed at blood pressure control. Antihypertensive therapy should be continued long term to guard against risks of recurrent dissection.

Currently, endovascular stent placement is undergoing evaluation in the management of type B dissections. Although highly attractive as a means of avoiding difficult and high risk surgery, the role of this approach is as yet uncertain.

ATYPICAL AORTIC DISSECTION

The advent of new imaging techniques has led to the recognition of two additional conditions closely related to aortic dissection:

- *Intramural haematoma* is a haemorrhage contained within the aortic media. The initiating event is believed to be rupture of the vasa vasorum. The condition is distinguished from traditional dissection by the lack of an associated intimal tear. Intramural haematoma may regress with time or may progress to aortic dissection. Because of a high incidence of progression, intramural haematomas should be managed in a similar fashion to conventional dissection.
- *Penetrating atherosclerotic ulcer* is a communication into the media from the aortic lumen which may extend for a few centimetres but which does not develop a false lumen. Such ulceration occurs almost exclusively in the descending aorta. The natural history is unclear but a substantial proportion progress to transmural rupture and for this reason, surgery should be considered. The placement of an intravascular stent may be an alternative to surgery in some patients.

AORTIC TRAUMA

Rupture of the aorta is a common cause of death following automobile accidents. Following sudden deceleration of the body, the heart and horizontal portion of the aortic arch continue to move forwards. The descending aorta is fixed to the spine by intercostal arteries. As a consequence a tear can arise in the aorta at the junction of the fixed descending aorta and the mobile aortic arch. The characteristic site is just beyond the origin of the left subclavian artery.

The diagnosis should be suspected in any chest injury that involves sudden deceleration of the body. A chest radiograph will commonly show widening of the upper mediastinum. In contradistinction to aortic dissection, CT and transoesophageal echocardiography may fail to detect the localized nature of an aortic tear, and aortography remains the investigation of choice. Treatment is surgical repair.

CHRONIC THORACIC ANEURYSMS

These are localized distensions of the wall of the thoracic aorta. They are less common than aneurysms of the abdominal aorta. They are described as being *fusiform* if the whole circumference of the vessel is involved and *saccular* if only part of it is affected. Aneurysms are commonest in the descending aorta, followed by the ascending, whereas aneurysms of the aortic arch are rare.

Pathology

These aneurysms may arise as a result of a number of pathological processes:

- *Atherosclerotic aneurysms* are commonest and are usually situated in the descending aorta. They result from atrophy of the media and adventitia with fibrous replacement.
- Aneurysms of the ascending thoracic aorta commonly result from *cystic medial necrosis*, a degenerative change in the media layer leading to weakening and expansion. These aneurysms commonly involve the aortic root and may be associated with aortic regurgitation. The commonest cause is *Marfan's syndrome* (see p. 354), but similar changes may be seen in other connective tissue disorders, including *Ehlers–Danlos syndrome*.
- *Syphilis*, formerly the major cause of aortic aneurysms, has become uncommon. Syphilitic aneurysms usually affect the ascending aorta and the aortic arch, as a result of inflammatory changes in the aortic wall and subsequent fibrosis and calcification.

Clinical features

The clinical features resulting from an aneurysm of the thoracic aorta depend upon its size and site:

- When the aneurysm is in the ascending aorta, there is often associated aortic regurgitation which leads to cardiac failure.

- As the aneurysm enlarges and encroaches upon neighbouring structures, there may be pain as a result of erosion of ribs and sternum. In extreme cases, a pulsating mass may be seen in the front of the chest and obstruction of the superior vena cava may occur.
- When the aneurysm is situated in the aortic arch, wheezing, cough and hoarseness may arise from compression of the trachea, bronchus or recurrent laryngeal nerves.
- Aneurysms of the descending aorta are most likely to produce symptoms as a result of encroachment on the vertebrae, ribs or spinal nerves.

Investigations

Often, however, an aneurysm of the thoracic aorta is first diagnosed in an asymptomatic patient by the radiographic demonstration of a localized dilatation of the aorta. The diagnosis can be confirmed and accurate sizing of the aneurysm achieved using other imaging methods, including CT, MRI, transthoracic and transoesophageal echocardiography and angiography. Choice of imaging modality depends on location and whether surgery is contemplated.

Natural history

The natural history of an aortic aneurysm is to continue to enlarge with eventual rupture. Rupture is in most cases fatal. However, prediction of prognosis and of rupture is difficult. Most patients with aneurysms of the aorta have associated disorders such as hypertension, ischaemic heart disease or cerebrovascular disease, and death often results from other intercurrent events rather than from the aneurysm.

The single most important determinant of rupture is aneurysm diameter.

Management

The optimal timing of surgical repair is difficult. Surgery carries a significant morbidity and mortality and consequently should only be considered when there is a significant risk of rupture which exceeds the surgical risk.

In general, surgical repair should be considered when an aneurysm measures 6 cm or more in diameter. However, surgery may be indicated earlier in aneurysms showing a rapid rate of expansion, those associated with aortic regurgitation and those with symptoms related to the aneurysm. Marfan's syndrome is also an indication for considering earlier surgery, as these patients are particularly susceptible to dissection and rupture. In adults with Marfan's syndrome, elective surgery should be considered if an aneurysm exceeds 5.5 cm in diameter. Even lower threshold for elective surgery may be considered in children with Marfan's syndrome or in adults with a family history of dissection. By contrast, in patients at high operative risk, surgery is likely to be deferred until the aneurysm is 7 cm or larger.

In general, surgery involves resection of the aneurysm and replacement with a prosthetic graft. In aneurysms involving the ascending aorta with significant aortic regurgitation, the aortic valve is frequently replaced as part

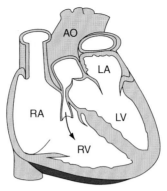

Fig. 15.4 Aneurysm of sinus of Valsalva rupturing into right atrium.

of the surgical repair. A composite graft comprising a Dacron tube with a suspended prosthetic aortic valve is sewn directly into the aortic annulus and the coronary arteries reattached to the Dacron graft.

ANEURYSM OF THE SINUS OF VALSALVA

This is most commonly caused by a congenital localized absence of the aortic media, but can result from syphilitic aortitis or infective endocarditis. The aneurysm forms a thin-walled sac which in most instances protrudes into the right ventricle or right atrium (Fig. 15.4). No symptoms or signs are produced until the aneurysm ruptures. When it does so a fistula is formed between the aorta and the relevant chamber. Congenital aneurysms of the sinus of Valsalva are often associated with other congenital lesions, particularly a ventricular septal defect.

Sudden death sometimes occurs; more often rupture causes the abrupt onset of chest pain and breathlessness. These symptoms subside over a period of days or weeks. Cardiac failure develops subsequently, but is very variable in its rate of progression.

Clinical features

- The patient may have a collapsing pulse due to the aortic diastolic leak,
- There is usually a continuous systolic and diastolic murmur, resembling that of a persistent ductus arteriosus, but loudest over the sternum at the level of the third or fourth interspace.
- The ECG may be normal initially, but the signs of right ventricular hypertrophy or right bundle branch block may develop later.
- The chest radiograph shows cardiac enlargement with pulmonary plethora.
- The aneurysm may be demonstrated by echocardiography, and the shunt by Doppler ultrasonography. The definitive diagnosis is made by showing the leak on aortography, and by the demonstration of a left-to-right shunt on cardiac catheterization.

The ruptured sinus of Valsalva should be treated by repair of the aortic wall.

FURTHER READING

Isselbacker, E. (2001) Diseases of the aorta. In: Braunwald, E., Zipes, D., & Libby, P. *Heart Disease. A Textbook of Cardiovascular Medicine*. Philadelphia: Saunders.

Khan, I., & Nair, C. (2002) Clinical, diagnostic and management perspectives of aortic dissection. *Chest* **122**: 311.

Prendergast, B., Boon, N., & Buckenham, T. (2002) Aortic dissection: advances in imaging and endoluminal repair. *Cardiovascular and Interventional Radiology* **25**: 85.

Treasure, T. (1993) Elective replacement of the aortic root in Marfan's syndrome. *British Heart Journal* **69**: 1062.

CHAPTER 16

Disorders of the lungs and pulmonary circulation

PULMONARY EMBOLISM

Pulmonary embolism is a major cause of morbidity and mortality. Diagnosis can be difficult and both underdiagnosis and overdiagnosis are common.

Pathophysiology

Pulmonary embolism, pulmonary thrombosis and pulmonary infarction are related conditions:

- *Pulmonary embolism* results from the obstruction of the pulmonary arterial vessels by thrombus or by material, such as fat or air, originating in some other site.
- *Pulmonary thrombosis* implies the formation of clot in situ. This is uncommon and implies the presence of pre-existing disease in the pulmonary arteries.
- *Pulmonary infarction* is the necrosis of a wedge of lung tissue resulting from pulmonary arterial occlusion.

Approximately 90% of pulmonary emboli originate in the leg veins. One or more of three mechanisms may contribute to their formation:

- *Venous stasis.* Venous stasis may result from prolonged immobilization or incompetent venous valves, possibly as a result of previous thromboembolism.
- *Blood hypercoagulability.* Blood hypercoagulability may be a result of drug therapy, including the oral contraceptive pill, hormone replacement therapy and steroids. In addition to this, there are a number of genetic abnormalities that predispose to thrombosis. The commonest involves resistance to an endogenous anticoagulant, activated protein C.
- *Injury to the vessel wall.* This may occur as a result of local injury or vascular endothelial damage, particularly previous thrombophlebitis.

In practice, several mechanisms may coexist. For example, there is an increased incidence of venous thromboembolism in pregnancy resulting both from venous stasis and a hypercoagulable state. The need to screen patients for possible underlying systemic hypercoagulability depends on clinical circumstances. Screening should be considered in young patients with no other identifiable predisposing factors, patients with a family history of thromboembolism and in patients with recurrent thrombosis.

The substantial majority of pulmonary emboli originate in the veins from the lower extremity. However, upper extremity venous thrombosis can also provide an embolic source and should be considered, particularly in patients with central venous catheters, pacing wires or intravenous drug abusers. In addition, the heart itself should be considered as a source of embolism in patients with atrial fibrillation, particularly in the presence of right heart failure.

Clinical features

The nature of the clinical presentation with pulmonary embolism depends on the size of the embolus:

- *A small embolus* may present with non-specific features such as dyspnoea or tiredness.
- *A medium-sized embolus* may cause the occlusion of a segment of the pulmonary arterial tree, causing pulmonary infarction. This may result in pleuritic pain, haemoptysis, a low-grade pyrexia and dyspnoea.
- *Massive pulmonary embolism* results from the occlusion of two-thirds or more of the pulmonary arterial bed. This causes right-sided failure, a low cardiac output and a rise in venous pressure.

The physical signs of pulmonary emboli vary with the size of the embolus. Small and even medium-sized emboli may be devoid of any abnormal clinical signs. Following pulmonary infarction, signs of a pleural effusion and pleural rub may be present.

Large emboli may cause:

- hypotension and shock
- tachycardia
- cyanosis
- elevation of the jugular venous pulse with a prominent V wave
- accentuation of the pulmonary component of the second heart sound due to pulmonary hypertension
- right ventricular third and fourth heart sounds
- occasionally continuous, systolic and diastolic murmurs due to turbulent flow caused by the embolus.

Massive pulmonary embolism should be suspected in any patient who suddenly develops the features of shock, syncope, acute dyspnoea or chest pain, particularly if the subject has evidence of a venous thrombosis or has been confined to bed during the preceding days.

Investigations

The range of clinical presentations of pulmonary embolism means that particular importance is placed on diagnostic investigations in confirming or refuting the diagnosis. Initial investigations should include:

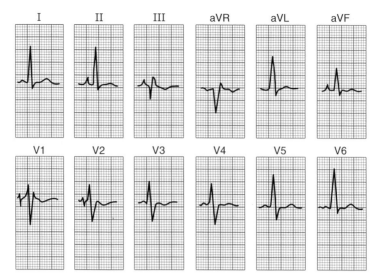

I   II   III   aVR   aVL   aVF

V1   V2   V3   V4   V5   V6

Fig. 16.1 ECG appearances in pulmonary embolism. Note tall, peaked P waves, partial right bundle branch block (rSr in V1), S in lead I, Q and negative T in III, and inverted T waves in V1 to V3.

- *Chest radiography.* This may show features of pulmonary atelectasis or pleural effusion which may accompany pulmonary embolism, but in many patients the chest X-ray is normal or shows only subtle changes. The chest X-ray is important to exclude other conditions, particularly pnueumothorax.
- *Electrocardiogram (ECG).* ECG changes accompanying pulmonary embolism are unreliable for diagnostic purposes. In cases of mild to moderate pulmonary embolism, the ECG is generally normal, except for demonstrating sinus tachycardia. In more severe pulmonary embolism, a number of ECG features may be observed (Fig. 16.1):
  - $S_1 Q_3 T_3$ pattern. A narrow Q wave and inverted T wave in lead III, accompanied by an S wave in lead I, all due to changes in the position of the heart caused by dilatation of the right ventricle and atrium
  - P pulmonale
  - right bundle branch block
  - 'right ventricular strain' pattern with T inversion in the leads of V1 to V4
  - atrial arrhythmias.
  The differential diagnosis from acute myocardial infarction may be extremely difficult. The ECG is of considerable value, but the patterns associated with massive pulmonary embolism are often misinterpreted as being those of a combination of inferior and anteroseptal infarction. The appearance of Q waves and negative T waves in lead III (but not in lead II) in association with inverted T waves from V1 to V4 strongly suggests pulmonary embolism.
- *Blood gases.* Characteristically pulmonary embolism causes a reduced arterial pO_2 due to shunting of blood through underventilated parts of the lung. Simultaneously pCO_2 is normal or reduced due to hyperventilation.

However, the sensitivity and specificity of these findings is relatively low.

- *D-dimer*. Plasma D-dimer is a useful screening test. The test is sensitive but not specific, that is D-dimer may be elevated in a number of conditions and D-dimer elevation does not confirm a diagnosis of pulmonary embolism However, a negative D-dimer virtually excludes pulmonary embolism and obviates the needs for additional tests.

Following these initial investigations, further investigations are likely to be required to confirm the diagnosis:

- *Pulmonary scintigraphy*. Using radioactive technetium, this is a sensitive technique for detecting perfusion abnormalities. A perfusion deficit might be due either to impaired blood flow to that segment of lung or to primary pulmonary problems, such as effusion or collapse. To improve the specificity of the method, it is generally combined with a ventilation scan using radioactive xenon gas. The demonstration of a non-perfused but ventilated zone is strongly suggestive of pulmonary embolism. However, in patients with existing lung disease, the diagnostic value of lung scanning is reduced.

- *Spiral pulmonary computed tomography (CT) scanning*. This involves the injection of contrast medium through a peripheral vein and enables the right and left pulmonary arteries to be visualized down to their segmental branches. The test is both sensitive and specific in diagnosing pulmonary emboli and is considered by many as the investigation of choice in patients unsuitable for a ventilation–perfusion scan or in whom a ventilation–perfusion scan gives equivocal results.

- *Pulmonary angiography*. Traditionally, pulmonary angiography has been regarded as the gold standard for diagnosis of pulmonary emboli. However, it is an invasive investigation which carries significant risk, particularly in this patient population who may already be critically ill. These risks can be reduced by selective injections into each lung in turn or by using digital subtraction angiography to enable the volume of contrast injected to be reduced. However, the advent of spiral CT scanning has largely superceded the need for pulmonary angiography.

- *Venous ultrasonography*. This may provide useful circumstantial evidence in cases in which the diagnosis remains uncertain following more direct imaging methods. If there is evidence of a deep venous thrombosis, this provides circumstantial evidence in favour of a diagnosis of pulmonary embolism. However, the converse does not apply and the absence of venous thrombosis in no way excludes pulmonary embolism.

- *Echocardiography*. Echocardiography is of value as a means of assessing pressure overload on the right ventricle which accompanies massive pulmonary embolism. Increase in afterload causes acute dilatation and hypokinesis of the right ventricle, with diastolic displacement of the septum towards the left ventricle and paradoxical movement of the septum. Pulmonary hypertension can be identified by Doppler ultrasound. Echocardiography may therefore provide a means of rapidly recognizing the most severely ill patients, most likely to benefit from intervention (see below).

Management

There are two major objectives in management:

- The prevention of further thromboembolism
- In severe cases, the detection and relief of right heart failure.

Anticoagulation

In the majority of patients the haemodynamic consequences of pulmonary emboli are not severe. The primary objective of treatment is the prevention of further emboli. Patients are treated initially with intravenous heparin, adjusted according to the patient's activated partial thromboplastin time. Warfarin therapy is commenced and heparin discontinued after 5–7 days. Heparin should be maintained for at least 2 days after achieving a therapeutic international normalized ratio (INR).

The recent introduction of low molecular weight heparins has substantially replaced the use of conventional heparin. Low molecular weight heparins carry several advantages:

- Predictable anticoagulation without the need for routine monitoring of anticoagulant status
- Subcutaneous administration
- A longer half-life than conventional heparin.

The target INR therapeutic range for the management of pulmonary embolism is generally 2.0–3.0. The duration of anticoagulation varies with clinical circumstances. If a predisposing factor can be identified and this factor no longer exists, treatment for 3 months may be adequate. If no predisposing factor can be identified, a minimum of 6 months anticoagulation is generally recommended. In patients with recurrent thromboembolism, lifelong anticoagulation is recommended. Similarly, in patients with a defined hypercoagulable state, lifelong anticoagulation may be necessary.

In exceptional patients who have recurrent pulmonary emboli while on warfarin, an inferior vena caval filter device can be considered. This device, inserted percutaneously via a catheter, traps clots preventing migration to the lungs.

Management of massive pulmonary embolism

In patients with massive pulmonary embolism, sufficient to cause severe haemodynamic compromise, thrombolytic therapy should be considered. Unlike thrombolytic treatment of acute myocardial infarction, there is no evidence-based consensus as to which patients should be treated. However, there is general agreement that patients with systemic hypotension should receive thrombolytic therapy, because the prognosis of this group if left untreated is so poor. The time window of possible benefit from thrombolytic therapy is similarly undefined, but is much wider than the time window of benefit in acute myocardial infarction; patients may benefit from treatment even days after their initial presentation.

General management and pain relief

Opiates such as diamorphine are appropriate, but care is needed in hypotensive patients. Hypoxaemia is likely and high concentrations of oxygen (at least 40%) should be administered. It is usual to have high right-sided filling pressures following pulmonary embolism. Any decrease in the right-sided filling pressure is likely to lead to a further decrease in cardiac output. For this reason, diuretics and vasodilators should be avoided. If right-sided pressure should fall, it may become necessary to give intravenous fluids to maintain cardiac output.

Anticoagulation

The patient should be heparinized to prevent further embolism. Therapy should be initiated with a bolus of 5000–10 000 units, followed by a maintenance infusion of 1000 units/h, adjusted according to the activated partial thromboplastin time (APTT). A low molecular weight heparin, such as enoxaparin 1.5 mg/kg every 24h given by subcutaneous injection can be used as an alternative.

Thrombolysis

In patients with severe haemodynamic compromise, thrombolytic therapy should be given to dissolve the embolus. A loading dose of 250 000 units of streptokinase should be given over 30 min, followed by a maintenance infusion of 100 000 units hourly, with subsequent adjustment in accordance with clotting parameters.

Embolectomy

Pulmonary embolectomy is rarely undertaken. Its use is confined to patients who continue to deteriorate despite thrombolytic therapy or patients in whom there is an absolute contraindication to the use of thrombolytic agents.

Recurrent pulmonary emboli and thromboembolic pulmonary hypertension

Recurrent pulmonary embolization, which is usually associated with chronic or recurrent venous thrombosis, may appear as massive emboli, as pulmonary infarction or be silent. Eventually, the vascular obstruction may become so widespread as to cause a substantial increase in the resistance of the pulmonary arteries and lead to pulmonary arterial hypertension. Once this has become established, the prognosis is poor and most patients die within a period of 5 years. The process may sometimes be reversed or prevented from progression by permanent anticoagulant therapy.

PULMONARY HYPERTENSION

The pulmonary circulation is a low pressure system. Pulmonary hypertension exists when the systolic pressure exceeds 30 mmHg. There are two types of pulmonary hypertension:

* Pulmonary hypertension is most commonly secondary to other cardiac or lung disease – this is termed *secondary pulmonary hypertension*.

• Less commonly, pulmonary hypertension occurs in isolation, unrelated to other heart and lung problems – this is termed *primary pulmonary hypertension*.

The normal pulmonary circulation

The pulmonary arterial pressure is determined by the pressure in the pulmonary capillaries, the pulmonary blood flow and the resistance of the pulmonary arteries (especially the arterioles).

The small pulmonary arteries of the fetus have a thick muscular media and the pulmonary vascular resistance of the non-aerated lung is high. This muscular layer regresses over the first 2–3 months of life. As a consequence, the pulmonary vascular resistance and arterial pressure start to fall shortly after birth and within a few weeks have declined to normal adult levels.

The pulmonary arteries in the adult are relatively thin-walled, the smaller vessels having considerably less muscle in their walls than corresponding systemic arterioles. The resistance to flow is much lower and the normal pressure in the pulmonary artery (about 20/10 mmHg) is approximately one-seventh that in the aorta. It is believed that many of the capillaries in the lung are closed at rest, particularly those of the upper parts of the lungs. When the cardiac output increases, as on exercise, the vascular resistance falls as capillaries open and small arteries dilate. As a consequence, blood flow through the lungs can increase threefold before any rise in pressure occurs.

Secondary pulmonary hypertension

Causes of secondary pulmonary hypertension

Pulmonary arterial hypertension (greater than 30/15 mmHg) may result from:

• an increase in pulmonary capillary pressure
• an increase in pulmonary blood flow
• an increase in pulmonary vascular resistance.

Elevated pulmonary capillary pressure

Passive pulmonary hypertension due to a raised pulmonary capillary pressure occurs in all conditions in which the left atrial pressure rises, such as mitral stenosis and left ventricular failure. The pulmonary artery pressure rises in proportion to the pulmonary capillary pressure.

Increased pulmonary blood flow

Pulmonary hypertension due to increased flow develops in disorders in which there are left-to-right shunts. These include:

• septal defects
• persistent ductus arteriosus
• atrial septal defect.

A large pulmonary blood flow of 10–15 L/min may be unassociated with pulmonary hypertension because there is a compensatory vasodilatation

Box 16.1	Causes of increased pulmonary vascular resistance
	Cor pulmonale
	Chronic thromboembolism
	Eisenmenger's syndrome
	Collagen vascular diseases
	Schistosomiasis
	Primary pulmonary hypertension

with a fall in vascular resistance. In many cases of ventricular septal defect and persistent ductus arteriosus, there is no vasodilatation, and the resistance remains normal. The pulmonary arterial pressure may therefore rise even with comparatively small shunts. With large shunts, pulmonary arterial pressure may reach systemic levels.

Increased pulmonary vascular resistance.

There are a number of causes of increased pulmonary vascular resistance (Box 16.1). These diverse causes lead to increased pulmonary vascular resistance through three basic mechanisms:

- *Pulmonary vasoconstriction*. Hypoxia is a potent pulmonary vasoconstrictor and is a factor in the pulmonary hypertension that occurs in respiratory disease.
- *Blockage* of the pulmonary arteries or arterioles by thrombosis and embolism, as in thromboembolism and schistosomiasis.
- *Arterial medial hypertrophy*. Proliferation of the muscular medial layer of the small pulmonary arteries which are the main determinants of the pulmonary vascular resistance. The muscular proliferation may progress to fibrosis. Medial hypertrophy plays a major role in primary pulmonary hypertension and in Eisenmenger's syndrome.

Combinations of the three mechanisms are common. In mitral stenosis, for example, the initial phase of passive pulmonary hypertension is often complicated by vasoconstriction and by the obliterative changes of pulmonary embolism. In many cases of ventricular septal defect, both high blood flow and pulmonary vascular disease contribute to pulmonary hypertension. In emphysema, obliteration of the vascular bed and hypoxia are contributory factors.

Clinical features of pulmonary hypertension

Independent of causation, certain clinical features are characteristic of severe pulmonary hypertension. The symptoms include:

- dyspnoea
- fatigue
- syncope
- haemoptysis
- chest pain
- symptoms of right-sided cardiac failure.

Abnormal features on clinical examination may include:

- elevation of the jugular venous pulse with a prominent 'a' wave
- features of tricuspid regurgitation
- a forceful right ventricular heave along the left sternal edge
- a right ventricular fourth-heart sound at the lower left sternal edge
- a loud pulmonary component to the second sound, which may be followed by an early diastolic murmur of pulmonary regurgitation (Graham Steell murmur).

Investigation

- The chest radiograph may show enlargement of the proximal pulmonary arteries, right ventricle and right atrium. The peripheral lung fields appear oligaemic.
- The ECG demonstrates features of right ventricular hypertrophy:
  - tall peaked P waves in lead II due to right atrial enlargement
  - right axis deviation
  - a predominant R wave in lead V1
  - inverted T waves in leads V1–V3.

Management

Both management and prognosis of pulmonary arterial hypertension depend upon its aetiology and on its severity. Passive pulmonary hypertension responds well if the underlying disorder can be corrected (e.g. mitral stenosis). Pulmonary hypertension due to high pulmonary arterial flow can usually be reversed by the correction of the underlying congenital abnormality. Increased pulmonary arterial resistance due to vasoconstriction can often be diminished by relieving hypoxia or by the successful treatment of mitral valve disease.

When pulmonary hypertension is due to severe pulmonary vascular disease, as in the Eisenmenger syndrome, the prognosis is poor and life is usually sustained for only a few years. In these cases, cardiac failure is progressive in spite of treatment and the only hope may lie in heart–lung transplantation.

Primary ('unexplained') pulmonary hypertension

Pulmonary hypertension is said to be primary when the aetiology cannot be determined. The pathology is complex and poorly understood. The diagnosis is made by exclusion in patients found to have the clinical features of pulmonary hypertension. Lung biopsy can aid diagnosis, but is potentially hazardous. Characteristic 'plexiform' lesions are present in approximately 70% of cases; these comprise a mass of disorganized vessels with proliferating endothelial cells and smooth muscle cells.

The condition, which is rare, is most common in young women. The onset of the disease is insidious. The first symptoms are usually fatigue and exertional dyspnoea. Chest pain, syncope and right heart failure may also occur. By the time symptoms occur, the disease is generally advanced with severe pulmonary hypertension.

Physical findings are generally subtle. A right ventricular lift and accentuation of the pulmonary component of the second sound may be evident. As the disease progresses, many patients develop tricuspid regurgitation and right heart failure.

Echocardiography is a particularly important diagnostic tool. The right atrium and right ventricle are generally dilated and tricuspid regurgitation often present. The right ventricular to right atrial pressure gradient can be calculated from the velocity of the regurgitant jet. Extensive additional investigations are then likely to be required to exclude secondary causes of pulmonary hypertension.

Management

Until recently the prognosis of primary pulmonary hypertension has been particularly poor, with a median survival of under 5 years. With modern therapies, in particular prostacyclin infusion, 4 year survival is approaching 75%.

A number of therapies should be considered:

- Thrombosis may contribute to the progression of hypertension and *anticoagulants* are recommended; oral contraceptives and pregnancy must be avoided.
- *Vasodilator therapy* may prove of value in some patients. Response is variable. Patients may be given a trial of an oral calcium channel blocker. Those responding with a lowering of pulmonary artery pressure and an improvement in symptoms are continued with long-term therapy. Amlodipine is commonly chosen, on account of its relative lack of negative inotropic effects.
- *Epoprostenol* (prostacyclin) causes vasodilatation and is of value in reducing pulmonary artery pressure. Epoprostenol has been shown to be effective in improving haemodynamic measures, exercise tolerance and survival. Unfortunately, the drug has a short half-life and continuous intravenous administration via an indwelling catheter is necessary. Currently, epoprostenol is considered to be the most effective therapy for patients with primary pulmonary hypertension, and most patients experience benefit. Newer prostacyclin analogues, not dependent on parenteral administration, are under development.
- *Endothelin-1 receptor antagonists*. Endothelin-1 is a potent vasoconstrictor of smooth muscle cells. Bosentan is an oral antagonist of endothelin-1 receptors and has been shown in preliminary studies to benefit exercise capacity in patients with primary pulmonary hypertension.
- *Phosphodiesterase inhibitors*. The endogenous vasodilator, nitric oxide, exerts its vasodilatory effects through the second messenger cGMP. Sildenafil is a selective inhibitor of cGMP-specific phosphodiesterase and hence potentiates vasodilatation. There are preliminary reports of a promising response to sildenafil in patients with primary pulmonary hypertension. Its full role awaits further evaluation.
- In patients failing to respond to conventional treatment, *transplantation* should be considered. This may be either lung transplantation or combined heart and lung transplantation.

PULMONARY HEART DISEASE

The understanding of pulmonary heart disease (*cor pulmonale*) has been made difficult by problems of nomenclature. Here it is defined as heart disease affecting the right ventricle secondary to disorders of ventilation and respiratory function. Right-sided heart failure due to pulmonary arterial disease or secondary to left-sided heart failure is not included in this definition, and is considered in the section on pulmonary hypertension (above).

The prevalence of pulmonary heart disease varies greatly between one geographical area and another. The commonest cause of cor pulmonale is chronic obstructive pulmonary disease (COPD) and this is reflected in its prevalence. There is abundant evidence that heavy cigarette smoking and air pollution are major factors in the production of COPD; cor pulmonale is commonest in those exposed to these influences. It is predominantly a disease of middle-aged and elderly men, and is uncommon in young men or in women of any age.

Pathogenesis of heart failure in lung disease

Lung disease causes heart disease mainly because of its effects on the pulmonary vessels. Due to a number of different mechanisms, there is an increase in pulmonary vascular resistance, leading to pulmonary hypertension, right ventricular hypertrophy and right heart failure.

These mechanisms include:

- *pulmonary arteriolar constriction* due to low alveolar oxygen tension in areas of underventilated lung
- *anatomical reduction of the pulmonary vascular bed* from rupture of alveolar walls and from fibrotic or thrombotic obliteration of capillaries
- *compression of pulmonary capillaries* by high intra-alveolar pressures when there is air trapping.

Pulmonary hypertension is seldom severe in pulmonary disease except when there is superadded respiratory infection.

Abnormalities in the blood gases nearly always precede the appearance of heart failure due to lung disease. Hypoxaemia is almost invariable. Even if the arterial oxygen tension is normal at rest, it is reduced on exercise. The hypoxaemia results either from disturbances in the ventilation–perfusion relationship or from interference with the diffusion of oxygen through the alveolar wall.

The carbon dioxide tension is raised when the heart failure is secondary to COPD and alveolar hypoventilation. If there is a rapid rise in carbon dioxide tension, the pH is low, but in the chronic stage of the disease the renal retention of bicarbonate maintains a normal or near normal acid–base balance.

These blood gas abnormalities are responsible for many of the characteristics of pulmonary heart disease:

- *polycythaemia* and increased blood volume due to hypoxaemia
- *peripheral vasodilatation*, due to high carbon dioxide tension, producing a large pulse and warm extremities
- *cerebral vasodilatation*, due to high carbon dioxide tension, which leads to a raised cerebrospinal fluid pressure, with tremor, confusion and papilloedema
- *impaired myocardial function* due to hypoxaemia.

The more advanced symptoms of carbon dioxide retention occur mainly, if not exclusively, in patients receiving oxygen in high concentration. Such treatment is dangerous if there is carbon dioxide retention because it abolishes the hypoxaemia which is a major stimulus to respiration.

Clinical features of pulmonary heart disease

Diseases causing pulmonary heart disease cover the full spectrum of pulmonary disease including obstructive pulmonary disease, emphysema, pulmonary fibrosis, pulmonary infiltration (e.g. sarcoidosis), pulmonary resection, skeletal abnormalities and disorders of the respiratory muscles.

The patient is commonly a cigarette-smoking middle-aged man with a long history of morning cough and sputum. There may have been recurrent attacks of winter bronchitis. These symptoms are slowly progressive until breathlessness becomes disabling. Overt cyanosis and peripheral oedema are usually late features but are sometimes the first clear manifestation of pulmonary disease. Recent worsening of cough and the production of purulent sputum is common.

The clinical features reflect pulmonary hypertension and right ventricular failure and include:

- dyspnoea
- cyanosis
- features of carbon dioxide retention
- an elevated jugular venous pulse, possibly with signs of tricuspid regurgitation
- peripheral oedema and hepatic enlargement.

Investigations

- The *ECG* is often normal but may show P pulmonale, right axis deviation, right ventricular hypertrophy, right bundle branch block, or an rS pattern across the chest. In emphysema the QRS complexes are often small.
- The *chest X ray appearance* depends upon the nature of the lung disease. When there is emphysema with an increased total lung volume, one may see a low diaphragm and a narrow heart. Enlargement of the main pulmonary artery and its major branches occurs when there is pulmonary hypertension. The radiograph is, however, often normal.
- *Pulmonary function tests* usually demonstrate a forced expiratory volume in 1 s (FEV_1) below 1.5 L and a peak expiratory flow rate less than 200 L/min. Blood gas analysis will usually show an arterial $pO_2 < 6$ kPa.
- *Echocardiography*. Patients are often poor echo subjects due to over inflation of the chest. The right ventricle is enlarged and there is generally evidence of tricuspid regurgitation, enabling the pressure gradient between the right atrium and the right ventricle to be estimated and hence giving an indirect estimate of pulmonary artery pressure.

Differential diagnosis

The pulmonary origin of cardiac failure is often overlooked, particularly when it coexists with known ischaemic, rheumatic or hypertensive heart disease. This is particularly the case with hypertension; mild hypertension is often blamed for heart failure which is secondary to chronic bronchitis and emphysema. The history of chronic cough with sputum and wheezing should suggest the possibility, as should poor chest movement and the presence of rhonchi. The diagnosis is usually best made by studies of ventilation and blood gases; carbon dioxide retention makes it almost certain that there is a pulmonary component in heart failure.

Prognosis and treatment

The prognosis is poor once cardiac failure has complicated pulmonary heart disease. COPD patients with elevated pulmonary artery pressure show decreased survival in comparison with COPD individuals with pulmonary artery pressure within the normal range. Treatment may overcome individual attacks, but the subject is liable to further episodes with recurrent infection and to acute exacerbations of heart failure.

When a patient is seen in cardiac failure due to pulmonary heart disease, the major objects of treatment should be to combat respiratory infection, correct hypoxaemia and carbon dioxide retention, and relieve airways obstruction.

- Acute chest infections should be promptly treated with *antibiotics*.
- *Beta$_2$-agonists*, such as salbutamol, may have some benefit in reducing pulmonary hypertension.
- *Corticosteroids* may be of benefit in patients with reversible airways obstruction.
- Some patients may also benefit from the provision of long-term *domiciliary oxygen*. This has been shown to lower mortality in patients with chronic obstructive airways disease and persistent hypoxaemia, although improvement in pulmonary hypertension has not been convincingly demonstrated.

Diuretics are widely used for the control of right heart failure, but should be used with caution as they may reduce cardiac output. In contradistinction to primary pulmonary hypertension, vasodilators have proved disappointing. The role of angiotensin-converting enzyme (ACE) inhibitors is uncertain.

FURTHER READING

American Heart Association (1996) Management of deep vein thrombosis and pulmonary embolism. A statement for healthcare professionals from the Council on Thrombosis, American Heart Association. *Circulation* 93: 2212.

Kearon, C. (2003) Natural history of venous thromboembolism. *Circulation* **107** (23 Suppl 1): 122.

Kroegel, C. (2003) Advances in the diagnosis and treatment of pulmonary embolism. *Respiration* 70: 4.

Rich, S. (2001) Pulmonary hypertension. In: Braunwald, E., Zipes, D. & Libby, P. *Heart Disease. A Textbook of Cardiovascular Medicine*. Philadelphia: Saunders.

Runo, J. & Loyd, J. (2003) Primary pulmonary hypertension. *Lancet* **361**: 1533.

Systemic disorders and the heart

INFECTIONS AND THE HEART

The heart may be involved in infections in a number of ways. There may be direct invasion of the endocardium, myocardium or pericardium. Alternatively the heart may be indirectly affected through toxin production or as a result of autoimmune mechanisms arising from the body's response to the infection.

Rheumatic fever

Acute rheumatic fever is a disease that follows infection by group A haemolytic streptococci and produces manifestations in many tissues and organs. Arthritis is often the most conspicuous feature, but cardiac involvement is of much greater importance. The duration of rheumatic activity is very variable; it may cease in 2 weeks or persist for many months. Recurrences are common. Death is rare in the acute phase but the sequelae of chronic rheumatic heart disease is responsible for a considerable morbidity and mortality.

Epidemiology

Over the last 50 years, rheumatic fever has been becoming progressively less frequent and is now rare in many countries, including the UK, the USA and Scandinavia. However, in the rapidly expanding cities of Asia, Africa and South America, rheumatic heart disease is the commonest cause of cardiac death. The decline of rheumatic fever in Western countries is not solely the result of the use of antibiotics for it preceded their discovery. It may be attributed both to a change in the virulence of streptococci and to improving social conditions. Rheumatic fever most commonly occurs between the ages of 5 and 15 years, with the peak about the age of 8. It is rare under the age of 4 and becomes progressively less common after the age of 15, although occasional cases are seen even after the age of 30.

Pathophysiology

Rheumatic fever seems to occur only after a group A streptococcal infection. It is a complication of less than 1% of episodes of streptococcal pharyngitis, developing some 10–20 days after the onset of the sore throat. No history of sore throat, however, can be obtained in some 30–50% of cases; nonetheless virtually all patients with acute rheumatic fever have a streptococcal antibody response.

The mechanism whereby group A streptococcal infection leads to rheumatic fever is uncertain. One theory is that antigenic proteins in the group A streptococci share structural similarities to cardiac myosin and sarcolemmal membrane proteins. As a consequence, antibodies produced in response to the streptococcal infection may cross-react with cardiac tissue and result in an autoimmune reaction.

Microscopic evidence of acute rheumatic fever is widespread, but particularly affects tissues lined by endothelium such as blood vessels, the endocardium, the pericardium and synovial membranes. The earliest lesion is one of swelling in and around collagen fibres, accompanied by oedema and lymphocytic infiltration. Later, and more specifically, granulomatous Aschoff nodules appear. These are formed by collections of round cells, fibroblasts and multinucleated giant cells, and are usually surrounded by an area of polymorphonuclear cells, lymphocytes and plasma cells.

The lesions of rheumatic fever are most obvious in relation to the heart valves and the pericardium. The valve cusps become thickened by oedema and by the infiltration of capillaries. Grey or yellow warty vegetations ('verrucae') form along the lines of closure. The mitral valve is most often affected, followed by the aortic. The tricuspid and pulmonary valves are involved less commonly. In the acute phase, dilatation of the mitral annulus may result in mitral regurgitation.

Chronic rheumatic heart disease is a sequel to acute rheumatic carditis, and many of its features are the result of fibrosis occurring during the healing of the acute lesion.

Clinical features

In most cases, some 2–3 weeks after the onset of acute pharyngitis, children begin to feel unwell, lose their appetite and complain of pains in the limbs. Fever is present, but it is not usually high. The major clinical features are:

- carditis
- polyarthritis
- subcutaneous nodules
- erythema marginatum
- chorea.

Carditis

The heart is involved in about half of the first attacks of rheumatic fever. The endocardium, myocardium and pericardium may all be involved to varying degrees.

Endocarditis. Endocarditis, with valvar involvement, is suggested by the appearance of cardiac murmurs:

- An apical pansystolic murmur indicates either mitral valve damage or functional mitral regurgitation associated with myocarditis.
- Rheumatic involvement of the mitral valve is also strongly suggested by the appearance of a low-pitched and short mid-diastolic apical murmur (Carey Coombs). This murmur is usually transient, but may persist for months or years until the characteristic features of mitral stenosis develop.

Midsystolic murmurs in the aortic or pulmonary area are less certain evidence of cardiac involvement, as they are common in febrile children without heart disease and usually disappear as recovery takes place. The diastolic murmur of aortic regurgitation is not uncommon, and usually persists after the acute rheumatic process has subsided.

Myocarditis. This is a common feature of acute rheumatic fever, but is difficult to diagnose with confidence. It is suggested by a tachycardia and by cardiac enlargement. More diagnostic is the appearance of left-sided or right-sided heart failure when this cannot be attributed to valve damage. The symptoms include dyspnoea, orthopnoea and oedema. A gallop rhythm is frequent.

Pericarditis. When clinical evidence of pericarditis is present, the carditis is usually severe and involves the myocardium and endocardium as well (pancarditis). Retrosternal pain and pericardial friction occur and there may be a pericardial effusion.

Polyarthritis

Characteristically, the joints become swollen, painful and hot, but in the younger child there may be only vague aches. The arthritis usually affects one joint after another, giving the impression of 'flitting'. The knees, ankles, shoulders, wrists and elbows are most commonly involved. The inflammation in each joint usually develops within a few hours and may take up to a week to subside. Even in the absence of treatment, the polyarthritis usually disappears within 3 weeks and leaves no residual abnormality.

Subcutaneous nodules

These seldom give rise to symptoms but are of diagnostic importance. They are firm painless structures which are attached to tendon sheaths, joint capsules and fascia, and the skin is movable over them. They occur mainly over the extensor surfaces of the wrists, elbows, knuckles, knees and Achilles tendons and also over the scalp. They usually last about a week.

Erythema marginatum

This consists of lesions which develop rapidly from small macules or papules into large circles with pink, slightly raised, sharply circumscribed edges and pale centres. As these circles intersect, a pattern of segments develops. These appear and disappear within a period of hours. Erythema marginatum affects the trunk and limbs, but never involves the face.

Chorea (St Vitus' dance)

This is a neurological manifestation of the acute rheumatic process. It often occurs without the other features, but cardiac involvement is common. The onset is usually insidious with the development of an apparent clumsiness in an otherwise healthy child. Jerky and non-repetitive movements occur and muscle tone is reduced.

Laboratory investigations

- In most cases there is a moderate leucocytosis of 12 000–15 000 white blood cells/mm^3, accompanied by a rise in acute phase reactants, including an increased erythrocyte sedimentation rate (ESR) and a raised level of C-reactive protein.

- In only about one-quarter of patients, can a group A streptococcus be grown from the throat. The presence of a raised or rising antistreptolysin 'O' (ASO) titre provides good evidence of recent infection, particularly if it rises and falls.
- A number of electrocardiographic abnormalities occur in acute rheumatic fever. Amongst these are a prolonged PR interval and, more rarely, more advanced degrees of atrioventricular block. Non-specific T wave changes are common and the ST and T wave changes characteristic of pericarditis may be seen.
- Echocardiography demonstrates mitral regurgitation in a minority of patients in the acute phase of the disease. This is generally secondary to prolapse of the anterior leaflet of the mitral valve.

Diagnosis of rheumatic fever

There is no certain way of establishing the presence of rheumatic fever, but the combination of certain clinical features and laboratory findings is highly suggestive. Criteria for diagnosis were originally suggested in 1944 by T. Duckett Jones and subsequently modified by the American Heart Association in 1992 (Box 17.1). The diagnostic criteria are divided into major and minor. Diagnosis is based on evidence of a recent streptococcal infection accompanied by two major criteria or one major and two minor criteria.

The absence of microbiological or serological evidence of group A streptococcal infection makes the diagnosis of acute rheumatic fever extremely unlikely. As an exception to this rule, chorea may on occasion be the only manifestation of rheumatic fever. In the absence of any other aetiology, rheumatic fever may be diagnosed, based on the presence of this finding in isolation.

Patients with a previous history of rheumatic fever are at increased risk of recurrent episodes. This should lead to an increased index of suspicion in considering possible recurrences.

Course and prognosis

The course of rheumatic fever is variable and unpredictable. In some apparently severely ill patients, complete recovery takes place within a few days, whereas in others the disease drags on for months.

Box 17.1

Modified Duckett Jones criteria for the diagnosis of rheumatic fever
(Revised Jones Criteria, American Heart Association, 1992.)

Major criteria
Carditis
Polyarthritis
Chorea
Erythema marginatum
Subcutaneous nodules

Minor criteria
Arthralgia
Fever
Raised ESR or C-reactive protein level
Prolonged PR interval

The first attack is seldom fatal, but recurrences may lead to increasing cardiac damage and heart failure. More than two-thirds of patients who have experienced rheumatic fever eventually develop chronic rheumatic valve disease.

There can be no doubt that many cases of rheumatic fever escape diagnosis because about half of the patients with proven chronic rheumatic disease give no history of an acute episode.

Treatment

During the acute phase of the disease the subject wants and needs bed rest. When the temperature, pulse rate and ESR have returned to normal and the evidence of acute arthritis and carditis has disappeared, the patient may be gradually mobilized and rehabilitated. Active carditis requires complete rest, and this may have to be continued for several weeks. Subsequent increases in activity must depend upon the individual response, and a full resumption of normal physical activity usually has to be delayed to 6 months from the time when the last signs of active carditis have resolved.

Both salicylates and corticosteroids have a dramatic effect on the fever and polyarthritis of rheumatic fever. Aspirin is effective in the relief of joint pain. It should be used in high doses. The value of steroids is controversial. They are similarly effective in reducing inflammation, but there is little objective evidence that they alter the course of the disease. It is nonetheless common practice to prescribe steroids to patients with a severe attack of rheumatic fever with carditis and heart failure.

Rarely, reumatic fever may be fulminant and it may be necessary to consider mitral valve surgery in the acute phase of the disease.

Prevention

Rheumatic fever may be prevented by the prophylaxis and treatment of acute streptococcal infections. However, many episodes of streptococcal pharyngitis are asymptomatic and even optimal treatment of symptomatic infections may fail to prevent recurrences of rheumatic fever. For this reason, continuous prophylaxis is indicated as the only means of preventing recurrent attacks.

All patients who have experienced acute rheumatic fever should receive long-term prophylactic therapy. It is not known how long prophylaxis should be continued, but it is common practice to recommend this up to the age of 25 years.

Chronic rheumatic heart disease

Chronic rheumatic heart disease is the result of damage produced by recurrent attacks of acute rheumatic carditis and the subsequent healing process. These changes are largely confined to the valve structures, although in some instances, myocardial damage may also be severe. Because valve damage predominates in patients with chronic rheumatic heart disease, this condition is considered in detail under the individual valve lesions (Ch. 12). Nevertheless, it is important to recognize that myocardial damage coexists and that correction of a valve abnormality will not necessarily restore normal cardiac function.

The pathological processes that cause valve deformity include thickening and distortion of the cusps at the time of rheumatic fever, contracture of the valve structures, fusion of the commissures, shortening of the chordae tendineae and, finally, calcification during the phase of healing. The nature of the valve lesion depends upon the relative importance of these factors in the individual case. Stenosis occurs if fusion of the cusps predominates; regurgitation is produced by shortening of the chordae tendineae and contracture of the valve leaflets.

The valve deformities may take many years to develop and, in particular, narrowing is not critical until the affected orifice is reduced to less than a quarter of its normal size. Regurgitation may be important from the time of the attack of acute rheumatic fever but its appearance as a symptomatic disorder, also, is likely to be delayed. Therefore, although the signs of mitral and aortic regurgitation may be present in childhood or early adult life, symptoms due to these lesions seldom develop until the third or fourth decade. The same is true for mitral stenosis; in aortic stenosis, symptoms are often postponed even longer.

Tuberculosis

Tuberculosis may cause pericarditis, with or without subsequent constriction (see p. 211). It may also be responsible for heart disease secondary to pulmonary fibrosis. Tuberculous myocarditis is very rare.

Virus infections

Viruses cause both pericarditis (p. 211) and myocarditis (p. 221). Coxsackie viruses of group B are probably the commonest organisms affecting the heart; most infections are subclinical. The clinical picture is usually one of fever, malaise and muscular pains, accompanied by evidence of pericarditis and, if there is myocarditis, tachycardia, gallop rhythm, cardiomegaly and cardiac failure. The electrocardiogram (ECG) usually shows non-specific abnormalities, but there may be ST and T wave changes suggesting pericarditis or myocardial infarction. Blood levels of myocardial enzymes (such as creatine kinase) may be raised transiently. The diagnosis can be made by isolating the organism from the stool or by demonstrating a rise or fall in serum antibodies. Rest is desirable during the acute phase, and return to vigorous activity should be progressive. The patient nearly always recovers completely, but there may be residual myocardial damage and recurrences are not unusual. Myocarditis may also be associated with infectious mononucleosis, acute anterior poliomyelitis and many other virus infections.

Acquired immune deficiency syndrome (AIDS)

Cardiac involvement is becoming more common in patients with AIDS as the prognosis in relation to other complications improves. It may take many forms:

- *Myocarditis*. In the majority of cases human immunodeficiency virus (HIV) itself is thought to be the cause of myocarditis, but in some cases, myocarditis may be due to other opportunistic pathogens.
- Myocarditis may progress to *dilated cardiomyopathy*.

- *Pericarditis* is relatively common. Many patients with small to moderate effusions may be asymptomatic and can be managed conservatively. In others, tamponade may occur and drainage may be required. Occasionally, pericarditis may be a manifestation of tuberculosis or *Kaposi's sarcoma*.
- *Accelerated atherosclerosis*. The use of protease inhibitors has prolonged patient survival. However, these drugs have adverse metabolic consequences, causing insulin resistance, hyperglycaemia and hyperlipidaemia. As a consequence of these metabolic effects and longer survival, patients may develop accelerated atherosclerosis.

Trypanosomiasis (Chagas' disease)

Myocarditis due to infection by *Trypanosoma cruzi* is common in South America, where about 20 million people are believed to be infected. It is transmitted by the bite of infected reduviid bugs. These live in the roofs and walls of houses, and drop down on to the face of a sleeping person below. There are two major forms, acute and chronic:

- *Acute Chagas' disease*, which occurs predominantly in childhood, may be asymptomatic but can produce tachycardia, cardiomegaly and cardiac failure.
- Much more important is *chronic Chagas' disease* which leads to cardiac failure of insidious onset and is a major cause of cardiac morbidity and mortality in South America.

The trypanosomes multiply in the digestive tract of the bug and are transmitted via its faeces. The organisms multiply near the site of a bite. They then enter the bloodstream, invading the heart, and other tissues. In the heart, they cause inflammation and fibrosis and may result, after several decades, in a dilated cardiomyopathy.

The left ventricle is enlarged, and there may be dyspnoea, chest pain and palpitation. Eventually, right-sided heart failure develops; this is frequently complicated by thromboembolic events. Arrhythmias are almost invariable and complete heart block common. The ECG usually shows right bundle branch block. Death is often sudden due to ventricular fibrillation or asystole. Echocardiography shows the features of a dilated cardiomyopathy.

Chagas' myocarditis should be suspected when patients who have lived in the tropical or subtropical areas of America develop arrhythmias, cardiac failure and right bundle branch block. A complement fixation test is useful in diagnosis. Specific treatment of Chagas' disease is not effective and treatment is essentially directed at the complications of heart failure, arrhythmias and heart block.

ENDOCRINE AND METABOLIC DISORDERS

Hyperthyroidism

Hyperthyroidism (thyrotoxicosis) is a syndrome due to an excess of the circulating thyroid hormones T4 and/or T3. This may result from diffuse hyperplasia of the thyroid gland (Graves' disease) or single or multiple hyperactive nodules. Thyroid overactivity is associated with increased oxygen consumption, heat production, and peripheral vasodilatation. The raised cardiac output which occurs in response to these demands, and to the direct effect of thyroid hormone on the heart, is achieved mainly by tachycardia and increased myocardial contractility rather than by an enlarged stroke volume.

The heart has to support the burden of a greatly enhanced cardiac output when its own metabolic requirements are increased. The normal heart may, in these circumstances, be unable to supply an adequate circulation; a diseased heart is likely to fail.

Clear manifestations of cardiac abnormality, such as cardiomegaly or heart failure, usually imply that the hyperthyroidism has aggravated underlying heart disease. This is most commonly ischaemic but it may be hypertensive or rheumatic. Occasionally, hyperthyroidism is the sole cause of heart failure.

Clinical features

Cardiac symptoms are common in hyperthyroid patients, even in the absence of cardiac disease:

- Palpitation is particularly frequent, and is usually attributable to the combination of sinus tachycardia and a vigorous cardiac action. Atrial fibrillation may be responsible for irregular palpitation. Sinus tachycardia is almost invariable if there is no atrial fibrillation, and is characterized by its persistence during sleep.
- Breathlessness is also common, and can be due to hyperventilation, anxiety or left ventricular failure.
- Hyperthyroidism may aggravate angina pectoris in those with coronary artery disease.
- The pulse is of large volume and may have a collapsing character. The systolic blood pressure is frequently high, whilst the diastolic is normal or low.
- There is often a pulmonary midsystolic murmur, due to high flow.
- Cardiac enlargement and the signs of left- or right-sided heart failure may develop if the thyroid disease is of long standing or if there is coexistent cardiac disease.

The classical features of hyperthyroidism such as weight loss, moist warm extremities, tremor, lid retraction, exophthalmos and goitre are usually present, but all these signs may be slight or absent in the older patient. There are no distinctive features on the ECG or chest radiograph.

Hyperthyroidism can be recognized easily if the characteristic features are present, but the diagnosis can be difficult if the abnormalities are largely confined to the cardiovascular system. It should be suspected whenever sinus tachycardia, atrial fibrillation or cardiac failure is unexplained.

The diagnosis of hyperthyroidism is established by finding abnormally high blood levels of T4 and/or T3 with suppression of levels of thyroid-stimulating hormone (TSH).

Hyperthyroidism may be treated by antithyroid drugs (such as carbimazole), radioiodine or partial thyroidectomy. Radioiodine is the most suitable therapy for most patients with thyrotoxic heart disease (except for women of child-bearing age), but surgery may be indicated if the gland is large or if there is a danger of tracheal compression.

When the rapid control of the tachycardia of hyperthyroidism is necessary, a beta-adrenoceptor blocking drug should be given.

The atrial fibrillation of thyrotoxicosis is difficult to slow adequately with digitalis alone; a beta-blocker should be added if not contraindicated. When thyroid overactivity is controlled, DC shock is usually effective in restoring sinus rhythm. Atrial fibrillation complicating thyrotoxicosis is an indication for anticoagulation.

One of the commonest situations in which hyperthyroidism is encountered amongst cardiac patients is in those treated with amiodarone. As this group of patients is by definition susceptible to arrhythmias and as they frequently have significant underlying left ventricular impairment, the development of hyperthyroidism can have particularly adverse consequences. Treatment of amiodarone-induced thyrotoxicosis is a particular problem. Amiodarone contains iodine which blocks the uptake of radioactive iodine by the thyroid. Initial treatment is with carbimazole, often with the addition of steroids and beta-blockers. Specialist referral is advisable.

Hypothyroidism

Hypothyroidism is associated with reduced levels of circulating T3 and T4, most often as a result of inflammatory destruction of the thyroid. It may, however, be secondary to reduced thyroid-stimulating hormone (TSH) secretion by the pituitary or hypothalamus. It is also frequently encountered as a side-effect of amiodarone.

Hypothyroidism affects the cardiovascular system in several ways:

- The reduced level of body metabolism is associated with a low cardiac output, a diminished peripheral blood flow, a reduction in venous return, and sinus bradycardia.
- The deficiency of thyroid hormone seems to be responsible for interstitial oedema and mucoid infiltration of the myocardium, and for a pericardial effusion.
- The hypercholesterolaemia characteristically present may be responsible for premature coronary atherosclerosis and ischaemic heart disease.
- 'Myxoedema coma' is associated with hypotension and bradycardia.

Clinical features
The patient with hypothyroidism seldom has cardiac symptoms, except for dyspnoea and angina pectoris due to coexistent coronary disease. The symptoms and signs of cardiac failure rarely, if ever, occur in the absence of some additional form of heart disease:

- The pulse rate is usually between 50 and 60/min. The sluggish apex beat is difficult to feel and the heart sounds are soft.
- Mild hypertension, particularly diastolic hypertension, is common.

- The ECG is abnormal in showing low voltage of all components of the PQRST complexes; the T waves are flattened or inverted.
- Echocardiography often reveals a pericardial effusion.

Hypothyroidism is usually suspected because of the general sluggishness, the cold and thickened skin, the husky voice, the coarse but scanty hair and the slow pulse, but minor forms of the disorder may easily escape detection. Blood levels of T4 and T3 are low. The most sensitive test for primary hyperthyroidism is the high serum level of TSH, but this is not raised if hypopituitarism is responsible.

Treatment with thyroid substances is effective but may provoke angina pectoris. For this reason, in those suspected of having coronary disease, small doses (e.g. thyroxine 0.025 mg daily) should be used initially and the dose should be increased very cautiously over several months to 0.1 to 0.15 mg daily. The serum TSH level can be useful as a marker of the adequacy of replacement therapy.

Management of hypothyroidism in patients with unstable angina is particularly difficult because of the risk of exacerbating the angina. Dosage increments should only be made very slowly. The addition of a beta-adrenoceptor blocking drug may help protect the patient from angina. Where appropriate, angioplasty or coronary bypass grafting should be considered and can be undertaken relatively safely even in the hypothyroid state.

Diabetes

Diabetes is a metabolic disorder due to the reduced availability or effectiveness of insulin.

In type I (insulin-dependent diabetes mellitus or IDDM), there is a defective secretion of insulin by the pancreas, probably consequent upon infective or autoimmune damage to the islet cells.

In adult-onset, type II diabetes, there is insulin resistance, hyperinsulinaemia and hyperglycaemia.

In both types, blood glucose is raised and there is glycosuria, but the major and most dangerous complications are predominantly cardiovascular.

Two types of vascular disease occur:

- *Macrovascular disease* results in stroke, myocardial infarction and heart failure.
- *Microvascular* disease causes retinopathy, nephropathy, neuropathy and small artery occlusion in the heart which can result in diabetic cardiomyopathy.

Clinical presentation
- Angina and myocardial infarction are common. Myocardial infarction is often painless, due to accompanying neuropathy.
- Congestive cardiac failure is common. It may be due to previous infarction or may occur in the absence of significant disease in the epicardial coronary arteries due to small vessel disease and diabetic cardiomyopathy.
- Autonomic dysfunction is common in diabetics and may result in a relative tachycardia which is fixed with limited variations in rate.

Diabetes is managed with diet, insulin and hypoglycaemic agents. In addition to diabetic control, particular attention is necessary in the management of:

- *Hypertension.* Associated hypertension is very common and vigorous management is indicated. ACE inhibitors are of particular value and have been shown to prolong life expectancy and to prevent myocardial infarction.
- *Hyperlipidaemia.* As diabetic patients are at particular risk of developing coronary disease, a rigorous approach to primary prevention is indicated with a low threshold for the administration of statins.

Carcinoid syndrome

Malignant carcinoid tumours with metastases in the liver may be associated with pulmonary stenosis and regurgitation, and with tricuspid stenosis or regurgitation, the valve cusps being fixed by fibrosis. The cardiac lesions are probably due to the actions of kinins or of 5-hydroxytryptamine (5HT, serotonin) secreted by the tumour. These substances are also responsible for the flushing attacks, telangiectasia, diarrhoea and bronchospasm characteristic of this syndrome.

The cardiac findings in the carcinoid syndrome are those of the particular valve lesion and of right-sided heart failure. The diagnosis is established either by identification of the tumour at laparotomy or by the detection in the urine of large quantities of 5-hydroxyindole acetic acid (5-HIAA), a breakdown product of 5-HT.

Treatment is unsatisfactory: the diarrhoea may be controlled by codeine, and the flushing by ketanserin (a 5-HT blocker); cardiac failure is treated on conventional lines, valve replacement occasionally being necessary.

Haemochromatosis

Haemochromatosis may be primary or secondary:

- *Primary* haemochromatosis is a primary autosomal recessive disorder of iron storage leading to iron overload.
- *Secondary* haemochromatosis arises due to exogenous iron overload in patients with congenital anaemias receiving repeated blood transfusions over a long period of time.

Excessive iron deposition occurs in a variety of tissues including heart, liver and pancreas. In the heart, this results in a cardiomyopathy with features of both systolic and diastolic dysfunction. Classically, patients present with features of cirrhosis of the liver, diabetes and pigmentation of the skin associated with heart failure. The heart failure is most typically right sided. Occasionally patients can present with heart block and require pacing. Diagnosis is based on the estimate of serum ferritin levels or transferrin saturation.

Heart failure is an important cause of mortality amongst patients with untreated haemochromatosis. Treatment consists of repeated phlebotomies and iron-chelating therapy.

Overweight and obesity

Overweight is associated with heart disease in a number of ways:

- Overweight is a risk factor for both coronary heart disease and hypertension; the hypertension in obesity needs to be distinguished from false high blood pressure readings in patients with fat arms due to use of an inappropriately small cuff.
- Obesity results in an increase in left ventricular mass, independent of hypertension.
- Obesity results in insulin resistance and is a major risk factor for type II diabetes.
- A specific Pickwickian syndrome of hypoventilation with carbon dioxide retention, hypoxia, somnolence, polycythaemia and right-sided heart failure is sometimes caused by obesity. The obesity is directly responsible for the hypoventilation because it restricts respiratory movement; improvement can be achieved by weight loss.
- Overweight is associated with sleep apnoea.

Obesity is important in patients with cardiac disease of any type because the demands on the heart are increased. Weight reduction is an essential component in the prevention and treatment of angina pectoris, hypertension and cardiac failure.

Beriberi

This disease is due to thiamine deficiency, which is usually the result of a diet with a high proportion of polished rice in Eastern countries but is associated with alcoholism in the USA and Europe. The deficiency leads to a lack of co-carboxylase which is necessary for the oxidation of pyruvic acid to acetyl coenzyme A. The citric acid cycle is inhibited and the accumulation of lactate and pyruvate may lead to peripheral vasodilatation and impaired cardiac function. The characteristic haemodynamic features are those of a low peripheral vascular resistance and a high cardiac output. Cardiac failure eventually occurs and, in the later stages, the cardiac output may fall.

The clinical features of beriberi heart disease include palpitation, fatigue, breathlessness and peripheral oedema. In some cases there may be acute circulatory failure with hypotension and syncope. There is usually sinus tachycardia with a large pulse and right-sided cardiac failure. The heart is enlarged and there may be a gallop rhythm and systolic murmurs.

The neurological features are those of an ascending peripheral neuritis, commonly accompanied by mental confusion. Paraesthesiae occur in the hands and feet and there is weakness of the legs. The calf muscles are tender and areas of anaesthesia occur.

Neither the ECG, which usually shows non-specific T wave changes, nor the chest radiograph, which reveals cardiomegaly, is helpful in diagnosis. This is usually achieved by obtaining a history of nutritional deficiency or of alcoholism, and by finding evidence of both peripheral neuritis and cardiac failure.

Most cases respond quickly to administration of thiamine.

Alcoholic cardiomyopathy

Heavy alcohol consumption, even in the absence of nutritional deficiency, can lead to cardiomyopathy. The initial symptom is either breathlessness or palpitation, due to ectopic beats or atrial fibrillation. The ECG may show low, dimpled T waves. In the early stages, abstinence may reverse the picture, but otherwise there is progression with increasing cardiac failure to death.

Treatment consists of complete abstinence from alcohol and use of conventional measures for controlling atrial fibrillation and cardiac failure.

MISCELLANEOUS DISORDERS

Systemic lupus erythematosus

This often affects the heart, although cardiac symptoms and signs seldom dominate the clinical picture:

- Acute or chronic pericarditis, with or without effusion, is usually the most obvious evidence of cardiac involvement.
- Myocarditis sometimes develops, and may be due to disease of the small coronary vessels.
- Endocarditis also occurs, with large warty excrescences which may involve any of the four heart valves. Endocardial involvement was originally described by Libman and Sacks and is referred to as Libman–Sacks endocarditis. The most common clinical lesions are mitral and aortic regurgitation.

Pseudoxanthoma elasticum

This is a familial disease affecting connective tissue associated with calcification and proliferation of the media of the coronary and peripheral arteries, which may give rise to ischaemic heart disease and hypertension. Initially, this is most evident in the radial and ulnar arteries and these pulses may be absent. The skin, particularly in certain areas such as the elbow creases and back of the neck, takes on a crepe-like appearance with much redundant tissue. Characteristic dark 'angioid' streaks occur in the fundi.

In addition, the heart may be affected by endocardial fibroelastosis which predominantly affects the atria. Mitral prolapse is also common.

Sarcoidosis

Cardiac involvement may be an accompaniment of systemic sarcoidosis. Symptomatic cardiac involvement is relatively rare, occurring in only 5% of cases of systemic sarcoidosis. However, it seems probable that subclinical involvement is more common, as postmortem studies demonstrate cardiac involvement in 25% of patients with known sarcoidosis. Such postmortem studies are of course subject to the reporting bias, that they may represent more severely affected individuals.

Cardiac involvement in sardoidosis has a number of manifestations:

- It may cause *heart failure*. Characteristically, there is granulomatous infiltration of the myocardium leading to scar formation and increased ventricular stiffness. This presents with the diastolic dysfunction of a restrictive cardiomyopathy. As the disease progresses, systolic dysfunction may additionally develop.
- *Heart block* may develop, due to infiltration of the A-V node.
- *Ventricular tachyarrhythmias* may develop. These may be life-threatening and patients with cardiac involvement are at increased risk of sudden death.

The diagnosis should be considered in patients with systemic sarcoidosis with evidence of heart failure, conduction disturbance or ventricular tachyarrhythmias. Endomyocardial biopsy is positive in approximately 50% of patients with cardiac involvement. However, a negative biopsy does not exclude the disease because of the patchy nature of the cardiac involvement.

Corticosteroids are frequently given in cases of cardiac involvement and may be associated with improved cardiac function. Pacing should be considered in patients with A-V conduction disturbance and an implantable defibrillator in patients with ventricular tachyarrhythmias.

Marfan's syndrome

This familial autosomal dominant disorder of connective tissue may result in many skeletal, cardiovascular and other abnormalities. These include:

- *skeletal abnormalities*, tall stature, long limbs with spidery fingers (arachnodactyly), a high arched palate and pectus carinatum and pectus excavatum
- *eye abnormalities*, dislocation of the lens, myopia
- *cardiovascular abnormalities*, aortic root dilatation, aortic regurgitation, mitral valve prolapse and mitral regurgitation.

Defects in the synthesis, secretion and assembly of fibrillin seem to be involved; the gene for fibrillin is closely identified with the site of the Marfan gene on chromosome 15. This results in a generalized defect in microfibrils, which for example, form part of the scaffolding upon which elastin is deposited to form elastic fibres.

Detection and diagnosis may be very difficult. Many families and individuals do not show the classical phenotype, but more subtle combinations of physical findings. In addition, there is a high rate of new mutations, accounting for approximately 30% of cases.

There are two serious cardiovascular complications – mitral valve and aortic root involvement:

- *Mitral valve involvement.* Mitral valve prolapse is very common amongst patients with Marfan's syndrome. The mitral leaflets have an elongated and redundant appearance. This may lead to mitral regurgitation and annular dilatation. Mitral regurgitation may become severe enough to warrant surgical repair.
- *Aortic root involvement.* (See also Ch. 15, p 324) A weakness of the aortic media is common and leads to dilatation, aneurysm formation, and

dissection. Aortic regurgitation may follow dilatation of the valve ring. The risk of aortic dissection and aortic regurgitation increase with the size of the aorta. These complications are uncommon with an aortic diameter below 55 mm in the adult. Patients with Marfan's syndrome require regular monitoring of aortic root diameter, generally by transthoracic echocardiography. An increase in diameter to 50 to 55 mm is frequently adopted as the criterion for elective surgery. Surgery involves replacement of the aortic root and aortic valve with a valved conduit.

General management

There is no specific treatment, but contact sports and isometric exercise should be avoided. The risk of aortic root dilatation and dissection can be reduced by the use of beta-blockers. Patients with valve problems should be advised of the need for antibiotic prophylaxis for dental and other procedures. Pregnancy is a particular concern as there is an increased risk of aortic dissection.

Cardiac tumours

Cardiac tumours are rare. The commonest is the *myxoma* which occurs most frequently in the left atrium, but occasionally in the other chambers. It varies from 1 to 8 cm in diameter, and is usually attached by a pedicle to the atrial septum. Because its position may vary with posture, transient or complete obstruction of the mitral valve may result. The tumour may prolapse into the left ventricle and cause mitral regurgitation.

The haemodynamic effects of left atrial myxoma usually resemble those of mitral stenosis. The tumour may also be responsible for embolic phenomena, and can produce constitutional effects such as fever, weight loss, anaemia, finger clubbing, raised plasma viscosity/ESR and abnormal serum protein levels. The obstruction of the mitral valve may lead to dyspnoea and, rarely, syncope or vertigo related to posture.

Variable mitral systolic and diastolic murmurs may be heard, and there may be a loud first sound and opening snap. The diagnosis should be suspected in patients with signs of mitral stenosis, who have a history of syncope, or variable murmurs, or unexplained fever with a high viscosity/ESR. The diagnosis can be most readily established by echocardiography which demonstrates a mass within the left atrium (Figs 17.1A and B). The tumour should be removed under cardiopulmonary bypass.

NORMAL PHYSIOLOGICAL STATES

Physical activity and the athlete's heart

Regular exercise has beneficial effects in preventing coronary heart disease and hypertension, but changes in trained athletes may simulate heart disease. The term *athlete's heart* refers to the cardiovascular changes in response to prolonged and repetitive exercise and includes the following changes:

- increased left ventricular volume
- reduction in resting heart rate

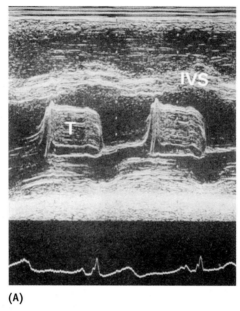

(A)

Fig. 17.1A Parasternal M-mode echocardiogram of a left atrial myxoma. Multiple echoes are seen behind the anterior mitral valve leaflet in diastole as the tumour prolapses downwards towards the left ventricle. (IVS : interventricular septum. T : tumour.)

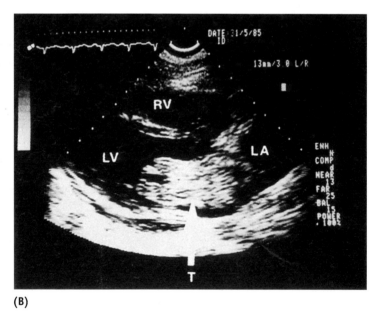

(B)

Fig. 17.1B Cross-sectional echocardiogram of myxoma. There is a large tumour (T) situated in the mitral valve orifice.

- slowing of A-V nodal conduction, with first degree block commonly seen and not infrequently, higher degrees of block
- voltage criteria of left ventricular hypertrophy on the ECG
- repolarization abnormalities in the ECG with ST segment or T wave abnormalities.

The physiological cardiac enlargement occurring in athletes can be difficult to distinguish from the pathological hypertrophy of hypertrophic cardiomyopathy. Echocardiography is particularly important in distinguishing between the two:

- Athletes show an increase in cavity size with a left ventricular end-diastolic dimension at or just above the upper limit of normal (55 mm). In hypertrophic cardiomyopathy, cavity size is generally reduced.
- In athlete's heart, any increase in wall thickness is symmetrical and generally does not exceed 14 mm. In hypertrophic cardiomyopathy, asymmetrical septal hypertrophy is common with wall thickness in excess of 14 mm.
- Athletes retain a normal left ventricular filling pattern, whereas in pathological hypertrophy, isovolumic relaxation is prolonged.

Sudden death in athletes is a topic of particular concern:

- Amongst younger age groups, hypertrophic cardiomyopathy is the commonest cause. Other causes include congenitally aberrant coronary arteries and right ventricular dysplasia (see p. 232).
- In older age groups, coronary artery disease predominates as the cause of sudden death.

Anaemia and the heart

Anaemia imposes increased demands upon the heart and, at the same time, impairs its function. It aggravates the symptoms of the patient with heart disease and has important circulatory effects, even in the individual with a normal heart.

The haemodynamic effects of anaemia probably result mainly from a decrease in blood viscosity and from tissue hypoxia, which is responsible for peripheral vasodilatation. As a consequence, the peripheral arterial resistance is diminished, the diastolic pressure falls and the pulse pressure widens. Ventricular afterload is decreased. The stroke volume and cardiac output are increased when the haemoglobin falls below 7 g/100 mL blood, and both respond to exercise to a greater degree than normal. The hypoxia produces coronary vasodilatation when this is possible, but in the patient with coronary heart disease, the ability to dilate is restricted. If anaemia is both severe and prolonged, fatty degeneration of the myocardium takes place.

For the reasons described, anaemia may precipitate or aggravate cardiac failure in the patient with pre-existing heart disease, and it may induce or exacerbate angina in those with coronary heart disease.

It is rare for either heart failure or angina to develop in anaemic patients with normal hearts, but signs and symptoms may occur in such patients which mimic those of heart disease. Dyspnoea, tachycardia and peripheral oedema are common in patients with chronic and severe anaemia.

Anaemia may produce:

- the warm skin and bounding arterial pulse of the high output state
- a venous hum in the neck

- cardiac enlargement in the advanced case
- very commonly, a systolic murmur in the second or third left intercostal space close to the sternum. This is probably due to turbulence resulting from increased flow and reduced blood viscosity
- a loud third heart sound
- in very severe cases, a short mitral mid-diastolic murmur, due to increased flow.

The ECG is usually normal, but non-specific ST and T wave changes may occur and the ST depression of myocardial ischaemia may develop.

The clinical features of anaemia are usually readily corrected either by appropriate drug therapy, or by blood transfusion. Rapid transfusion is dangerous, particularly if there is heart failure; in this situation, it is advisable to use packed cells. If whole blood only is available, a diuretic such as intravenous furosemide (frusemide) 40 mg should also be given.

Pregnancy and the heart

Pregnancy imposes a substantial load on the heart and circulation. The cardiac output and blood volume increase from the sixth week onwards, until/about the 30th week when they are some 30–50% above normal levels, at which they remain during the rest of pregnancy. During the last 8 weeks, the inferior vena cava may be obstructed by the uterus when the subject is supine; as a consequence, the cardiac output may fall when this position is assumed. Other factors affecting the cardiovascular system are an increased metabolic rate, a corresponding rise in oxygen consumption, the arteriovenous shunt in the uterus and an elevation in the venous pressure due to the increased blood volume.

Cardiovascular symptoms and signs of normal pregnancy

Dyspnoea, orthopnoea and syncope are not uncommon in the normal pregnancy. The circulatory changes of pregnancy produce characteristic signs:

- The hands are warm and the pulse is large.
- A tachycardia is present and the venous pressure slightly raised.
- The apex beat is vigorous and may be displaced outwards, partly as a consequence of cardiomegaly and partly by the high diaphragm.
- The high flow almost always produces a soft pulmonary midsystolic murmur and a third heart sound. These are often mistaken for cardiac disease.
- The ECG often shows an axis shift and minor ST segment and T wave changes.

Heart disease in pregnancy

The circulatory burden of pregnancy frequently reveals pre-existing heart disease for the first time. Symptoms may start at about week 12 and tend to progress until they may become severe from week 24 onwards. A period of particular danger occurs after delivery, when the sudden reabsorption of blood from the uterus into the circulation may precipitate pulmonary oedema.

Valvular heart disease

Mitral stenosis is the commonest valve lesion in women of child-bearing age and is the most serious lesion encountered. Patients with tight mitral stenosis may become breathless in early pregnancy and progress to pulmonary oedema or right-sided cardiac failure. Even those with less severe lesions may develop symptoms during the last months or shortly after delivery.

Where possible, haemodynamically significant mitral stenosis should be corrected prior to pregnancy. When significant mitral stenosis is encountered in a patient who is already pregnant, the patient should be assessed for her suitability for balloon mitral valvuloplasty. This procedure can be safely performed in pregnancy, although it is best delayed until late in the second trimester to reduce the risks of radiation exposure to the fetus. Formal valve surgery during pregnancy carries a high risk both to the fetus and to the mother.

Balloon pulmonary valvuloplasty can also be safely carried out during pregnancy. Patients with mild mitral stenosis, mitral regurgitation and aortic regurgitation usually tolerate pregnancy well, although they may become increasingly breathless. Mild or moderate aortic stenosis is similarly generally well tolerated. Severe aortic stenosis is rare in pregnancy, but is a major cause for concern when it is encountered and may be an indication to consider termination.

Prosthetic heart valves

Prosthetic heart valves pose a special problem in pregnancy. Warfarin, particularly in the first trimester, may induce congenital abnormalities, but the discontinuation of anticoagulants exposes the patient to an increased risk of thromboembolism. Heparin may be preferable for this early phase as well as for the last few weeks of pregnancy. However, it is difficult to achieve a stable pattern of anticoagulation with subcutaneous heparin and patients are at increased risk of thromboembolic events.

The role of low molecular weight heparin as a substitute for warfarin in anticoagulation in pregnancy remains uncertain. Low molecular weight heparin carries a number of theoretical advantages including longer half-life and once daily dosing. In addition, its pharmacokinetics are more predictable and as a consequence monitoring for anticoagulant status is not required. However, these drugs are currently not licensed for use in pregnancy and should only be used at the physician's discretion.

Congenital heart disease

Patients who were born with congenital heart disease are being seen with increasing frequency in pregnancy, but the cardiac abnormality is usually mild or has been corrected by surgery prior to conception. Pregnancy is tolerated well if there is an uncomplicated septal defect or persistent ductus arteriosus. Severe pulmonary hypertension of whatever aetiology is extremely hazardous, with a 25–50% risk of maternal death during the pregnancy or in the puerperium; termination in early pregnancy is to be strongly recommended. In cases of complex congenital heart disease, each case should be considered individually by an expert in adult congenital heart disease to assess maternal and fetal risk.

Cardiac arrhythmia

The normal heart rate increase during pregnancy is about 10 beats/min above baseline. Greater degrees of sinus tachycardia are common and may be difficult to distinguish from abnormal rhythms.

The commonest arrhythmias encountered in pregnancy are paroxysmal supraventricular tachycardias. It is common for the frequency of attacks to increase during pregnancy. Where appropriate, definitive treatment by radiofrequency ablation should be considered prior to pregnancy.

When troublesome arrhythmias are encountered during pregnancy, ablation is contraindicated because of the radiation risks to the fetus. Drug treatment is also problematic because of the potential teratogenicity of antiarrhythmic agents, particularly during the first trimester. When antiarrhythmic agents are required, beta-blockers are the treatment of choice. There is widespread experience in the use of propranolol and atenolol. However, beta-blockers may cause intrauterine growth retardation and for this reason expert advice and monitoring is advised.

Hypertrophic obstructive cardiomypathy

Most patients with hypertrophic obstructive cardiomyopathy do well in pregnancy because they are young enough not to have developed significant diastolic dysfunction, and left ventricular volumes are able to increase to meet the demands of pregnancy. Endocarditis prophylaxis should be considered at the time of delivery. During delivery and in the early post-partum period, it is important to pay particular attention to avoiding blood loss and to fluid replacement to maintain left ventricular volume and cardiac output.

Peripartum cardiomopathy

Cardiomyopathy ('peripartum') of unknown aetiology sometimes develops during later pregnancy or the puerperium. There is a wide spectrum of severity ranging from mild to severe heart failure. Management is to exclude other causes of heart failure. Treatment is supportive with diuretics, ACE inhibitors and, if appropriate, inotropes. Over half of the patients have a complete or near complete recovery. However, there is a risk of relapse in future pregnancies.

FURTHER READING

American Medical Association (1992) Guidelines for the diagnosis of rheumatic fever. Jones Criteria 1992 update. *Journal of the American Medical Association* **268**: 2069.

Braunwald, E., Zipes, D. & Libby, P. (2001) *Heart Disease. A Textbook of Cardiovascular Medicine*. Philadelphia: Saunders.

Mitha, A.S. (1994) Acute rheumatic fever. In: Julian, D.G., Camm, A.J., Fox, K.M. et al (eds) *Disease of the Heart*, 2nd edn. London: Saunders.

CHAPTER 18

Psychological aspects of heart disease

The relationship between psychological factors and heart disease is complex. Many anxious individuals believe, erroneously, that they have heart disease; anxiety and depression often complicate and aggravate organic heart disease.

PSYCHOLOGICAL FACTORS IN THE GENESIS OF HYPERTENSION AND CORONARY DISEASE

Both hypertension and coronary heart disease are clearly related to psychosocial factors. In the earlier part of the twentieth century, coronary heart disease was perceived as being particularly common in those, such as doctors and business executives, in 'stressful' jobs. But more recent surveys have shown that there is a progressive decrease in the prevalence of coronary disease as one ascends the socioeconomic scale. Some have attributed this to the 'job strains' to which less skilled workers are exposed, such as lack of control of one's workload. Others have failed to confirm this, but point to depression, social isolation and poor social support as important factors both in the genesis and in the prognosis of coronary heart disease.

Associations have also been made between certain personality traits and cardiovascular disease, of which the so-called Type A behaviour pattern has attracted most attention. Type A individuals are aggressive, ambitious, impatient and preoccupied with deadlines. Evidence has been produced both in favour and against this hypothesis, but certain elements of it, such as the tendency to hostility and suppressed anger, seem more convincing as risk factors.

On the other hand, there can be no doubt of the importance of emotional stress in precipitating episodes of angina pectoris. Rarely, there is strong circumstantial evidence that emotional stress has been a contributory factor in causing myocardial infarction or fatal arrhythmias.

ANXIETY STATE AND THE HEART

Individuals with an anxiety state often have complaints suggestive of heart disease. A large number of labels have been applied to the complex of symptoms of such patients, including *effort syndrome*, *cardiac neurosis* and *neurocirculatory asthenia*. It was particularly common in the armed services during war-time, and has therefore been called 'soldier's heart', but it also occurs frequently in civilians.

Breathlessness, palpitation and fatigue are almost invariable, and are usually accompanied by feelings of faintness and dizziness. Chest pain is less common, but is often the reason for referral to a physician.

The breathlessness may be related to exertion, but also occurs at rest. Frequent complaints are that 'I can't take a deep breath' or 'I can't get enough air'. The palpitation is usually the awareness of a sinus tachycardia, but can be due to ectopic beats which cause the patient to think that the heart is about to stop.

The chest pain of anxiety state is usually situated in the left submammary region but may be elsewhere in the left chest and may radiate to the left arm. It is sometimes provoked by effort, but tends to come on after exercise rather than during it; it can develop at rest and at night time. It often takes the form of a persistent ache lasting for hours or days; sharp momentary stabs of pain are also frequent. The patient will often say that the pain is 'in my heart' and the muscles in the area may be tender.

Whilst recounting the history, the patient gives an impression of distress, and is tense or rather withdrawn in manner. Sighing respiration is common and there may be hyperventilation. Sinus tachycardia is usual, and palpation reveals a hyperdynamic heart. The hands are often sweaty but cool; there may be a coarse tremor.

The ECG confirms sinus tachycardia and may show non-specific flattening or slight inversion of T waves.

The diagnosis can usually be made from the characteristic symptoms and from observing the patient. The poor relationship of the breathlessness and pain to exertion, and the site, character and duration of the chest discomfort differentiate the syndrome from angina pectoris. The palpitation can be distinguished from that of paroxysmal tachycardia by the lack of sudden onset and by the relationship to emotion.

The prognosis with regard to the relief of symptoms is poor if it is a chronic condition or if there is a serious personality derangement. If the complaints have occurred in response to an obvious emotional stress, the outlook is relatively good. When anxiety about the heart has been induced by the thoughtless or ill-informed comments of physicians, it is particularly difficult to eradicate.

Psychiatric treatment is necessary for the more severe cases, but strong reassurance by the physician may be effective in those patients in whom cardiac symptoms predominate, particularly when an unfounded fear of organic heart disease provoked them. The patient should be instructed to embark upon a programme of gradually increasing physical activity. Sometimes, it may be necessary to give tranquillizers such as diazepam 2–5 mg three times a day. Beta-blockers may be helpful if the palpitation of sinus tachycardia is distressing.

Psychological disturbances in patients with heart disease

Many individuals equate heart disease with total disability and death. Patients with cardiac disorders may regard themselves and be considered by others as 'invalids', even though the lesion may be of little importance or be correctable.

Fear of sudden death is common in those who experience angina and palpitation. Anxiety and depression are important causes of symptoms and disability in patients who have sustained a myocardial infarction or have undergone coronary surgery. Headache in hypertensive patients is usually due to tension and only rarely to the high blood pressure.

Excessive anxiety can be prevented by thoughtful management of patients and their relatives. Frankness should be combined with optimism. One must be careful in one's choice of words; if such terms as angina, murmur or heart failure are to be used, they must be explained in such a way that they do not cause alarm.

Advanced heart disease can cause confusion and delirium as a result of hypoxia or hypotension or, when associated with pulmonary disease, carbon dioxide retention. Similar symptoms may arise from lidocaine (lignocaine) overdosage, or following cardiac surgery. Depression may result from a number of cardiac drugs. Fatigue is common in patients on beta-blocking drugs. These psychological disturbances, which are secondary to medical disorders, should be treated by correcting the underlying cause.

CHAPTER 19

Surgery and the heart

ANAESTHESIA AND GENERAL SURGERY IN PATIENTS WITH HEART DISEASE

Anaesthesia is potentially hazardous in patients with heart disease. Problems may arise due to the direct cardiovascular effect of the anaesthetic agent or indirectly through autonomic reflexes. The interplay of these factors can produce profound effects on blood pressure, cardiac output and heart rhythm and may lead to myocardial ischaemia, myocardial infarction and serious arrhythmias. However, with modern anaesthetic agents and skilled anaesthetic management, these risks can be minimized.

The period of induction of anaesthesia is a time of particular risk. Induction agents generally lower blood pressure. In addition, vagal reflexes initiated by endotrachael intubation may result in bradycardia, heart block or even asystole. These problems can once again be minimized with good anaesthetic management.

Although regional anaesthesia, for example with a spinal or epidural anaesthetic, avoids direct cardiac depressant effects, this does not necessarily reduce the risks of the procedure, as these techniques are particularly prone to hypotension, which may provoke myocardial ischaemia.

Ischaemic heart disease

Ischaemic heart disease is a major determinant of operative mortality. Hypotension may provoke serious arrhythmias or result in myocardial infarction. The risks are greatest in patients with a recent myocardial infarction. Operation within 3 months of infarction carries a 30% risk of reinfarction or cardiac death. From 3 to 6 months, this risk falls to 15%, and thereafter to 5%.

Elective surgery should therefore be avoided in the first 6 months following a myocardial infarction. If surgery is unavoidable, risks can be reduced by invasive monitoring and careful regulation of oxygenation, electrolytes and volume status.

In patients with symptoms of stable angina, surgery is in general well tolerated. Once again hypotension should be avoided. Severity of ischaemia can be assessed non-invasively before operation by exercise testing. Maximum workload achieved on exercise testing is an important prognostic indicator – patients who can achieve higher workloads have fewer postoperative complications. In patients with severe symptoms of angina, with symptoms occurring at rest or with minimal provocation, the risks of surgery increase considerably. Similarly, if a patient has experienced symptoms of unstable angina in the last 6 months, risks are appreciably increased and are equivalent to the risks amongst patients with a myocardial infarction in the last 6 months.

Patients undergoing surgery for peripheral vascular disease pose a particular problem for two reasons. Firstly, this patient population has a high incidence of serious underlying coronary disease. Secondly, patients may be incapable of performing an exercise stress test because of the development of claudication. Nuclear perfusion imaging (p. 66) is of particular value in this patient group as a means of predicting postoperative complications. Patients with a positive myoview scan should undergo coronary angiography to determine the need for a coronary revascularization procedure prior to their peripheral vascular surgery. Investigation with stress echocardiography represents another approach (p. 64).

Antianginal therapy should, in general, be maintained preoperatively. For beta-blockers in particular, there is a risk of rebound phenomena if the drugs are discontinued. Oral medication should be continued up to and including the morning of the operation. Postoperatively, oral medication should be resumed as soon as possible. If there is a delay in resuming oral medication, parenteral alternatives should be considered.

Hypertension

Patients with hypertension are at increased risk of major perioperative cardiac complications. This risk is related to associated ischaemic heart disease and left ventricular impairment. Where possible, hypertension should be controlled preoperatively. Antihypertensive medications should be continued up to the time of operation.

Congestive heart failure

Congestive heart failure is a major determinant of perioperative risk. Both the symptomatic functional class, determined according to the New York Heart Association functional criteria (p. 19), and the presence of clinical signs of heart failure, such as a third sound or pulmonary crepitations, are predictive of outcome. When such features are present, treatment regimens should be optimized before undertaking elective surgery. Care should be taken to avoid excessive diuresis which may cause hypovolaemia and hypotension.

Arrhythmias

The risks associated with surgery in patients with arrhythmias are related to the risks of the underlying heart disease, rather than to the arrhythmias per se. There is, therefore, no evidence that simple suppression of ventricular ectopics, for example, will lower risk. The best approach for such patients is careful intraoperative and postoperative monitoring, with management of any haemodynamically compromising rhythm disturbances as they occur.

Conduction defects are a source of concern during anaesthesia, because of the possibility of progression to complete heart block. Temporary pacing is required for patients in established complete heart block or with Mobitz II second-degree AV block (p. 183). Pacing is in general not required for Mobitz I second-degree AV block (Wenckebach) or for patients with bifascicular block.

In patients with an implanted permanent pacemaker, special care is needed in the use of electrocautery. There is a danger that the electrical fields caused by diathermy may cause inappropriate suppression of a demand pacemaker. Bipolar diathermy is preferable to unipolar. When unipolar diathermy is used, the indifferent electrode should be placed as far from the pacemaker generator as possible. A magnet should be available in the theatre to convert the pacemaker to fixed rate, if pacemaker inhibition should occur. Similar interference can occur in the case of implantable defibrillators. Antitachycardia functions should be turned off prior to surgery to guard against inappropriate therapy delivery intraoperatively, and turned on again after the operation.

Valvular heart disease

Major surgery should, if possible, be avoided in patients with severe heart valve disease; it is better to defer general surgery until the valve lesion has been corrected. However, if prosthetic valve surgery is contemplated, it may be preferable to carry out general surgery first in order to avoid operating on a patient receiving anticoagulants.

Short-term withdrawal of anticoagulants in patients with valve prostheses is relatively safe. Oral treatment can be discontinued a few days before surgery, and patients maintained on intravenous heparin until the day of surgery. Heparin should then be resumed as early as is considered safe postoperatively, and maintained until the adequate anticoagulation on oral therapy is established once again.

In emergency operations, clotting can be restored to normal using fresh frozen plasma. Vitamin K reversal is best avoided, as this creates difficulties in re-establishing anticoagulant control postoperatively.

Estimation of risk

Attempts have been made to quantify the cardiac risk in patients undergoing general surgical procedures (Table 19.1). The most important factors in this risk table are a history of myocardial infarction in the last 6 months, and signs of heart failure. Patients can be stratified into four risk groups according to the number of points scored.

More complex algorithms are also available incorporating, for example, anginal symptoms and their severity, and in addition adjusting risk for the nature of the proposed operation (see Detsky et al., 1986 in Further Reading). Such tables are a useful adjunct in predicting cardiac risk, particularly for those less experienced in patient assessment. They are not a substitute for experience or for clinical judgement.

Table 19.1 Multifactorial index score to estimate cardiac risk (Source: Goldman, L., Caldera, D.L. & Nussbaum, S.R. et al [1977] Multifactorial index of cardiac risk in noncardiac surgical procedures. *New England Journal of Medicine* **297**: 845.)

Criteria	Point score
History: Age > 70 years	5
Myocardial infarction in last 6 months	10
Examination: S_3 or raised jugular venous pressure	11
Significant aortic stenosis	3
Electrocardiogram: Rhythm other than sinus	7
> 5 ventricular ectopic beats/min	7
General: Any of the following:	
Respiratory failure, K^+ <3.0 mmol, HCO_3 <20 mmol,	3
renal failure, liver dysfunction, immobilization	
Surgery: Abdominal, thoracic, aortic	3
Emergency	4
Total possible	53

Group	Points total	Non-fatal complications (%)	Cardiac death (%)
I	0–5	0.7	0.2
II	6–12	5	2
III	13–25	11	2
IV	>26	22	56

SURGERY FOR HEART DISEASE

Indications and contraindications

Most types of congenital and rheumatic heart disease are amenable to surgical treatment (for discussion of individual lesions, see Chs 12 and 13). Surgery also has a major part to play in the management of ischaemic heart disease, infective endocarditis, pericardial constriction and in diseases of the aorta. In deciding whether surgery is necessary in an individual case, one must weigh up the prognosis of the patient without surgery and the risks of morbidity and mortality imposed by surgery. For example, most patients with atrial septal defects or persistent ductus arteriosus are asymptomatic, but have a life expectancy reduced to about 40 years. Surgery in childhood is justified in these cases because the mortality is very low. At the other end of the symptomatic scale, severe aortic stenosis carries a very poor prognosis and surgery should be undertaken in spite of a high operative mortality.

Unfortunately, it is often the case that the patients who stand to derive greatest benefit from surgery are also those at greatest risk. This may create great difficulty in deciding whether to undertake surgery, particularly in an era of surgical audit when individual surgeons are understandably protective of their operative mortality.

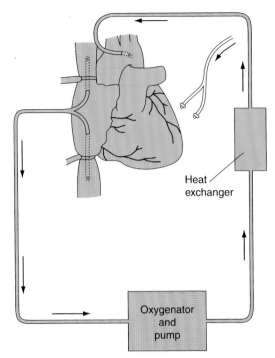

Fig. 19.1 Cardiopulmonary bypass. Venous blood drains from cannulae in the venae cavae into an oxygenator, and is then returned to the femoral artery or aorta by a pump. The temperature of the perfusing blood can be controlled with a heat pump.

Cardiopulmonary bypass

The vast majority of cardiac operations in the adult require cardiopulmonary bypass. In cardiopulmonary bypass, the heart and lungs are completely excluded from the circulation. Venous blood is drained by gravity into an oxygenator through cannulae inserted into the inferior and superior venae cavae. A pump is used to recirculate the blood through a cannula positioned in the aorta (Fig. 19.1). When operations are undertaken on the mitral valve, the aortic valve prevents regurgitation into the left ventricle of the blood pumped into the aorta by the artificial heart–lung apparatus. When operations are being carried out on the aortic valve, the aorta must be cross-clamped below the origin of the innominate artery to permit a dry surgical field.

The ischaemic myocardium is protected during cross-clamping by a combination of cooling and electromechanical dissociation. Electromechanical dissociation can be achieved either by instilling a potassium-containing, crystalloid, cardioplegic solution into the aortic root (and hence into the coronary tree), or by fibrillating the heart so that contraction ceases. Cross-clamping is also necessary during the construction of coronary anastomoses in coronary artery bypass grafting.

With total cardiopulmonary bypass, the cerebral circulation is maintained, and operations on the open heart lasting up to 5 h can be performed. The potential risks are considerable; the major hazards are cerebral air embolism, trauma to blood by the pump-oxygenator, and electrolyte and acid–base disturbances. The lungs often become abnormally stiff in the postoperative phase, and pulmonary atelectasis and infection are common. If perfusion has been inadequate, renal failure may occur. In the first few days after operation, arrhythmias are frequent.

Much of the risk associated with cardiopulmonary bypass relates to problems in maintaining adequate cerebral perfusion. Patients with a history of previous stroke are at risk of further cerebral damage, particularly if their stroke was in the last 6 months. In addition, there is a high incidence of more covert cerebral damage following cardiopulmonary damage with many patients noting deterioration of intellectual function post bypass.

Open heart surgery with total bypass is suitable for all surgically treatable lesions. In the best hands, the mortality rate of the bypass technique itself is less than 1%.

Cardiac surgery without cardiopulmonary bypass

Because of the morbidity associated with cardiopulmonary bypass, there is currently great interest in developing minimally invasive techniques to enable cardiac surgery to be undertaken without the need for bypass. One such example is the *Minimally Invasive Direct Coronary Artery Bypass* (MIDCAB) procedure. This can be used as an alternative to cardiopulmonary bypass (and to PTCA) for single vessel disease of the left anterior descending coronay artery.

In a MIDCAB operation the heart is exposed through a 10 cm transverse parasternal incision. This provides exposure of the underlying left anterior descending artery. The left internal mammary artery is then grafted to the coronary artery directly without bypass.

Techniques are under development to allow off-pump access to the other coronary arteries.

Types of conduit for coronary grafting

Coronary bypass surgery accounts for a substantial majority of the heart surgery undertaken in the UK. The two common types of graft are:

- *Venous grafts.* A length of saphenous vein is grafted between the aorta and a coronary artery, beyond the stenotic area of the artery (see p. 103).
- *Left internal mammary graft.* The left internal mammary artery is freed and anastomosed to the left anterior descending coronary artery. More rarely, the right internal mammary artery may be used to graft the right coronary artery.

Internal mammary arterial grafts have the advantage over saphenous vein grafts of higher long-term patency rates. Because of the greater long-term patency of arterial over venous grafts, there has been interest in exploring other types of arterial grafts, such as the radial artery. However, these other types of conduit are rarely used and generally restricted to situations in which saphenous grafts and the internal mammary arteries cannot be used.

MEDICAL MANAGEMENT OF PATIENTS UNDERGOING CARDIAC SURGERY

Preoperative medical assessment and risk evaluation

The overall medical condition of the patient should be assessed, paying particular attention to major determinants of outcome and complications of surgery. These include:

- *Left ventricular function*. This is the most important single determinant of outcome following cardiac surgery.
- *Pulmonary function*. Patients with severe respiratory impairment are likely to require prolonged ventilatory support following surgery.
- *Renal function*. Patients with renal impairment are likely to suffer further deterioration of renal function following surgery with a possible need for dialysis in the postoperative period.
- *Cerebrovascular disease*. Patients with cerebrovascular disease are at increased risk during cardiopulmonary bypass and are at high risk of developing or extending a stroke due to cerebral ischaemia.
- Other risk factors include the need for emergency operation, age, repeat operation, diabetes and peripheral vascular disease.

In many cases, these risk factors cannot be modified, but form part of the overall assessment of the risks and benefits of surgery. Where risk factors are modifiable (e.g. treatment of a chest infection), the patient's condition should be optimized before surgery.

Postoperative management

Ventilation

Most patients require 6–24 h on a ventilator following cardiac surgery, but substantially longer periods may be required with underlying pulmonary disease.

Low output states

Low cardiac output is common particularly in patients with poor preexisting left ventricular function. In others, intraoperative myocardial infarction may contribute to a low cardiac output. Such patients require prolonged haemodynamic monitoring, including measurements of pulmonary and systemic arterial pressures together with cardiac output. Filling pressures (preload) should be optimized with administration of intravenous fluid or blood as appropriate. Many patients will require *inotropic support*, while in a few, circulatory support with an *intra-aortic balloon pump* (see below) may be necessary.

Hypertension

Postoperative hypertension is common, particularly in patients with a previous history of hypertension. It is important that hypertension should be treated, both to reduce cardiac workload (afterload) and to reduce the risk of postoperative bleeding.

Arrhythmias

Postoperative arrhythmias occur frequently. Atrial flutter and atrial fibrillation are the commonest, occurring in approximately 30% of patients undergoing surgery with cardiopulmonary bypass. There is no single management strategy and optimal management will depend on the patient's haemodynamic status. Possibilities include DC cardioversion, pharmacological cardioversion or pharmacological control of ventricular rate. Management strategies should take consideration of the need for prior anticoagulation to minimize embolic risk in patients with a duration of atrial fibrillation of more than 24 h. Sinus rhythm should be the goal in all patients, although in some patients a decision may be taken to delay this for 6 weeks following surgery until the risks of recurrent atrial fibrillation have diminished. In such cases anticoagulation is essential.

Intra-aortic balloon pumping (counterpulsation)

Mechanical support may be given to the circulation by a balloon introduced via a femoral artery into the descending thoracic aorta which is inflated in diastole and deflated in systole by an external pump (Fig. 19.2). This reduces afterload and increases coronary and peripheral diastolic blood flow. It greatly improves the patient with poor cardiac performance, particularly immediately after cardiopulmonary bypass surgery. It is of value in cardiogenic shock, as after myocardial infarction, only if it allows the patient to survive until some corrective surgical procedure can be undertaken.

Longer-term mechanical assistance

A number of left ventricular assist devices can be used for longer-term support. These devices share the common principle of taking blood from

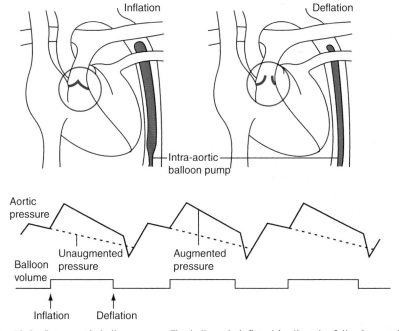

Fig. 19.2 Intra-aortic balloon pump. The balloon is inflated in diastole, following aortic valve closure. Balloon inflation augments aortic pressure without adding to cardiac workload. The balloon is deflated in late diastole. The resulting reduction in aortic pressure reduces left ventricular afterload.

the left heart and pumping it to the aorta, thereby both contributing to cardiac output and off-loading the left ventricle to enable it to perform more efficiently as a pump. The devices are implanted, but are powered by an external power supply. They can be used for periods of up to several months and patients are able to be ambulant during this time.

There are a number of problems associated with their use. These include:

- infection
- thromboembolic complications
- trauma to blood components with consequent haemolysis.

Currently available devices cannot be used to provide indefinite support to the failing heart. Consequently, their use should be restricted to situations in which there is reasonable likelihood of recovery of ventricular function or to patients under consideration for cardiac transplant.

THE REPLACEMENT OF HEART VALVES (SEE ALSO CH. 12)

Valve replacement has proved highly successful in the management of serious valvular disease. In appropriately selected patients, valve replacement ameliorates or abolishes symptoms and causes striking haemodynamic improvement.

Replacement valves are of two types, mechanical and tissue. Mechanical prostheses take a variety of forms (Fig. 19.3):

- ball valves (e.g. Starr–Edwards)
- tilting disc valves (e.g. Bjork–Shiley)
- bi-leaflet valves (e.g. St Jude).

Most tissue valves are isolated, sterilized animal valves (heterografts). The Carpentier–Edwards prosthesis (Fig. 19.4), for example, is prepared from pig valves.

Choice of prosthesis – mechanical or tissue?

Mechanical tissue prostheses differ in their types of complications and in the need for anticoagulants. For tissue valves, the thromboembolic complication rate is low and there is no requirement for long-term anticoagulation. However, tissue valves are prone to failure due to a stiffening and subsequent tearing of the valve leaflets. Over a 10-year period, 20–30% of patients require repeat valve replacement for this reason. Deterioration of tissue valves occurs at an accelerated rate amongst young patients under the age of 35.

For mechanical valves the incidence of thromboembolic complications is greater. Consequently patients require long-term anticoagulation. This in itself carries a small risk of serious haemorrhagic complications. Set against this disadvantage, the incidence of valve failure is very much lower for mechanical valves than for tissue valves. Hence the likelihood of reoperation for valve failure is considerably less.

Prosthesis selection needs to be tailored to the individual patient. In a young individual with no contraindication to anticoagulation, a mechanical prosthesis is preferable. In patients in whom anticoagulants are contraindicated, tissue prostheses will be preferred. In elderly patients, in whom

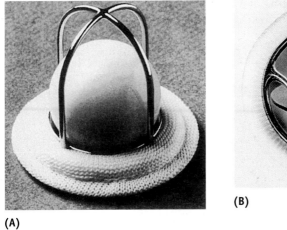

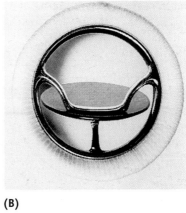

(B)

(A)

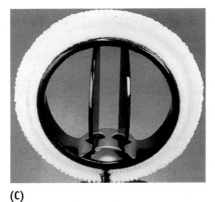

(C)

Fig. 19.3 Mechanical valve prostheses. (A) Starr–Edwards; (B) Bjork–Shiley; (C) St Jude.

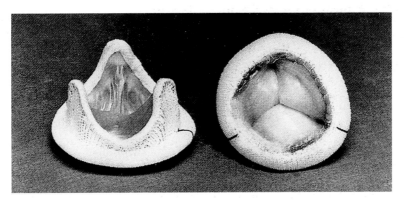

Fig. 19.4 Carpentier–Edwards tissue prosthesis.

anticoagulants are relatively contraindicated and who are unlikely to live long enough to require a second valve replacement, tissue prostheses are once again preferable.

Complications of prosthetic valves

Thromboembolism

The annual incidence of thromboembolic events in a patient with a metal prosthesis receiving anticoagulant therapy is approximately 1–2%. The risk of thromboembolism is generally greater following mitral than following aortic replacement. The risk of embolic problems is related to the adequacy of anticoagulant control. The international normalized ratio (INR) should be maintained between 3 and 4.5.

Anticoagulant-related complications

The risk of serious haemorrhagic complications related to anticoagulation is of the order of 1% per annum. For tissue valves, this is greater than the thromboembolic risk and for this reason anticoagulants are unnecessary, unless there is some additional indication for anticoagulation, such as atrial fibrillation.

Primary valve failure

Valve failure is rare with mechanical prostheses. On the rare occasions when failure does occur, it is generally sudden and results in disastrous haemodynamic consequences, frequently resulting in the death of the patient.

In contrast, primary valve failure is common with tissue valves. The incidence of valve failure in 10 years is approximately 20–30% but an accelerated rate of failure is probable after this time. Failure is generally gradual with adequate forewarning, allowing valve replacement to be undertaken before serious haemodynamic consequences ensue.

Endocarditis

Endocarditis is a particularly serious complication in prosthetic valves, because eradication of the infection with antibiotics alone is difficult. Endocarditis frequently results in the development of a paraprosthetic leak, with consequent haemodynamic deterioration. Prosthetic valve endocarditis is further discussed on page 267.

Valve repair as an alternative to replacement

Despite the great success of valve replacement, the problems and complications of prosthetic valves are well recognized. In recent years there has been an increasing emphasis on conservative surgery, when feasible, as an alternative to replacement.

The mitral valve presents the greatest scope for conservation. In patients with mitral stenosis, balloon valvuloplasty is the operation of choice for patients with a non-calcified valve and minimal regurgitation.

Valve conservation is also possible for some regurgitant mitral lesions. Valve repair involves a variety of techniques as appropriate to the particular case, including:

- annuloplasty to reduce the diameter of the mitral ring, often involving the insertion of a ring prosthesis
- resection of a prolapsing segment of leaflet

- repair of the subvalvar apparatus involving elongation or shortening of chordae tendineae.

These techniques are used increasingly because of the avoidance of the need for a valve prosthesis. Patients with rigid, calcified or severely deformed valves are unlikely to be suitable and are more likely to require valve replacement.

Conservative procedures have also proved successful in the management of tricuspid disease – this generally involves the insertion of a ring prosthesis.

FURTHER READING

Adams, D. & Antman, E. (2001) Medical management of the patient undergoing cardiac surgery. In: Braunwald, E., Zipes, D. & Libby, P. (eds) *Heart Disease. A Textbook of Cardiovascular Medicine.* Philadelphia: Saunders.

Detsky, H.S., Abrams, H.B., McLaughlin, J.R. et al (1986) Predicting cardiac complications in patients undergoing non-cardiac surgery. *Journal of General Internal Medicine* **1**:211–219.

Goldman, L., Caldera, D.L., Nussbaum, S.R. et al (1977) Multifactorial index of cardiac risk in non-cardiac surgical procedures. *New England Journal of Medicine* **297**:845–850.

Goldman, L. & Adler, J. (2001) General anaesthesia and non-cardiac surgery in patients with heart disease. In: Braunwald, E., Zipes, D. & Libby, P. (eds) *Heart Disease. A Textbook of Cardiovascular Medicine.* Philadelphia: Saunders.

Miller, R. & Treasure, T. (1995) *Explaining Cardiac Surgery.* London: BMJ Publishing Group.

Index

A

Abciximab, 99
ACE inhibitors
    cardiomyopathy, 226
    heart failure, 147–8
    hypertension, 315
    myocardial infarction, 128, 131
Acute circulatory failure *see* Cardiogenic
        shock
Acute coronary syndrome, 105
Acute pericarditis, 116, 208–12
    aetiological diagnosis, 211
    causes, 209
    clinical features, 209–10
    differential diagnosis, 210–11
    investigations, 210
    treatment, 211–12
Adams-Stokes attacks, 23, 182, 187
Adult congenital heart disease, 298–9
Advanced life support, 203–7
AIDS, 346–7
Alcohol, 88, 133, 170
Alcoholic cardiomyopathy, 224, 226, 353
Aldosteronism, primary, 307–8
Allergic pericarditis, 211
Alpha-adrenoceptor blockers, 316
Amiloride, 146
Aminophylline, 153
Amiodarone, 171, 198, 199, 201
Amlodipine, 96, 316
Amoxicillin, 270
Ampicillin, 270
Amyloidosis, 223, 231
Anacrotic pulse, 26
Anaemia, 159, 357–8
Anasarca, 21
Aneurysms
    atherosclerotic, 324
    atrial septal, 59
    chronic thoracic, 324–6
    dissecting, 116–17, 320–3
    left ventricular, 129
    mycotic, 171
    sinus of Valsalva, 326
    syphilitic, 324
    ventricular, 128–9

Angina, 19–20, 81, 90–105
    characteristics, 90–2
    definition, 90
    diagnosis, 92–3
    differential diagnosis, 93–4
    prognosis, 94
    revascularization, 97–104
    treatment, 94–7, 104–5
    unstable, 105–8
Angiography, 72, 73–6
    aortic, 319, 322
    mitral regurgitation, 250–1
    pulmonary, 331
    tetralogy of Fallot, 287–8
Angiotensin, 146–7
Angiotensin converting enzyme inhibitors
        see ACE inhibitors
Angiotensin receptor antagonists, 148
    hypertension, 316
Ankylosing spondylitis, 259
Annuloplasty, 374
Antiarrhythmic drugs, 197–8
Antibiotics, 270
Anticoagulant therapy
    atrial fibrillation, 172
    atrial flutter, 169
    cardiomyopathy, 226
    infective endocarditis, 172
    myocardial infarction, 121
    pulmonary embolism, 332, 333
    pulmonary hypertension, 337
Antidiuretic hormone, 138
Anxiety states, 361–3
Aorta, 319–27
    aneurysm of sinus of Valsalva, 326
    atypical aortic dissection, 323
    chronic thoracic aneurysms, 324–6
    coarctation *see* Coarctation of aorta
    dissecting aneurysm, 320–3
    imaging, 319–20
    normal, 319
    trauma, 324
    see also Aortic
Aortic endocarditis, 53
Aortic regurgitation, 40, 259–63, 321,
        355
    aetiology, 259

Aortic regurgitation—(*Continued*)
  with aortic stenosis, 263
  clinical course, 262
  clinical features, 260
  differential diagnosis, 262
  investigations, 260–2
  pathology, 259
  pathophysiology, 259
  prognosis, 262
  treatment, 262–3
Aortic stenosis, 38, 39, 72, 253–9
  aetiology and pathology, 253
  with aortic regurgitation, 263
  complications, 258
  diagnosis/differential diagnosis, 258
  investigations, 256–8
  pathophysiology, 253–5
  physical signs, 255
  prognosis, 258
  symptoms, 255
  treatment, 258–9
Aortography, 73
Apex beat, 31, 110
Arginine vasopressin *see* Antidiuretic
      hormone
Arrhythmias, 77
  atrial *see* atrial fibrillation; atrial flutter
  carotid sinus, 173–4
  conduction disorders, 180–5
  heart failure, 140, 152
  investigation of, 185–6
  late, 129
  paroxysmal, 20
  postoperative, 370–1
  in pregnancy, 360
  reperfusion, 122
  sinus node abnormalities, 159–61
  supraventricular, 161–73
  surgery, 365–6
  syncope, 23–4, 160
  ventricular, 122–3, 174–80
  see also individual arrhythmias
Arrhythmogenic right ventricular
      dysplasia, 232–3
Arterial medial hypertrophy, 335
Arterial pulse, 25–7
Arteriosclerosis, 80
Ascites, 21–2, 142
Aspirin, 172, 317–18
  angina, 95, 99
  myocardial infarction, 118, 132
  unstable angina, 107
Asystole, 206
Atenolol, 120
Atheroma *see* Atherosclerosis
Atherosclerosis, 80–9, 309
  AIDS-related, 347
  pathogenesis, 82–3
  pathology and complications, 80–2
  response to injury hypothesis, 83–4
Atherosclerotic aneurysms, 324
Athlete's heart, 355–7
Atorvastatin, 86
Atrial arrhythmias, 123
Atrial ectopic beats, 161–2

Atrial fibrillation, 21, 169–73, 173, 237, 239,
      349
  management, 200–2
Atrial flutter, 6, 167–9, 173
  management, 201
Atrial natriuretic peptide, 139, 141
Atrial septal aneurysm, 59
Atrial septal defects, 38, 39, 72, 275–9
  clinical signs, 277–8
  investigations, 278
  physiology, 277
  symptoms, 277
  treatment, 278–9
Atrial tachycardia, 167
Atrioventricular (heart) block, 181–3
  complete, 183
  first-degree, 181
  second-degree, 182–3
Atrioventricular node, 1, 2
  reentry tachycardia, 163
Atrioventricular valves, 40
Atypical aortic dissection, 323
Auscultation, 32–42
Austin Flint murmur, 40
Azathioprine, 156

B

Bacterial pericarditis, 212
Basic life support, 202–3
Beriberi, 352
Beta-2 adrenoceptor agonists, 340
Beta-adrenoceptor blockers
  angina, 96
  arrhythmias, 171
  cardiomyopathy, 226, 230
  heart failure, 149–50
  hypertension, 315
  myocardial infarction, 120–1, 131
  unstable angina, 108
Bigeminy, 174
Bile acid sequestrants, 86
Bisoprolol, 120, 150
Bjork-Shiley prosthetic valve, 373
Blood gases, 330–1
Blood pressure
  ambulatory monitoring, 311–12
  measurement, 27–8, 303
  normal, 301–2, 303
  and risk, 302
  screening, 301
  see also Hypertension
Bosentan, 337
Brachytherapy, 100
Bradyarrhythmias, 123–4
  management of, 187–93
Brain natriuretic peptide, 141
Bretylium, 198
Broad complex tachycardias,
      199–200
Brugada syndrome, 184, 185
Bumetanide, 145, 245
Bundle branch block, 8, 124, 183–5
Bundle of His, 2

C

C-reactive protein, 171
Cachexia, 143
Calcium antagonists
  angina, 96–7
  cardiomyopathy, 230
  hypertension, 316
  unstable angina, 108
Candesartan, 316
Cannon waves, 29–30
Captopril, 315
Capture beats, 176
Carcinoid syndrome, 231, 351
Cardiac arrest, 202–7
Cardiac catheterization, 70–3
  aortic regurgitation, 261–2
  aortic stenosis, 257–8
  cardiomyopathy, 225, 228
  mitral regurgitation, 250–1
  mitral stenosis, 243–4
  pericardial constriction, 217
  pulmonary vascular disease, 285
  ventricular septal defects, 281
Cardiac catheters, 74
Cardiac contour, 43–4
Cardiac dilatation, 136–7
Cardiac hypertrophy, 137, 309
Cardiac neurosis, 361
Cardiac output, 72, 137–8
Cardiac pain, 19–20
Cardiac rupture, 126–7
Cardiac surgery see Surgery
Cardiac transplantation, 155–7
  complications, 157
  immunosuppression, 156
  rejection, 156
Cardiac tumours, 61, 355
Cardiogenic shock, 124–5, 153–5, 370
  clinical features, 154
  management, 154–5
Cardiomyopathy, 61, 62, 223–33
  arrhythmogenic right ventricular
    dysplasia, 232–3
  dilated, 223–6
  hypertrophic, 226–31
  peripartum, 360
  restrictive, 218, 231–2
  restrictive/infiltrative, 231–2
Cardiopulmonary bypass, 368–9
Cardiovascular pressures, 71
Cardioversion, 171
Carditis, 342
Carey Coombs murmur, 40, 342
Carotid sinus arrhythmias, 173–4
Carotid sinus hypersensitivity, 173
Carotid sinus massage, 164
Carotid sinus syncope, 24
Carpentier-Edwards tissue prosthesis, 373
Carvedilol, 150
Catheter ablation, 194, 196–7
Cerebral vasodilatation, 338
Cerebrovascular accidents, 127
Cerebrovascular disease, 370
Chagas' disease, 347
Chest
  auscultation, 32–42
  inspection, 30
  palpation, 31–2
Chest pain, 221
Chest X-ray see Radiography
Cheyne-Stokes respiration, 19
Cholesterol-lowering drugs see Statins
Cholestyramine, 86
Chordae tendineae rupture, 247
Chorea, 343
Chronic thoracic aneurysms, 324–6
Chronotropic incompetence, 191
Ciclosporin, 156
  nephrotoxicity, 157
Clopidogrel, 99, 107
Clubbing, 42, 268
Coarctation of aorta, 290–3, 299, 308
  investigations, 292
  physiology, symptoms and signs,
    291–2
  treatment, 292–3
Coffee intake, 88
Collagen vascular disease, 335
Collapsing pulse, 27, 260, 348
Colour flow doppler
    echocardiography, 48–50
Complete heart block, 183
Computed tomography
  aorta, 319
  dissecting aneurysm, 322
  spiral pulmonary, 331
Conduction disorders, 180–5
Congenital heart disease, 61, 274–300
  classification of, 274–5
  in pregnancy, 359
  see also individual conditions
Congenital mitral regurgitation, 247
Congenital subaortic stenosis, 229
Congestive heart failure, 171
  surgery, 365
Conn's syndrome, 311
Constrictive pericarditis see Pericardial
    constriction
Continuous wave Doppler
    echocardiography, 47–8
Cor pulmonale, 218, 335, 337–40
  clinical features, 339
  differential diagnosis, 339–40
  investigations, 339
  pathogenesis, 338–9
  prognosis and treatment, 340
Cor triatriatum, 244
Coronary angiography see Angiography
Coronary angioplasty, myocardial
    infarction, 120
Coronary arteries, 61, 78
Coronary artery bypass surgery, 101–4,
    369
Coronary artery disease, 79–89
  atherosclerosis, 80–9, 309
  dietary fat, 86–7
  family history, 87
  prevention, 88–9
  psychological factors, 88, 361–2

Coronary circulation, 78–9
Coronary occlusion, 80
Coronary thrombosis, 80
Corticosteroids, 156, 340
Counterpulsation, 371
Coxiella burnetti, 267
Creatine kinase, 113, 115
Cushing's syndrome, 306–7, 311
Cyanosis, 22, 42, 238, 286–90, 293,
      339
   central, 22
   differential, 285
   peripheral, 22
Cystic medial necrosis, 324

D

D-dimer, 331
Delteparin, 107
Diabetes mellitus, 88, 350–1
Diamorphine, 153
Diastolic pressure, 28, 303, 313
Diazoxide, 316
Dicrotic notch, 25
Diet
   and essential hypertension, 304
   fat in, 86–7
   post-myocardial infarction, 133
Differential cyanosis, 285
Digitalis, 10, 150, 169, 201, 245
Digoxin *see* Digitalis
Dilated cardiomyopathy, 223–6, 346
   alcoholic, 226
   causes, 224
   clinical features, 225
   investigation, 225
   prognosis, 226
   treatment, 225–6
Diltiazem, 96, 316
Dilutional hyponatraemia, 139
Direct current shock therapy, 193–4
Directional atherectomy, 100
Disopyramide, 198
Dissecting aneurysm, 116–17, 320–3
   classification, 321
   clinical features, 321
   investigations, 321–3
   management, 323
Diuretics
   cardiomyopathy, 226
   cor pulmonale, 340
   heart failure, 145–6, 153
   mitral stenosis, 245
Dobutamine, 155
Dopamine, 155
Doppler echocardiography, 45–50
   persistent ductus arteriosus, 283
   ventricular septal defects, 280–1
Doppler ultrasonography, 278
Doxazosin, 316
Dressler syndrome, 209
Drug-eluting stents, 100–1
Ductal dependency, 293
Dyspnoea, 17–19, 255, 260, 339, 348

exertional, 18
paroxysmal, 18

E

Ebstein's anomaly, 263
Echocardiography, 44–60
   acute pericarditis, 210
   aorta, 319
   aortic regurgitation, 49, 261
   aortic stenosis, 49, 256–7
   atrial septal defects, 278
   cardiomyopathy, 225, 228
   coarctation of aorta, 292
   contrast media, 57–9
   cor pulmonale, 339
   Doppler, 45–50
   fetal, 294
   hypertension, 312
   left heart failure, 141
   mitral regurgitation, 249–50
   mitral stenosis, 240–4
   myocarditis, 221
   pericardial effusion, 213
   pericardial tamponade, 214
   pulmonary embolism, 331
   pulmonary hypertension, 337
   pulmonary stenosis, 296
   pulmonary vascular disease, 285
   stress, 64–5
   tissue doppler, 60
   transoesphageal *see* Transoesophageal
      echocardiography
   transposition of great arteries, 290
   utility of, 51–3
   ventricular septal defects, 50
Ectopic beats, 20
Effort syndrome, 361
Effusive-constrictive pericarditis, 208
Ehlers-Danlos syndrome, 324
Eisenmenger complex, 280
Eisenmenger syndrome, 284–6, 335
Ejection sounds, 35–6
Ejection systolic murmurs, 37
Electrical alternans, 213
Electrocardiogram, 1–16
   acute pericarditis, 210
   angina, 92
   aortic regurgitation, 260
   aortic stenosis, 256
   arrhythmogenic right ventricular
      dysplasia, 232–3
   atrial septal defects, 278
   cardiomyopathy, 225, 228
   coarctation of aorta, 292
   cor pulmonale, 339
   dissecting aneurysm, 321
   electrodes and leads, 1–4
   hypertension, 310–11
   interpretation, 14–15
   left bundle branch block, 12
   left heart failure, 141
   left ventricular hypertrophy, 10–11
   mean frontal QRS axis, 12–14

mitral regurgitation, 249
mitral stenosis, 239
myocardial infarction, 110–12
myocarditis, 221
normal, 4–10
pathways of conduction, 1
persistent ductus arteriosus, 283
pulmonary embolism, 330
pulmonary stenosis, 296
pulmonary vascular disease, 285
right bundle branch block, 12, 14
right ventricular hypertrophy, 11–12
tetralogy of Fallot, 287
transposition of great arteries, 290
unstable angina, 106
ventricular septal defects, 280
ventricular tachycardia, 175
Wolff-Parkinson-White syndrome,
165–7
Electromechanical dissociation, 206
Electrophysiological testing, 76–7
Embolectomy, 333
Enalapril, 315
End-diastolic volume, 136–7
Endocarditis, 56, 299, 342–3
aortic, 53
infective see Infective endocarditis
mitral, 53
prosthetic valves, 267, 374
Endocrine disease, 347–53
Endomyocardial fibrosis, 231
Endothelial derived relaxing factor, 139
Endothelin, 139
Endothelin-1 receptor antagonists, 337
Endothelium, 83
Enoxaparin, 107
Epoprostenol, 337
Eptifibatide, 99
Erythema marginatum, 343
Essential hypertension, 304–5
Exercise, 87–8, 132–3, 144, 355–7
and angina, 91
and essential hypertension, 304
Exercise electrocardiogram, 61
Exercise testing, 130
Exertional syncope, 23–4
Extrasystoles, 174
Exudation, 212

F

Faint see Syncope
Family history, 87
Fat intake, 86–7
Fatty streak, 80
Fibrates, 86
Fibrillation, 6
see also Atrial fibrillation
Fibro-lipid plaque, 81
Flecainide, 171, 198, 201
Fluvastatin, 86
Foam cells, 83
Fontan circulation, 299
Friedreich's ataxia, 223

Frusemide see Furosemide
Functional capacity, 19
Furosemide (Frusemide), 145, 153, 245
Fusion beats, 177

G

Gallop rhythm, 35
Gentamicin, 270
Giant 'a' wave, 29
Glutamic-oxalo-acetic transaminase, 115–16
Glyceryl trinitrate, 95–6
Glycogen storage disease, 223, 231
Glycoprotein IIb/IIIa inhibitors, 99–100,
107
Graham Steell murmur, 40, 266, 336
Graves' disease, 347

H

Haematuria, 268
Haemochromatosis, 223, 231, 351
Haemoptysis, 22–3, 238
Heart block, 123, 354
Heart failure, 135–58, 221, 354
acute left ventricular failure, 152–3
arrhythmias, 140, 152
cardiac and circulatory responses, 136
cardiac dilatation, 136–7
cardiac hypertrophy, 137
cardiac output, 137–8
cardiac transplantation, 155–7
cardiogenic shock, 153–5
causes, 135–6
cellular changes, 137
drug therapy, 145–50
left heart failure, 140–2
management, 143–5
neuroendocrine response, 138–9
raised venous pressure, 139–40
regional circulations, 139
right heart failure, 142–3
salt/water retention, 139
ventricular resynchronization
therapy, 150–2
Heart murmurs, 268
Heart rate, 15
Heart sounds, 33–6
Heart valves
repair, 374–5
replacement, 372–3
see also Prosthetic valves
Heart-lung transplantation, 157
Heparin, 107
Hepatomegaly, 142
Hereditary long QT syndrome, 179
High-density lipoprotein, 85
HMG CoA reductase inhibitors see Statins
Human immunodeficiency virus, 222, 224
Hydralazine, 148–9, 316
Hypercholesterolaemia, 85, 132, 349
Hypercoagulability, 328
Hypercyanotic attacks, 287

Hypereosinophilic syndrome, 231
Hyperkalaemia, 146, 206
Hyperlipidaemia, 85–6, 351
Hypertension, 170, 301–18
    aetiology, 303–4
    classification, 303
    and coronary artery disease, 87
    decision to treat, 312–14
    definitions of, 303
    and diabetes, 351
    essential, 304–5
    examination and investigation, 309–12
    and ischaemic heart disease, 87
    malignant, 312
    measurement of blood pressure, 303
    normal blood pressure, 301–2
    pathophysiology, 309
    postoperative, 370
    psychological factors, 361
    secondary, 305–9
    surgery, 365
    treatment, 314–18
    white coat, 311–12
    see also Pulmonary hypertension
Hyperthyroidism, 159, 168, 170, 347–9
    clinical features, 348–9
Hypertrophic cardiomyopathy, 52, 226–31,
        357
    clinical features, 228
    differential diagnosis, 229–30
    genetics, 227–8
    investigations, 228–9
    management, 230–1
    pathogenesis, 227
    pathophysiological consequences, 228
    in pregnancy, 360
Hyperventilation, 17
Hypocalcaemia, 224
Hypokalaemia, 307
Hyponatraemia, 139
Hypophosphataemia, 224
Hypoplastic left heart, 293–4
Hypotension, 214
Hypothermia, 10
Hypothyroidism, 349–50
Hypovolaemia, 155, 159
Hypoxaemia, 17
Hysteresis, 190

I

Immunosuppression, 156
Implantable defibrillators, 176, 194, 195
Infections, 341–7
    AIDS, 346–7
    rheumatic fever, 341–6
    trypanosomiasis, 347
    tuberculosis, 346
    virus, 346
Infective endocarditis, 237, 247, 259, 266–73
    anticoagulation, 272
    clinical features, 268
    complications, 271
    diagnostic criteria, 269

intravenous drug abusers, 266
    investigations, 268–9
    native valve, 266
    pathology, 267–8
    prevention, 272–3
    prognosis, 272
    prosthetic valves, 267
    surgical treatment, 271–2
    treatment, 269–71
Infiltrative cardiomyopathy, 231–2
Inotropic agents, 155
Inoue balloon, 245–6
Insulin resistance, 88
Intra-aortic balloon pumping
        (counterpulsation), 371
Intracardiac abscess, 171
Intramural haematoma, 323
Investigations
    invasive, 70–7
    non-invasive, 43–69
Ischaemia
    assessment, 130
    recurrent, 127
Ischaemic cardiomyopathy, 223
Ischaemic cascade, 63–4
Ischaemic heart disease, 80, 168, 170
    incidence and prevalence, 84
    prevention, 88–9
    risk factors, 84–8
    surgery, 364–5
    see also Atherosclerosis

J

Janeway lesions, 268
Judkins catheter, 74
Jugular venous pressure, 142
Junctional bradycardia, 123
Junctional (nodal) rhythm, 162–3

K

Kaposi's sarcoma, 347
Kerley's B lines, 239
Korotkoff sounds, 28, 303
Kussmaul's sign, 214, 232

L

Lactate dehydrogenase, 116
Lanecteplase, 118
Laplace's Law, 136
Large volume pulse, 26
Laser angioplasty, 100
Late systolic murmurs, 39
Law of Laplace, 136
Left atrial ball valve thrombus, 244
Left atrial myxoma, 244
Left axis deviation, 13
Left bundle branch block, 12
Left heart failure, 140–2
Left ventricular aneurysm, 129

Left ventricular failure, 124, 152–3
  effect on lungs, 140
Left ventricular function, 51, 72, 370
  assessment, 130
Left ventricular hypertrophy, 10–11, 311
Lidocaine, 198, 199
Life support
  advanced, 203–7
  basic, 202–3
Lignocaine see Lidocaine
Lipid, 83
Lipid disorders, 84–5
Lipid lowering drugs, 317
Lisinopril, 315
Losartan, 316
Low output state see Cardiogenic shock
Low-density lipoprotein, 83, 85

M

Macrophages, 83
Magnetic resonance imaging, 60–1, 67
  dissecting aneurysm, 322
  persistent ductus arteriosus, 283
Malignant hypertension, 312
Marfan syndrome, 247, 259, 320, 324, 325,
  354–5
Metabolic disease, 347–53
Methaemoglobinaemia, 22
Metoprolol, 120, 150
Mexiletine, 198
Micturition syncope, 23
Midsystolic murmurs, 37–8
Minimally Invasive Direct Coronary Artery
  Bypass (MIDCAB), 369
Minoxidil, 316
Mitral endocarditis, 53
Mitral regurgitation, 38, 39, 247–52
  causes, 247–8
  complications, 248
  course and prognosis, 251
  differential diagnosis, 251
  echocardiography, 50
  investigations, 249–51
  medical treatment, 251
  pathophysiology, 248
  physical signs, 249
  surgery, 251–2
  symptoms, 248–9
Mitral stenosis, 40, 41, 72, 235–47
  combined valve disease, 244
  complications, 237
  course and prognosis, 244
  differential diagnosis, 244
  interventional treatment, 245–6
  investigations, 239–44
  medical treatment, 245
  pathology, 235
  pathophysiology, 235–7
  physical signs, 238–9
  in pregnancy, 359
  surgical treatment, 246–7
  symptoms, 237–8
Mitral valve prolapse, 247, 354

Mobitz type 1 block, 182
Mobitz type 2 block, 182
Murmurs, 36–42
  continuous, 41
  diastolic, 40–1
  pansystolic, 38–9
  pericardial friction rub, 41–2
  systolic, 37–9
Muscular dystrophy, 223
Mycotic aneurysm, 171
Myocardial biopsy, 222, 225, 232–3
Myocardial contrast echocardiography, 58
Myocardial infarction, 19–20, 62, 80,
  108–32, 210
  anticoagulant therapy, 121
  clinical features, 109
  complications, 122–9
  diagnosis, 110–16
  differential diagnosis, 116–17
  electrocardiogram, 110–15
  expansion of, 128
  mortality, 121–2
  non-Q wave, 105
  non-ST segment elevation, 105
  pain relief, 117
  pathology, 81–2
  physical signs, 109–10
  prognosis, 121–2
  recurrent, 127
  rehabilitation, 132–4
  reperfusion therapy, 118–20
  risk stratification, 130–1
  serum enzymes, 112–13, 115–16
  ST segment, 9
  T wave, 8
  thrombolysis, 118–20
  treatment, 117–21, 131–2
Myocardial ischaemia, 19–20
  ST segment, 10
  T wave, 8
Myocarditis, 168, 220–2, 343
  AIDS-related, 346
  clinical features, 221
  HIV-associated, 222
  investigations, 221–2
  pathology, 220–1
  viral, 222
Myofibrillar disarray, 227
Myotonic dystrophy, 223
Myxoedema, 212
Myxoedema coma, 349
Myxoma, 355

N

National Institute of Clinical Excellence
  (NICE) guidelines, 176
Native valve endocarditis, 266
Neisseria gonorrhoeae, 267
Neonatal cardiology, 293–4
Neonatal coarctation, 293–5
Neurocirculatory asthenia, 361
Nicardipine, 96, 316
Nicorandil, 97

Nicotinic acid, 86
Nifedipine, 96, 316
Nitrates, 95–6, 108, 148, 153
Nitric oxide, 83
Nitroprusside, 316
Non-Q wave myocardial infarction, 105–8
Non-ST segment elevation myocardial
    infarction, 105–8
Nuclear cardiology *see* Single photon
    emission computerized tomography

O

Obesity, 87, 352
Obstructive lesions, 290–6
Oedema, 21, 142
Oesophageal tumour, 54
Oral contraception, and
    hypertension, 308–9
Orthopnoea, 18
Osler's nodes, 42, 268
Overweight, 352
Oxygen therapy, 153, 340

P

P wave, 1, 5–6
    absent, 6
    broadened/notched, 5–6
    interpretation, 15
    inverted, 5
    tall/peaked, 6
Pacing, 123, 187–93
    choice of pacemaker, 192
    dual-chamber, 190–1
    external, 188
    indications, 192–3
    modes, 191–2
    permanent, 189–93
    rate-responsive, 191
    temporary, 188–9
Palpation, 31–2
Palpitations, 20–1, 348, 362
Pancarditis, 343
Pansystolic murmurs, 38–9
Papillary muscle rupture, 126
Paracentesis, 213
Paravalvar abscess, 172
Paroxysmal supraventricular
    tachycardia, 163–5, 173
    management, 201
Patent foramen ovale, 59, 275
Penetrating atherosclerotic ulcer, 323
Penicillin, 270
Percussion, 32
Percutaneous coronary
    intervention, 97–101
Pericardial aspiration, 215
Pericardial constriction, 30, 61, 62, 216–19
    clinical features and diagnosis, 216
    differential diagnosis, 218
    investigations, 216–17
    treatment, 218–19

Pericardial disease, 208–19
    pathology, 208
Pericardial effusion, 54
Pericardial friction rub, 41–2, 209
Pericardial infusion, 212–13
Pericardial tamponade, 212, 213–15
Pericarditis, 20, 128, 343
    acute *see* Acute pericarditis
    AIDS-related, 347
    allergic, 211
    effusive-constrictive, 208
    ST segment, 9
Pericardium, 53
Perindopril, 315
Peripartum cardiomyopathy, 360
Peripheral vasodilatation, 338
Persistent ductus arteriosus, 41, 70, 282–4
    clinical signs, 282–3
    investigation, 283
    physiology and symptoms, 282
    treatment, 284
Petechiae, 268
Phaeochromocytoma, 308
Phosphodiesterase inhibitors, 337
Pigtail catheter, 74
Platelet-derived growth factor, 83
Platelets, 83
Pleural effusion, 321
Pleurisy, 211
Plexiform lesions, 336
Pneumothorax, 189, 211
Polyarteritis, 209, 223
Polyarthritis, 343
Polycythaemia, 338
Post-pericardiotomy syndrome, 209
Postural syncope, 24
Potassium-sparing diuretics, 146
PR interval, 1, 6
    interpretation, 15
    progressive prolongation, 183
Pravastatin, 86
Prazosin, 316
Pregnancy, 299, 358–60
Premature beats, 174
Pressure load, 136
Primum atrial septal defects, 275–6, 277
Prinzmetal's angina, 80
Procainamide, 198
Propafenone, 198
Prostacyclin *see* Epoprostenol
Prosthetic valves
    complications, 374
    endocarditis, 267, 374
    failure, 374
    in pregnancy, 359
    selection of, 372–3
Proteinuria, 143, 268, 311
Pseudoxanthoma elasticum, 353
Psychosocial factors, 361
Pulmonary angiography, 331
Pulmonary arteriolar constriction, 338
Pulmonary artery wedge pressure, 125
Pulmonary artery wedge tracing, 71
Pulmonary blood flow, 334–5
Pulmonary capillary pressure, 334

Pulmonary circulation, 334
Pulmonary embolism, 127, 143, 237, 328–33
  clinical features, 329
  investigations, 329–31
  management, 332, 332–3
  pathophysiology, 328–9
  recurrent, 333
Pulmonary function tests, 339, 370
Pulmonary heart disease *see* Cor pulmonale
Pulmonary hypertension, 52, 333–7
  primary, 334, 336–7
  secondary, 333, 334–6
  thromboembolic, 333
Pulmonary oedema, 18–19
Pulmonary regurgitation, 40
Pulmonary scintigraphy, 331
Pulmonary stenosis, 38, 39, 294–5
Pulmonary thrombosis, 328
Pulmonary valve disease, 265–6
Pulmonary vascular disease, 284–6
  clinical signs, 285
  investigations, 285
  natural history, 285
  physiology and symptoms, 284–5
  treatment, 285–6
Pulmonary vascular resistance, 335
Pulmonary vasoconstriction, 335
Pulse
  amplitude and character, 26–7
  peripheral, absence of, 27
  rate, 26
  respiratory variation, 27
  rhythm, 26
  see also Venous pulse
Pulse wave Doppler echocardiography, 47
Pulsus alternans, 27
Pulsus bisferiens, 26
Pulsus paradoxus, 27, 214
Purkinje system, 1, 2

Q

Q fever, 171, 267
Q waves, 7–8
QRS complex, 1, 6–7, 15
QT interval, 8, 15
Quinidine, 198

R

Radiofrequency ablation, 172, 176
Radiography, 43–4, 225
  aortic regurgitation, 260
  aortic stenosis, 256
  atrial septal defects, 278
  coarctation of aorta, 292
  cor pulmonale, 339
  dissecting aneurysm, 321
  mitral regurgitation, 249
  mitral stenosis, 239, 240
  pericardial effusion, 212–13
  persistent ductus arteriosus, 283
  pulmonary embolism, 330

  pulmonary stenosis, 296
  pulmonary vascular disease, 285
  tetralogy of Fallot, 287
  transposition of great arteries, 290
  ventricular septal defects, 280
Raised venous pressure, 139–40
Ramipril, 315
Rehabilitation, 132–4
Reiter's disease, 259
Renal artery stenosis, 305–6
Renal disease, 305–6
Renal failure, 171
Renal function tests, 370
Renin-angiotensin system, 306
Renin-angiotensin-aldosterone system, 138
Reperfusion arrhythmias, 122
Rescue angioplasty, 120
Response to injury hypothesis, 83–4
Restrictive cardiomyopathy, 218, 231–2
Reteplase, 118
Return to work, 133
Rheumatic endocarditis, 247
Rheumatic fever, 209, 341–6
  clinical features, 342–4
  course and prognosis, 344–5
  diagnosis, 344
  epidemiology, 341
  pathophysiology, 341–2
  prevention, 345–6
  treatment, 345
Rheumatic heart disease, 168, 170, 342, 345–6
Rheumatoid arthritis, 209
Rhythm, 15
Right axis deviation, 13
Right bundle branch block, 12, 14
Right heart failure, 142–3
Right ventricular abnormalities, 51
Right ventricular failure, 125–6
Right ventricular hypertrophy, 11–12
Right ventricular impulse, 31
Right ventricular outflow tachycardia, 178
Rotational atherectomy, 100
Roth's spots, 268

S

St Jude prosthetic valve, 373
St Vitus' dance, 343
Salbutamol, 340
Salt retention, 139
  management, 144–5
Salvage angioplasty, 120
Sarcoid, 209
Sarcoidosis, 223, 231, 353–4
Schistosomiasis, 335
Scleroderma, 209, 223
Secundum atrial septal defects, 275, 276
Sestamibi, 66
Sexual problems, 133
Shock, 214
  see also Cardiogenic shock

Sick sinus syndrome, 160–1
Sildenafil, 337
Silent ischaemia, 80
Simvastatin, 86
Single photon emission computerized
        tomography (SPECT), 66–7
Single ventricle, 296–7
Sinoatrial block, 180–1
Sinus arrest, 180–1
Sinus arrhythmia, 161
Sinus bradycardia, 123, 160
Sinus node, 1, 2
Sinus tachycardia, 159–60, 173, 214
        ST segment, 10
Sinus of Valsalva, aneurysm, 326
Sleep apnoea, 352
Small volume pulse, 26
Smoking, 87, 133
Smooth muscle cells, 83
Sotalol, 198
Spiral pulmonary computed
        tomography, 331
Spironolactone, 146, 226
Splenomegaly, 268
Splinter haemorrhages, 42, 268
Spontaneous contrast, 240
ST segment, 9–10
        interpretation, 15
Staphylococcus aureus, 267
Staphylococcus epidermidis, 267
Starr-Edwards prosthetic valve, 373
Statins, 86, 132
Streptococcus bovis, 267
Streptococcus faecalis, 267
Streptococcus viridans, 267
Streptokinase, 118
Stress, 88, 361–2
Stress agents, 64
Stress echocardiography, 64–5
Subclavian artery puncture, 189
Sudden dropped beats, 183
Sulphaemoglobinaemia, 22
Superior vena cava obstruction, 218
Supraventricular arrhythmias, 161–73
Supraventricular tachycardia, 176–7
Surgery, 364–75
        cardiopulmonary bypass, 368–9
        coronary grafting, 369
        indications and contraindications, 367
        intra-aortic balloon pumping, 371
        mechanical assistance, 371–2
        postoperative management, 370–1
        preoperative medical assessment, 370
        risk quantification, 366–7, 370
        valve repair, 374–5
        valve replacement, 372–4
        without cardiopulmonary bypass, 369
Swan-Ganz catheter, 72
Sympathetic nervous system, 137
Syncope, 23–4, 160, 187, 255
Syphilitic aneurysms, 324
Syphilitic aortitis, 259
Systemic arterial embolism, 127
Systemic lupus erythematosus, 209, 223,
        353

Systolic pressure, 28, 303, 313
Systolic venous pulsation ('v' wave), 30

T

T wave, 1, 8, 15
Tachyarrhythmias, 193–4
        ventricular, 354
Tenectaplase, 118
Terazosin, 316
Tetralogy of Fallot, 286–8, 298
        clinical signs, 287
        hypercyanotic spells, 287
        investigations, 287–8
        physiology, 286
        symptoms, 286–7
        treatment, 288–9
Tetrofosmin, 66
Thiamine deficiency, 224, 352
Thiazide diuretics, 145–6
        hypertension, 315
Thrills, 31–2
Thromboembolic pulmonary
        hypertension, 333
Thromboembolism, 374
Thrombolytic therapy
        complications, 119–20
        indications, 118–19
        myocardial infarction, 118–20
        pulmonary embolism, 333
        timing, 119
Thyrotoxicosis see Hyperthyroidism
Tietze's syndrome, 93
Tirofiban, 99
Tissue plasminogen activator, 118
Torsades de pointes, 177, 179, 200
Transoesophageal echocardiography, 53–7
        atrial septal defects, 278
        dissecting aneurysm, 321–2
        mitral stenosis, 246
Transposition of great arteries, 289–90
        Mustard/Senning repair, 299
Transudation, 212
Travel, 133–4
Triamterene, 146
Tricuspid atresia, 297–8
Tricuspid regurgitation, 38, 39, 142, 218,
        244, 264–5
Tricuspid stenosis, 40, 41, 218, 244, 263–4
Troponins, 105, 112–13
Trypanosomiasis, 347
Tuberculosis, 346
Tuberculous pericarditis, 208, 211

U

U wave, 10
Ultrasonography
        Doppler, 278
        venous, 331
Unstable angina, 105–8
Urea, 311
Urinalysis, 311

V

Valsalva manoeuvre, 165, 229
Valsartan, 316
Valvar aortic stenosis, 228
Valvular heart disease
  in pregnancy, 359
  surgery, 366
Vaso vasorum, 319
Vasodilators, 337
Vasomotor/vasodepressor syncope, 23
Vasospastic angina see Prinzmetal's angina
Venous hum, 41
Venous pressure, 29
Venous pulse, 28–9
Venous stasis, 328
Venous ultrasonography, 331
Venous waveform, 29–30
Ventilation, 370
Ventricular aneurysm, 128–9
Ventricular arrhythmias, 122–3, 174–80, 354
Ventricular ectopic beats, 174
Ventricular fibrillation, 122–3, 179–80
Ventricular hypertrophy
  ST segment, 10
  T wave, 8
Ventricular resynchronization
        therapy, 150–2
Ventricular septal defects, 39, 72, 126,
        279–82
  clinical signs, 280
  investigation, 280–1
  physiology, 279–80
  symptoms, 280

treatment, 281–2
Ventricular tachycardia, 122, 173
  benign, 178–9, 197
  management, 198–9
  non-sustained, 178
  sustained, 174–6
Ventriculography, 73
Verapamil, 96, 198, 230, 316
Verrucae, 342
Viral myocarditis, 222, 224
Viral pericarditis, 211
Virus infections, 346
Vital capacity, 17
Volume load, 135

W

Warfarin, 172, 332
Water retention, 139
  management, 144–5
Waterhammer pulse, 27, 260, 348
Wenckebach block, 182
White coat hypertension, 311–12
Williams' syndrome, 253
Wolff-Parkinson-White syndrome, 6, 76, 77,
        163, 165–7, 196
  management, 201–2

X

Xanthelasma, 42
Xanthomata, 42